The Wrong Prescription for Women

The Wrong Prescription for Women

How Medicine and Media Create a "Need" for Treatments, Drugs, and Surgery

**Maureen C. McHugh and
Joan C. Chrisler, Editors**

Foreword by Paula J. Caplan

Women's Psychology
Michele A. Paludi, Series Editor

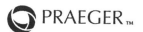 PRAEGER ™

An Imprint of ABC-CLIO, LLC
Santa Barbara, California • Denver, Colorado

Library of Congress Cataloging-in-Publication Data

The wrong prescription for women: how medicine and media create a need for treatments, drugs, and surgery / Maureen C. McHugh and Joan C. Chrisler, editors; foreword by Paula J. Caplan.
    p.; cm.—(Women's psychology)
  Includes bibliographical references and index.
  ISBN 978-1-4408-3176-8 (alk. paper)—ISBN 978-1-4408-3177-5 (ebook)
  I. McHugh, Maureen C., editor.   II. Chrisler, Joan C., editor.
  [DNLM: 1. Women's Health.   2. Body Image—psychology.
3. Medicalization—methods.   4. Stereotyping. WA 309.1]
  RS57
  615.1'4082—dc23   2015005594

ISBN: 978-1-4408-3176-8
EISBN: 978-1-4408-3177-5

19 18 17 16   3 4 5

This book is also available on the World Wide Web as an eBook.
Visit www.abc-clio.com for details.

Praeger
An Imprint of ABC-CLIO, LLC

ABC-CLIO, LLC
130 Cremona Drive, P.O. Box 1911
Santa Barbara, California 93116-1911

This book is printed on acid-free paper ∞
Manufactured in the United States of America

"First, do no harm."

—attributed to the surgeon Thomas Inman (1820–1876),
based on precepts from the Hippocratic Oath

Contents

Series Foreword

Michele A. Paludi

Because women's work is never done and is underpaid or un-
paid or boring or repetitious and we're the first to get fired and
what we look like is more important than what we do and if we
get raped it's our fault and if we get beaten we must have pro-
voked it and if we raise our voices we're nagging bitches and if
we enjoy sex we're nymphos and if we don't we're frigid and if
we love women it's because we can't get a "real" man and if we
ask our doctor too many questions we're neurotic and/or pushy
and if we expect childcare we're selfish and if we stand up for
our rights we're aggressive and "unfeminine" and if we don't
we're typical weak females and if we want to get married we're
out to trap a man and if we don't we're unnatural and because
we still can't get an adequate safe contraceptive but men can
walk on the moon and if we can't cope or don't want a pregnancy we're made to feel guilty about abortion and . . . for lots of
other reasons we are part of the women's liberation movement.

Author unknown, quoted in *The Torch*, September 14, 1987

This sentiment underlies the major goals of Praeger's Book Series
"Women's Psychology":

1. Valuing women. The books in this series value women by valuing
   children and working for affordable child care; valuing women by

respecting all physiques, not just placing value on slender women; valuing women by acknowledging older women's wisdom, beauty, aging; valuing women who have been sexually victimized and viewing them as survivors; valuing women who work inside and outside of the home; and valuing women by respecting their choices of careers, of whom they mentor, of their reproductive rights, their spirituality and their sexuality.
2. Treating women as the norm. Thus the books in this series make up for women's issues typically being omitted, trivialized, or dismissed from other books on psychology.
3. Taking a non-Eurocentric view of women's experiences. The books in this series integrate the scholarship on race and ethnicity into women's psychology, thus providing a psychology of all women. Women typically have been described collectively; but we are diverse.
4. Facilitating connections between readers' experiences and psychological theories and empirical research. The books in this series offer readers opportunities to challenge their views about women, feminism, sexual victimization, gender role socialization, education, and equal rights. These texts thus encourage women readers to value themselves and others. The accounts of women's experiences as reflected through research and personal stories in the texts in this series have been included for readers to derive strength from the efforts of others who have worked for social change on the interpersonal, organizational and societal levels.

A student in one of my courses on the psychology of women once stated:

I learned so much about women. Women face many issues: discrimination, sexism, prejudices . . . by society. Women need to work together to change how society views us. I learned so much and talked about much of the issues brought up in class to my friends and family. My attitudes have changed toward a lot of things. I got to look at myself, my life, and what I see for the future. (Paludi, 2002)

It is my hope that readers of the books in this series also reflect on the topics and look at themselves, their own lives, and what they see for the future.

Michele A. Paludi
Series Editor

REFERENCE

Paludi, M. (2002). *The psychology of women* (2nd ed.). Upper Saddle River, NJ: Prentice Hall.

Foreword

Paula J. Caplan

Like many women who came of age in the late 1960s, on the cusp of the Second Wave of the Women's Movement, I was transformed by two related kinds of learning as many of us began to speak out about our lives. One was learning how many of my confusing, uncomfortable, perplexing, and humiliating experiences were not unique to me and, in fact, seemed to happen to most girls and women. The other was learning how many girls and women had horrific experiences that I had not had, such as having been sexually abused as children or adolescents or having been shamed or even threatened by family members when growing up or later by their husbands when they wanted to continue their education. Both were about manifestations of sexism, which ran like a sewer through every realm of life. After learning about one form of mistreatment of women and girls after another after another after another, it struck me: *In a sexist society, anything that can be used against women will be used against women.*

The Wrong Prescription for Women is an essential remedy for myriad kinds of harm done to women by the medicalizing of so much about us, including, but not limited to, sexuality, menstruation and menopause, pregnancy and childbirth, many features of physical appearance, and emotions. With their long and stellar histories of illuminating works about the effects of sexism on women's bodies and feelings as the subjects of research and clinical practice, Maureen McHugh and Joan Chrisler were ideally positioned to conceive and recognize the importance of the subject of this book.

The decades since the late 1960s have been marked by massive up-surges in medical research and the use of mass media to publicize medical theories, case studies, and empirical research. Unfortunately, laypeople often learn from talk shows, print media, and broadcast news what is happening in medicine, but no critical perspective is offered by most hosts and reporters, and even many professionals and academics fail to think critically about this work.

The intimate connection between medicalizing women's bodies and pathologizing women's emotions appears in what is sometimes called diagnostic creep. That is, after a long history of regarding menopausal women as unfeminine, emotionally and physically "dried up," and given to irrational behavior (which was often actually justified rage at the way women, especially older women, are treated), suddenly some people in the medical and mental health fields started to talk about "perimenopausal" problems, which supposedly foreshadow the menopausal problems and supposedly need treatment with hormones or psychiatric drugs. Diagnostic creep sometimes reaches absurd proportions, to the point that some professionals tell women in their thirties or even late twenties that their feelings, thoughts, moods, and behavior are not normal human variations but rather pathological early versions of the uncontrolled emotions that supposedly characterize menopausal women. When we add to that the pathologizing of women through premenstrual dysphoric disorder (PMDD), which can even be applied just before their first period, as early as age 10 to 12, it would not be surprising if soon physicians and drug companies claim to have discovered a mental disorder called "*pre*-PMDD" that can be diagnosed in girls from birth up to the moment they qualify for ordinary PMDD. Who knows, maybe pre-PMDD can begin in the birth canal or even at conception! If this seems far-fetched, it is pertinent to consider the way that everything unique to women is so often medicalized and pathologized: When the enormous physical and emotional demands on a woman's body in pregnancy lead to her being tired, distracted, or overwhelmed, she is often described as having "pregnancy brain" if she is forgetful or feels vulnerable. When men forget things or become agitated because they are under enormous work pressures or they experience mood changes or distractibility because of worries about the responsibilities of impending fatherhood, they tend not to be pathologized and are often regarded with indulgence. When a woman has a new baby and experiences the enormous physiological changes that come with giving birth and breastfeeding (or the pressures of deciding whether or not to breastfeed), and when, as often happens in dominant Western culture, she is socially isolated and receives little support while overwhelmed by the demands of caring for a vulnerable baby, her upset in the face of all of this is frequently considered purely physiological or chemical in ways related to being a woman. Then she is diagnosed with postpartum depression and put on psychiatric drugs but not given the support, understanding, and validation she needs to function well in her new role.

The pathologizing of the feelings and behavior of women and girls is part of the larger phenomenon that I call the *psychiatrizing* of society, that is, the movement toward classifying nearly every emotion, thought, and kind of behavior as a form of mental illness. Of course it is not only psychiatrists but also many other professionals (psychologists, social workers, counselors, marriage and family therapists, even clergy) and the general public (thanks to media messages) who participate vigorously in *psychiatrizing*. This has led to the following outcome: *Psychiatrizing of society + thriving sexism = medicalizing and pathologizing of anything a girl or woman might do.* One of the most disturbing features of this equation is the totally unwarranted presentation of mental health treatment as objective and scientific. In response to the well-documented findings that women are more likely than men to be diagnosed as mentally ill even when their behavior is the same (Ali, Caplan, & Fagnant, 2010; Caplan & Cosgrove, 2004), anyone wishing to deny that bias against women is in play can point to widely believed advertisements and poorly conceived and irresponsibly interpreted research to support their response that "We're not being sexist. This is science. Women just happen to have more mental illnesses than do men."

As a member of two committees that were tasked to write the fourth edition of the *Diagnostic and Statistical Manual of Mental Disorders* (DSM; American Psychiatric Association, 1995), I went from believing the portrayal of the manual as scientifically based to learning, to my shock, that: (a) good research was variously ignored, distorted, or lied about when the results did not support what the *DSM* committee heads wanted to include in their new edition; and (b) junk science was portrayed as legitimate research when it fit with their aims. I resigned from the committees after learning that psychiatric diagnosis is not scientific and that those at the top of the *DSM* hierarchy knew that was the case, knew that assigning someone a psychiatric label did not help to reduce her or his suffering, and knew that assigning a label carried enormous risks of harm. Not only did these serious problems fail even to slow their march to create the manual they wanted, but many in the most influential positions publicly denied these truths. I wrote an exposé of what I learned as a *DSM-IV* insider, a book titled *They Say You're Crazy: How the World's Most Powerful Psychiatrists Decide Who's Normal* (Caplan, 1995). Then, because I believed it was important for the public to know what went on in the enterprise of creating categories of mental disorder, I wrote a comedy-drama with music titled *CALL ME CRAZY.*[1]

The numbers of psychiatric categories in various editions of the *DSM* have ballooned over time, which has increasingly made it possible to classify as a mental illness almost anything that anyone does. In the absence of scientific, objective standards, what swoops into that vacuum is every conceivable kind of bias. My belief in the public's need to know how sexism, racism, homophobia, classism, and ageism affect the creation of psychiatric labels; how the labels are applied; and the harm that often comes to those who are labeled[2] led me to coedit the book *Bias in Psychiatric Diagnosis* (Caplan & Cosgrove, 2004). Maureen McHugh and Joan Chrisler arranged for the book to be published as a project of the Association for Women in Psychology (AWP).

In the mid-2000s, as work heated up on the fifth edition of the *DSM* (American Psychiatric Association, 2013), a group of us formed an ad hoc committee of AWP members, and each wrote a short paper to express concern about what might be retained in that next edition or created anew for it. Topics of the papers included the lack of science in preparations for *DSM-5* regarding anorexia nervosa, borderline personality disorder, female sexual dysfunction, gender identity disorder, parental alienation syndrome, racial bias, social class bias, and a much-discussed proposal to classify obesity as a mental disorder. The collection was published on the AWP website.[3]

There is a myth for every occasion that can be used to cast women in a bad light. After all, if you are the group in power, then it is a threat to your power if a member of a scapegoated group does something good. That makes it harder to conceal your own responsibility for social ills and blame them on others instead. It is striking to observe the use of psychiatric diagnosis and myths about mothers to cast in a negative light whatever women might do. And it is done increasingly through the route of medicalizing or psychiatrizing, a way of pathologizing everything about women. As a consequence, intolerable burdens are placed on way too many women. This happens increasingly to women who are related in some way to the military. As the wars in Iraq and Afghanistan have wound down and more new veterans have returned home, the psychiatrized problems of women are becoming more visible. The high probability that a woman serving in the military will be sexually assaulted has become well known, but what is far less known is that nearly every such woman (as well as male assault victims) who, because of feeling devastated by the assault, goes to see a therapist in the military is diagnosed as mentally ill. Instead of being told that she is devastated because that is how rape affects people, all the more when the rapist serves with her in an entity whose members have been trained to trust and rely on each other in life-and-death situations, she is almost always diagnosed with posttraumatic stress disorder, which is simply a way to recast a typical, deeply human response to trauma as a mental illness. On the all too rare occasions when a report of sexual assault in the military is investigated and the perpetrator is brought to trial, the victim's credibility is often damaged because she has been diagnosed as mentally ill, whereas the perpetrator is not considered mentally ill and is almost never dishonorably discharged. The victims not infrequently *are* discharged on the basis of their label of mental illness, which makes it harder for them to obtain employment and may make them feel forever emotionally damaged.

Although anyone can be harmed by rampant medicalization, it is essential to resist especially the more common pathologizing of women that is such a powerful tool for maintaining the status quo and the mistreatment of women. Resistance needs to include constant vigilance by all of us to spot the ways that pathologizing is used to oppress women, as well as the increased likelihood of such consequences for women who belong to racialized groups, those who are poor or old or not heterosexual, and those who are victims of physical, sexual, or financial violence. Resistance is essential in both the public and the professional realms. In the personal realm, resistance can mean speaking up when someone says that a battered woman must be a masochist because she stayed with her children's father, the batterer; one can point out that battered women often stay with the abuser because they cannot support their children on their meager salaries, because they know they will be cast as the villain for "deserting" him or failing to teach him to control his violence, because therapists have warned that she will harm the children by depriving them of a male role model, or because the batterer has threatened to kill her or to kidnap the children if she leaves. In the professional realm, resistance can include similar types of challenges as well as educating one's colleagues and students to step out of the medicalized perspective and consider how people look when we acknowledge the refreshing possibility that there are ways to understand and help women and girls more effectively when we stop rushing to call their normal experiences a physical or mental illness.

Paula J. Caplan

NOTES

1. Available to view at https://www.youtube.com/watch?v=6myXKiXGuUA.

2. See also psychdiagnosis.weebly.com and the Facebook page called Stop Psychiatric Diagnosis Harm.

3. Available at http://awpsych.org/index.php?option=com_content&view =article&id=102&Itemid=126.

REFERENCES

Ali, A., Caplan, P. J., & Fagnant, R. (2010). Gender stereotypes in diagnostic criteria. In J. C. Chrisler & D. R. McCreary (Eds.), *Handbook of gender research in psychology* (vol. 2, pp. 91–109). New York: Springer

American Psychiatric Association. (1994). *Diagnostic and statistical manual of mental disorders* (4th ed.). Washington, DC: Author.

American Psychiatric Association. (2013). *Diagnostic and statistical manual of mental disorders* (5th ed.). Washington, DC: Author.

Caplan, P. J. (1989). *Don't blame mother: Mending the mother-daughter relationship.* New York, NY: Harper and Row.

Caplan, P. J. (1995). *They say you're crazy: How the world's most powerful psychiatrists decide who's normal.* Reading, MA: Addison-Wesley.

Caplan, P. J., & Cosgrove, L. (Eds.). (2004). *Bias in psychiatric diagnosis.* Lanham, MD: Jason Aronson.

Chrisler, J. C., & Caplan, P. J. (2002). The strange case of Dr. Jekyll and Ms. Hyde: How PMS became a cultural phenomenon and a psychiatric disorder. *Annual Review of Sex Research, 13,* 274–306.

Introduction

The Medicalization of Women's Bodies and Everyday Experience

Maureen C. McHugh and Joan C. Chrisler

We are pleased to offer you this book, a book designed for every woman who is exposed to media messages about women's lives, women's bodies, and the potential of drugs, surgeries, or other "prescriptions" to address women's psychological and social problems. Here a series of experts address some of the aspects of women's lives that have been targeted as deficient in order to support the multibillion dollar profits of the medical-pharmaceutical industry. The authors challenge the medicalization (i.e., the marketing of "science" for profit) that increasingly renders women's bodies and experiences as a series of symptoms, diseases, and dysfunctions that require treatment by medical professionals who prescribe pharmaceutical and surgical interventions. Our contributors are psychologists, sociologists, and other health experts who explain the "real" scientific evidence about women's experiences and question the (mis)information that is marketed toward women to sell drugs, surgery, and other products (e.g., antiaging creams, diet pills, hormones). Each chapter in the book addresses the marketing of a specific "condition" that has been constructed to convince a woman that her body is inadequate or that her experience and behavior are not good enough.

An important objective of this book is to challenge "accepted" information often presented as science and fact in popular media. Other authors have also challenged Big Pharma, the industrial complex that includes pharmaceutical companies; medical research conducted with funds from corporate sponsors; and the public relations firms, advertising agencies, and media outlets that publicize new illnesses and new treatments (Abramson, 2004; Cosgrove & Wheeler, 2013; Goldacre, 2010, 2013; Moynihan & Cassels, 2005; Tiefer, 2001). Moynihan and Cassels (2005) documented the objectives and successes of pharmaceutical companies who want to sell drugs to everyone, not just to sick people. According to Abramson (2004), the scientific evidence doctors and laypeople use to make health care decisions is increasingly based on false or distorted "science" that has been sponsored and spun by the pharmaceutical industry. Other authors (e.g., Campos, 2005; Moynihan & Cassels, 2005) have commented on the difficulty of disputing widely shared misinformation about "health conditions" such as obesity. Today, in addition to traditional sources (e.g., magazines, newspapers, television), the general public, especially adolescents and young adults, is exposed to (mis)information on Internet sites (e.g., Wikipedia, blogs, Big Pharma, marketing that is disguised as unbiased "health information"). This book will contribute to the public's scientific literacy by helping our readers become more critical consumers of health-related media messages.

This book differs from others that critically challenge the medical-pharmaceutical industry in one important way. In addition to providing a scientific critique of the available literature, we provide a gender critique. The authors are all gender experts and feminist scholars who recognize the ways in which gender is an important aspect of the human experience and an important factor in how medical decisions are framed. Feminist authors (e.g., Bordo, 1993; Chrisler, 2011; Leyser-Whalen, 2014; Martin, 1987; Ussher, 1989) have suggested that women's bodies are more likely than men's to be subjected to medicalization because our bodies are seen as weaker than men's, as abnormal (i.e., men's bodies are the "standard" in medicine), and, in some ways (e.g., menstruation, lactation), as base, appalling, or pathetic. For example, the labeling of menstrual cycle–related experience as a syndrome (premenstrual syndrome [PMS]) or a psychiatric disorder (premenstrual dysphoric disorder [PMDD]) is based on a culturally pejorative perspective on women's bodies and bodily processes, which has resulted in the widespread experience of reproductive shame (Chrisler & Caplan, 2002; Johnston-Robledo, Sheffield, Voigt, & Wilcox-Constantine, 2007; Ussher, 2006). Similarly, the shame about being fat in a culture that embraces the thin ideal is a different experience for women than for men because women's social worth is primarily determined by their appearance (Chrisler, 2012; Fikken & Rothblum, 2012). Feminist criticism of the way that the biomedical model has viewed women's bodies has been published previously, and the authors in this book based their work on that foundation. Other authors have tended to focus on one particular aspect of medicalization in women's lives. For example, Bacon (2008) and Campos (2005) challenged the medicalization of obesity, and Caplan (1995; Caplan & Cosgrove, 2004) criticized the medicalization of anxiety, sadness, and other common psychological experiences as psychiatric disorders. Here we offer a collection of chapters that take a more diverse approach to various aspects of women's experience, including reproduction, appearance, sexuality, and mental health. We hope that this broader focus will result in greater insight and a more nuanced and complex understanding of how medicalization can negatively impact women's lives.

The biomedical perspective, the basis for medicalization, has often been criticized for its reductionistic approach and its single-minded focus on basic biology (e.g., cells, genes, hormones) to the exclusion of contextual factors (e.g., socioeconomic, psychological, and cultural factors). The biomedical approach also concentrates on illness (rather than on both health and illness) and encourages the prescription of pharmaceutical solutions to every problem, including everyday experiences such as stress and unhappiness. In contrast, the biopsychosocial model, which has been increasingly adopted in studies of chronic illness (e.g., diabetes, heart disease, cancer), acknowledges the role of psychosocial factors (e.g., mental health, spirituality, cultural beliefs about health and illness) in producing well-being and dis-ease. Both the biopsychosocial and feminist perspectives emphasize the ways in which women's lives are also influenced by factors such as relationships, community, environment, identity, sociohistorical context, and culture. The biomedical model also homogenizes women: It treats women who are diverse in age, race, ethnicity, social class, physical ability, religion, and sexual orientation as "just bodies." Yet, women's experiences and their understanding of themselves and their experiences are impacted by these and other factors. In this book, each of the authors argues for the importance of a feminist perspective on the biopsychosocial model.

MEDICALIZATION

Medicalization is the term used to refer to the process whereby everyday experiences and problems become framed as "illness" (Conrad, 1980, 2007). In the course of this process, behaviors or conditions take on medical meanings or are defined (or redefined) in terms of health and illness (Riessman, 1983). The term *disease mongering* similarly refers to the expansion of the boundaries of illness and disease in pursuit of financial profits

(Payer, 1992). The medical-pharmaceutical complex is widely viewed as expanding conceptions of disease in order to expand the markets for treatment, including drugs, surgery, and visits to hospitals and physicians (Brownlee, 2008; Cosgrove & Wheeler, 2013; Goldacre, 2013; Moynihan & Cassals, 2005; Watters, 2010). There is a lot of money to be made by telling healthy people they are sick (Moynihan & Cassals, 2005). Marketing and public relations efforts are characterized by Big Pharma as raising public awareness of underdiagnosed conditions, but, in reality, the medical-pharmaceutical alliance promotes a view of those "conditions" as widespread, serious, and treatable (Moynihan, Heath, & Henry, 2002). The industry's influence over medical practice, medical education, and scientific research is widespread, and it has multiple negative impacts on health care, perhaps especially in the United States (Abramson, 2004; Moynihan & Cassels, 2005), which has unusually high health care costs. Below we discuss the impact of medicalization on health care services and on society.

Defining Disease and Disorders

In some cases, representatives from the pharmaceutical industry, or experts who receive funds from the drug companies, serve as members of government panels or professional association task forces that set the criteria that define a disease or illness. When the criteria that mark the boundaries of the disease are reset (i.e., lowered), a larger number of individuals become eligible for treatment, which results in larger profits for the pharmaceutical industry. For example, a recent decision to lower the "acceptable" blood cholesterol level led to a huge increase in the number of people prescribed statins, drugs that have been largely tested in men and have been shown to have negative side effects in women (Rabin, 2014). When the body mass index (BMI) that serves as the cutoff for "overweight" and "obese" was lowered, the obesity rate in the United States increased dramatically, as millions more individuals became "too fat" overnight and were then subjected to increased pressure to lose weight (Bacon, 2008).

Enforcing Social Norms

In both medicalization and disease mongering, "medical practice becomes a vehicle for eliminating or controlling problematic experiences that are defined as deviant, for the purpose of securing adherence to social norms" (Riessman, 1983, p. 4). For example, the medicalization of grief creates unrealistic expectations for how bereavement should look and feel and how long it should last (see Chapter 13), and the adoption of clinical criteria for hypoactive sexual arousal disorder suggests that there is a normative level of sexual desire for women (McHugh & Interligi, 2015). Conrad (1980, 2007) and other sociologists have examined the impact of medicalization on many aspects of everyday life, such as mood, sleep, appetite, emotions, alcohol use, activity level, weight, aging, pregnancy, menstruation, child development, drug use, mental state, and sociability.

Increasing Health Care Costs

Whenever clinical criteria are manipulated, large numbers of new individuals are categorized as ill or in need of treatment. Common experiences become recast as symptoms of serious conditions. For example, the feelings that can accompany being shy or old or short may be difficult to handle at times, but they are not symptoms of a disease; only disease-mongers suggest otherwise (Parens, 2011). Medicalization *does not* improve the quality of health care; in some cases patients are actually exposed to ineffective medication or drugs with serious side effects. What medicalization *does* do is increase health care costs substantially. When medicalization expands our diagnostic categories, disease constructs, and recommended pharmaceutical or surgical treatments, the cost of medical care grows exponentially (Abramson, 2004; Parens, 2011).

Undermining Patients' Agency

In addition to the astronomical direct costs of such interventions, there are the indirect costs accrued when medicine reduces human beings to objects in need of repair. The medicalization process potentially undermines seeing ourselves as subjects (Parens, 2011); and our sense of ourselves as agents of our own health deteriorates. People are viewed as increasingly less competent as experts begin to "manage" and "mystify" human experiences (Riessman, 1983, p. 4). For example, Dillway (see Chapter 5) notes that perimenopausal women now consult experts to understand developmental experiences that historically women understood better than doctors. Increasingly, both physicians and patients believe that good health is a product of medical science rather than the consequence of a healthy lifestyle and environment (Abramson, 2004). As long as attention remains focused on drugs, we are less likely to consider alternative, equally or more effective, and less expensive ways to achieve health or prevent illness.

Ignoring Diversity and Intersectionality

The medical model ignores diversity; it reduces all women to a single set of physiological responses, symptoms, dysfunctions, and causes. In contrast, feminist approaches within sociology, anthropology, nursing, psychology, and sexology recognize that women are not a homogenous group. For example, understanding and experience of sexual desire, attraction, arousal, and satisfaction are complex, develop in a sociohistorical context, and are impacted by race or ethnicity, age, religion, sexual orientation, culture, class, and even neighborhood norms (McHugh, 2006). A medical model that views genital and physiological processes as identical across women (and as basically the same for both men and women) ignores the implications of inequalities related to gender, social class, race or ethnicity, age, and sexual orientation. Social, political, and economic conditions can limit women's access to sexual health, pleasure, and satisfaction (McHugh, 2006; Tiefer, 2001, 2006), and no drug can change that.

Distorting Medical Science

Medicalization is distinct from the science and practice of medicine. Physicians and medical researchers have contributed extensively to women's health, through, for example, the development and application of vaccines, surgical techniques, and necessary medications. Yet, medicalization has negatively impacted both medical science and practice. Abramson (2004) contended that medicalization in the United States, driven by profit and greed, has challenged the integrity of medicine, disrupted the physician–patient relationship, and presented a threat to public health. Abramson, a physician himself, documented how the pharmaceutical industry has undermined the integrity of medical science through funding of certain types of research (e.g., the development of drugs that can make a lot of money, rather than drugs to treat rare diseases or diseases common in countries that cannot afford to buy expensive drugs) and then issuing selective and misleading reports of research findings. The scientific knowledge on which decisions to develop and prescribe tests and drugs rests is currently funded primarily by Big Pharma, and they advertise the (selected) results to physicians and to the public in misleading ways. Hospitals, journals, physicians, advocacy groups, charities, and researchers are all under the sway of the pharmaceutical industry. Even the U.S. Food and Drug Administration (FDA), the federal agency that is supposed to regulate the drug industry, makes its decisions about drug safety and effectiveness based on research funded by the pharmaceutical industry and testimony from drug companies and the researchers they have funded. It is standard operating procedure for the pharmaceutical industry to attempt to influence medical research, to withhold unfavorable findings, to misrepresent research results, and to spin the research results (Abramson, 2004). Increasingly, both the education of physicians and the information presented to consumers are in the hands of Big Pharma.

Advertising and Manipulation

Moynihan and Cassels (2005) exposed the modus operandi of the billion-dollar pharmaceutical industry: Big Pharma uses advertising and "awareness" campaigns to construct new "disorders" (e.g., attention deficit disorder, PMDD) and to convey health concerns as "diseases" (e.g., runny noses are now allergic rhinitis, socially awkward or eccentric children are now on the autism spectrum) that require pharmaceutical prescriptions. Moynihan and Cassels demonstrated effectively the problems with the corporate sponsorship of medical research and the production and dissemination of (mis)information by the pharmaceutical industry. Direct to consumer advertising (DTCA) is a problematic aspect of medicalization in the United States, but not in most other countries, where it is prohibited. Patients increasingly request, or even demand, prescriptions for heavily advertised medicine ("Ask your doctor if . . . is right for you!") (Kravits, Epstein, Feldman, Franz, & Rahman, 2005). In Abramson's (2004) opinion, DTCA has undermined the doctor–patient relationship; it is an important factor in medicalization and in producing high-cost, drug-oriented, low-quality health care in the United States.

THE IMPACT OF MEDICALIZATION ON WOMEN

Medicalization can have a serious impact on women's health and well-being because it teaches us to doubt our bodies' wisdom and abilities and to think of ourselves as unable to withstand common experiences (e.g., birthing, menopause, bereavement) without medical supervision or management. Changes in the body (e.g., stretch marks, wrinkles, weight gain, water retention) that women have always expected and coped with on their own or by sharing their experiences with other women are now seen as defects in need of repair by experts. If women come to see their bodies (and themselves) as weak, abnormal, ugly, or debased, can they ever see themselves as strong, attractive, and capable? Can they have happy relationships, take good care of themselves, and enjoy life? Sometimes a medicalized view of the self is simply the wrong prescription for women.

The chapters in this book discuss medicalized views of women's bodies and everyday experiences. The chapters address three main areas that have been a focus of the medical-pharmaceutical industry: reproduction and women's sexuality; women's size, shape, and appearance; and women's moods. Of course, other areas have been medicalized, but the areas covered here are specific to, or more often targeted at, women, so much so that many women accept the medicalized view of their bodies and everyday experience as the way things are or should be. It is our hope that this book will cause our readers to reevaluate the conventional wisdom and learn new ways to see themselves and to cope with everyday concerns.

REPRODUCTION AND WOMEN'S SEXUALITY

The book begins with a consideration of pregnancy and birth, perhaps the most "natural" and powerful things a woman's body can do. Yet these processes have become thoroughly medicalized in developed nations. Although a few generations ago, most American women gave birth at home with a midwife or female relative to assist them, now almost everyone gives birth in a hospital with medical personnel managing and directing the action. We even speak about birth from the point of view of the medical attendants, who are said to "deliver" the baby, rather than from the point of view of the woman who "births" (or "gives birth to") her child. In Chapter 1, Ruthbeth D. Finerman, Adriane M. F. Sanders, and Lynda Sagrestano describe and discuss the benefits (e.g., life-saving techniques such as cesarean sections) and drawbacks (e.g., far more cesarean sections than are necessary) of medicalized pregnancy and birth, and they consider the irony that some women (in wealthy nations) get too much medical treatment, whereas others (in poor nations or neighborhoods) get too little. This chapter should help to reempower women to take control of their reproductive experiences.

Does every woman who wants a child have a "right" to become pregnant and give birth? If a couple does not conceive, are they ill? If there is something that can be done to assist with conception, should it be done, despite the cost, pain, and stress involved? If the inability to conceive is the man's fault, should the woman's body be subject to medical "treatment"? These are some of the provocative questions raised by Emily Breitkopf and Lisa R. Rubin in Chapter 2. The authors discuss "Fertility Inc.," the medical-pharmaceutical industry that has focused on developing and marketing techniques to treat infertility. This is a booming area of medicine that draws doctors away from other areas where the need is greater but the profits are lower (e.g., family medicine, internal medicine); it is also an area of medical practice that is fraught with ethical issues that have not been adequately addressed by practitioners or consumers.

Most women menstruate for three to four decades of their lives, an experience that is considered by many to be part of what it means to be a woman. Although managing menstrual hygiene can be a hassle and some menstrual cycle–related symptoms (e.g., uterine or pelvic cramps, headaches, water retention) can be distressing, women have always been able to cope with menstruation and to manage their cycles without medical intervention. There are positive aspects of menstruation: Experiencing and complaining to one another about cycle-related symptoms has been a bonding experience for women, there can be no pregnancy (or maternal joy) without menstrual cycles, and the public health initiative Project Vital Sign promotes the view that menstruation is a sign of a healthy woman. However, in the 1990s, a Brazilian gynecologist published a best-selling and much-translated book titled *Is Menstruation Obsolete*? In Chapter 3, Jessica Barnack-Tavlaris shows us how the use of that book in the service of medicalization has changed society's view of menstruation from a healthy process to an unnecessary risk factor; in effect, menstruation is now considered a disorder in and of itself. Medications to suppress menstruation are being sold to girls and women, despite the fact that we know little about their long-term effects on the body.

Prior to 1980, few people had ever heard of PMS, and most premenstrual symptoms were the phenomenological equivalent of a bad hair day; yet today most American women who menstruate think they have PMS. The biomedical approach is dominant in both the professional and popular literature, where premenstrual women's hormones are often described as "raging" or "unbalanced." Yet, few have stopped to consider how it is possible that the hormones of millions of women could suddenly be so unbalanced that they require medical treatment (Laws, 1983). In Chapter 4, Joan C. Chrisler and Jennifer A. Gorman discuss the medicalizing (PMS) and psychiatrizing (PMDD) of the premenstrual phase of the menstrual cycle. They emphasize the importance of a feminist biopsychosocial approach to premenstrual symptoms and suggest ways that self-care and coping strategies can alleviate symptoms and help women to avoid the wrong prescription.

Menopause, the close of menstrual life, has been viewed as a disorder rather than a normal developmental transition. The medicalization of menopause is usually traced back to the publication of Wilson's (1966) best-selling book *Feminine Forever*. Wilson's work was subsidized by Big Pharma, which also manufactured the "cure" for menopause: hormone replacement therapy (HRT). In Chapter 5, Heather Dillaway traces the medicalization of menopause and discusses the (sometimes outrageous) claims about the ways that women's aging bodies betray them and the "miracle cure" that HRT is said to be. Despite considerable scientific evidence to the contrary, menopause continues to be seen as needing medical attention, monitoring, and treatment. She also considers side effects of hormone therapy and suggests other, nonmedical ways to cope with bothersome symptoms that sometimes accompany the menopausal transition.

One of the ways that Wilson (1966) frightened women into wanting a "cure" for menopause was that he blamed menopause for every aspect of women's aging, with special emphasis on attractiveness and sexuality. Menopause, he wrote, makes attractive women ugly by causing wrinkles, drooping breasts, and dowager's hump, and the lower levels of sex hormones postmenopause turn women into "neuters" who are no longer interested in sex and unable to be sexually responsive to their partners. Although some women do find sex less enjoyable after menopause, others find it more enjoyable (perhaps because they no longer have to worry about an accidental pregnancy), and some notice little change. Sexuality, like almost everything else, is contextual. In Chapter 6, Jane M. Ussher, Janette Perz, and Chloe Parton discuss the medicalization of sexuality at midlife, and they share stories from women who have participated in their research projects. These women's stories illustrate the complexity and variability of women's sexual experiences at midlife, and they suggest ways to cope with changes and rethink, if necessary, what it means to be sexual.

In Chapter 7, Leonore Tiefer tells us that sexuality has been medicalized at every age and every stage of sexual experience. From early sex manuals (how to do it "right") to the research of Kinsey (what is "normal") and Masters and Johnson (how the body "should" respond) to the construction of sexual disorders and dysfunctions (e.g., hypoactive sexual desire disorder) to the search for the "female Viagra," sexologists have joined the medical-pharmaceutical industry to convince people that medical assistance is required even in the most intimate of acts. Tiefer exposes the marketing techniques of Big Pharma (including celebrity spokeswomen and cooptation of feminist rhetoric) and urges readers to take a "new view" (i.e., a complex and contextualized view) of women's (and men's) sexuality.

Women's Appearance

One of most women's everyday experiences is body dissatisfaction, which has been described as a "normative discontent" (Rodin, Silberstein, & Striegel-Moore, 1984). This discontent derives in large part from the ubiquitous images of idealized beauty in the media and popular culture. Thinness is now a key component of how beauty is evaluated in Western and Westernized countries. In Chapter 8, Mindy J. Erchull examines the thin ideal as perpetrated by the media and fashion industry and internalized and reinforced by women themselves. She also critically explores the complex relation between thinness and health and notes that the media rarely publicize the negative health effects of the extreme thinness they promote. Erchull establishes the thin ideal as the basis for both women's desire to be thin and their belief that thin is both "good" and healthy. This is the foundation for women's concern about body weight, their obsession with dieting, and their willingness to use often-dangerous diets, drugs, and surgeries in pursuit of weight loss.

In Chapter 9, Ashley E. Kasardo and Maureen C. McHugh examine the negative effects of the thin ideal, including the stigmatizing and shaming of fat women who are seen as violating beauty standards. Women are encouraged to lose weight through dieting, under the mistaken medical belief that dieting is a route to weight loss and better health. They discuss research that challenges the beliefs that diets work and that being thin or of average weight is the same as being healthy. Rather, fat prejudice and fat shaming often result in psychological and physical harm, and health care professionals' bias against fat people is a barrier that prevents fat women from receiving appropriate health care. The authors describe an alternative approach—Health at Every Size—which emphasizes self-acceptance, intentional eating, and positive movement, rather than highly restrictive regimens that are impossible to follow and decrease quality of life.

In Chapter 10, Julie Konik and Christine A. Smith examine two medicalized approaches to weight loss: diet pills and bariatric surgery. If Big Pharma could produce a weight-loss pill that works, the profits would be enormous, given that many (if not most) women would want to try it. However, the available pills are the wrong prescription for women. Konik and Smith describe and discuss research that indicates no long-term efficacy for either diet pills or bariatric surgery, both of which have potentially serious side effects that are much worse than maintaining a heavy body weight. The authors also present a critical analysis of the BMI both as a measure of "appropriate" and "inappropriate" weight and as an indicator of an individual's health. They also introduce "the obesity paradox": being "overweight" is actually a health and mortality advantage; this idea obviously is only a paradox to the extent that one accepts the medicalized view that fat is inherently and always unhealthy.

Body dissatisfaction extends beyond weight to many (if not every) other aspects of women's bodies. Thus, it is not surprising that cosmetic surgery is one of the fastest growing medical specialties in many countries around the world. The United States is a leader in both the development and the application of cosmetic surgeries (e.g., breast augmentation, face lifts, nose jobs) and procedures (e.g., botox, dermabrasion, liposuction), which are often marketed to women as "cures" for aging, low self-esteem, and body dysmorphic disorder (a psychiatric diagnosis for the tendency to obsess about a body part that causes dissatisfaction). In Chapter 11, Charlotte N. Markey and Patrick M. Markey examine the history of the medicalization of body dissatisfaction, the risks of the procedures, and the evidence for the marketing claims. Although short-term studies often show a rise in self-esteem after a "successful" procedure, studies of long-term effects are rarely published, perhaps because they show that dissatisfaction returns or becomes focused on another body part, which results in more procedures. That is good for the surgeons' profits, but it is the wrong prescription for women's negative body image. The authors suggest other, less risky and less expensive ways to feel better about our bodies and our selves.

Women's Moods

There are several excellent books about the psychiatrization of everyday experience (see, for example, Caplan, 1995; Caplan & Cosgrove, 2004; Watters, 2010). Here we focus on mood-related "disorders" because of the greater tendency for women rather than for men to be diagnosed with them.

The common belief that the body (especially its reproductive processes) is responsible for women's negative moods (see Chapter 4) is one reason why mental health professionals, the general public, and women themselves are likely to see women's moods as in need of medical management.

In Chapter 12, Alisha Ali considers the widespread diagnosis of depression among women in light of the "fundamental incompatibility between what is 'known' by those who claim expertise in the field of depression and what is lived by women who are diagnosed as depressed." Given that much of women's reported depression is connected to life circumstances that are difficult to bear (e.g., violence, poverty, trauma, discrimination, marginalization, strained relationships), could medication really be the "cure"? The medicalized view of depression as caused by a chemical imbalance in the brain (i.e., a deficiency of serotonin) promotes the use of drugs (e.g., selective serotonin reuptake inhibitors [SSRIs]) as the best treatment. However, as Ali points out, drugs might make a woman's moods less dark, but they cannot change her history and circumstances. The diagnosis and treatment of depressed women has important implications for both the patients and society. In addition to large profits for Big Pharma, Ali suggests that the medicalized approach is an effective way to distract our attention away from poverty, violence, discrimination, and other barriers to women's mental health and well-being. Thus, drug therapy may serve to silence women's protest of abuse and inequality, and it may limit resistance to the status quo.

In Chapter 13, Leeat Granek discusses a common experience—bereavement—that has recently become the subject of medicalization. In traditional societies, people are expected to grieve the loss of a loved one for a significant length of time (e.g., 6 to 12 months, or even longer). However, in contemporary societies, where cultural messages urge people to seek "closure" or "bounce back" or "move on" after losses of all types, grief has become pathologized if it lasts more than a few weeks. Furthermore, as Granek points out, given that women have traditionally been responsible for expressing grief (e.g., as "professional mourners," as funeral planners, as responders to letters of sympathy), the distinction between grief and depression has become blurred, which makes a much larger number of women eligible for antidepressant medications. She also makes the important point that a medicalized view of grief diminishes the range of what is considered acceptable human emotion and places "arbitrary limits around how long our grief can last, how intensely we can feel it, and the modes by which we can express our mourning."

CONCLUSION

We hope it is clear that we are not saying that it is always bad to fill a prescription for a drug or agree to surgery or seek other types of medical treatment. We assure you that we would have a tumor removed, a cavity filled, and a broken leg set. If we were diagnosed with type 1 diabetes or schizophrenia or cancer, we would want to take insulin or an antipsychotic drug or chemotherapy, despite those medications' side effects. If the result of not seeking treatment is death or severe discomfort, the benefit outweighs the cost. Today, however, many people, especially many women, are seeking treatments whose costs outweigh the benefits. The costs include side effects more dangerous than the "condition" the drug is meant to treat, enforcement of the status quo (e.g., women as weak, women's bodies as inherently defective), the redefinition of normal experience as illness, the reduction of women's personal agency, the massive increase in our society's health care costs, and the manipulation of science in the service of Big Pharma's profits.

The authors of the chapters in this book aimed to be provocative and to cause readers to question the increasing medicalization of women's bodies and everyday experiences. Readers can use information in the chapters to initiate dialogue with their health care providers about the treatment they have received and the advice they have been given. The knowledge that the medicalized view is not the only view can be empowering and lead to an increase in women's agency to make their own decisions and stand by them. It is our hope that our readers will ask themselves whether the next prescription they receive is the right one or the wrong one for them.

REFERENCES

Abramson, J. (2004). *Overdosed America: The broken promise of American medicine.* New York: Harper Perennial.

Bacon, L. (2008). *Health at every size: The surprising truth about your weight.* Dallas, TX: BenBella Books.

Bordo, S. (1993). *Unbearable weight: Feminism, western culture, and the body.* Berkeley, CA: University of California Press.

Brownlee, S. (2008). *Overtreated: Why too much medicine is making us sicker and poorer.* London: Bloomsbury Books.

Campos, P. (2005). *The diet myth: Why America's obsession with weight is hazardous to your health.* New York: Gotham Books.

Caplan, P. J. (1995). *They say you're crazy: How the world's most powerful psychiatrists decide who's normal.* Reading, MA: Addison-Wesley.

Caplan, P. J., & Cosgrove, L. (Eds.). (2004). *Bias in psychiatric diagnosis.* Lanham, MD: Jason Aronson.

Chrisler, J. C. (2011). Leaks, lumps, and lines: Sigma and women's bodies. *Psychology of Women Quarterly, 35,* 202–214.

Chrisler, J. C. (2012). "Why can't you control yourself?" Fat *should* be a feminist issue. *Sex Roles, 66,* 608–616.

Chrisler, J. C., & Caplan, P. J. (2002). The strange case of Dr. Jekyll and Ms. Hyde: How PMS became a cultural phenomenon and a psychiatric disorder. *Annual Review of Sex Research, 13,* 274–306.

Conrad, P. (1980). *Deviance and medicalization: From badness to sickness.* Philadelphia, PA: Temple University Press.

Conrad, P. (2007). *The medicalization of society.* Baltimore: Johns Hopkins University Press.

Cosgrove, L., & Wheeler, E. E. (2013). Drug firms, the codification of diagnostic categories, and bias in clinical guidelines. *Journal of Law, Medicine, and Ethics, 41,* 644–653.

Fikkan, J. L., & Rothblum, E. D. (2012). Is fat a feminist issue? Exploring the gendered nature of weight bias. *Sex Roles, 66,* 575–592.

Goldacre, B. (2010). *Bad science: Quacks, hacks, and big pharma flacks.* New York: Faber and Faber.

Goldacre, B. (2013). *Bad pharma: How drug companies mislead doctors and harm patients.* New York: Faber and Faber.

Johnston-Robledo, I., Sheffield, K., Voight, J., & Wilcox-Constantine, J. (2007). Reproductive shame: Self-objectification and young women's attitudes toward their reproductive functioning. *Women & Health, 46*(1), 25–39.

Kravits, R., Epstein, R., Feldman, M., Franz, C., & Rahman, A. (2005). Influence of patients' requests for direct to consumer advertised antidepressants. *Journal of the American Medical Association, 293,* 1995–2002.

Laws, S. (1983). The sexual politics of premenstrual tension. *Women's Studies International Forum, 6,* 19–31.

Leyser-Whalen, O. (2014). "Crazy woman juice": Making sense of women's infertility treatment with clomiphene. *Women's Reproductive Health, 1,* 73–89.

Martin, E. (1987). *The woman in the body: A cultural analysis of reproduction.* Boston: Beacon Press.

McHugh, M. C. (2006). Women and sex at midlife: Desire, dysfunction, and diversity. In V. Muhlbauer & J. C. Chrisler (Eds.), *Women over 50: Psychological perspectives* (pp. 26–52). New York: Springer.

McHugh, M. C., & Interligi, C. (2015). Sexuality and older women: Desirability and desire. In V. Muhlbauer, J. C. Chrisler, & F. L. Denmark (Eds.), *Women and aging: An international, intersectional power perspective* (pp. 89–116). New York: Springer.

Moynihan, R., & Cassels, A. (2005). *Selling sickness: How the world's biggest pharmaceutical companies are turning us all into patients.* New York: Nation Books.

Moynihan, R., Heath, I., & Henry, D. (2002). Selling sickness: The pharmaceutical industry and disease mongering. *British Medical Journal, 324,* 886–891.

Parens, E. (2011). On good and bad forms of medicalization. *Bioethics, 27,* 28–35.

Payer, L. (1992). *Disease mongers: How doctors, drug companies, and insurers are making you sick.* New York: Wiley.

Rabin, R. C. (2014, May 5). A new women's issue: Statins. *New York Times.* Retrieved from http://well.blogs.nytimes.com/2014/05/05/a-new-womens -issue-statins/?_r=0.

Riessman, C. K. (1983). Women and medicalization: A new perspective. *Social Policy, 14,* 3–18.

Rodin, J., Silberstein, L., & Striegel-Moore, R. (1984). Women and weight: A normative discontent. In T. B. Sonderegger (Ed.), *Nebraska symposium on motivation* (pp. 267–307). Lincoln, NE: University of Nebraska Press.

Tiefer, L. (2001). The selling of "female sexual dysfunction." *Journal of Sex and Marital Therapy, 27,* 625–628.

Tiefer, L. (2006). Female sexual dysfunction: A case study of disease mongering and activist resistance. *PLOS Medicine, 3*(4), 178.

Ussher, J. (1989). *The psychology of the female body.* New York: Routledge.

Ussher, J. M. (2006). *Managing the monstrous feminine: Regulating the reproductive body.* London: Routledge.

Watters, E. (2010). *Crazy like us: The globalization of the American psyche.* New York: Free Press.

Wilson, R. (1966). *Feminine forever.* New York: M. Evans.

Chapter 1

Pregnancy and Birth as a Medical Crisis

Ruthbeth D. Finerman, Adriane M. F. Sanders, and Lynda M. Sagrestano

Throughout history, women have managed to carry a pregnancy to term and give birth with support from family and social systems, but without requirement for medical intervention. So why have pregnancy and birth become so heavily medicalized, and is this transition to greater intervention good or bad? We argue that medicalization is a double-edged sword with both benefits and costs. A number of factors, including medical advancement, but also historic shifts toward paternalistic control of medicine, fear-inducing media, market-driven insurance, and litigation have driven the shift toward increased medicalization. This shift has occurred at a rate that has not afforded space to reflect on medicalization's broader implications, both positive and negative (Sagrestano & Finerman, 2012).

THE LURE OF MEDICALIZATION

Medicalization is credited with saving the lives of women and newborns, providing a sterile environment and pain relief, and making childbearing both safer and more comfortable. Between 1920 and 1950, maternal deaths in the United States fell by nearly 75% due to improvements in public health and medical science (Loudon, 1991; Omran, 1977). For instance, contemporary cesarean sections have been credited with reducing postpartum complications in high-risk cases, saving mothers' lives, and resolving fetal distress (Villar et al., 2006). Similarly, prematurity, low birth weight, and infant mortality have decreased in the industrialized world, where infant deaths now average just 4 per 1,000 live births (OECD, 2013).

At the same time, interventions often introduce unnecessary risk of complications in what would otherwise be routine pregnancies and births (Chen & Wang, 2006; Spong, Berghella, Wenstrom, Mercer, & Saade, 2012; Tracy, Sullivan, Wang, Black, & Tracy, 2007; Villar et al., 2006). Despite ever-increasing technological and medical interventions, maternal mortality in the United States has doubled over the past three decades and complications have increased; for instance, serious complications (severe maternal morbidity) more than doubled between 1998 and 2011 (from 78 cases to 163 cases per 10,000 pregnancies) (CDC, 2014a, 2014b). The United States also has one of the highest rates of maternal death among all industrialized nations (CIA, 2013; Hogan et al., 2010; WHO & UNICEF, 2012a). Similarly, declines in U.S. infant death rates have been slower than in other industrialized nations, and rates have actually increased in some years. Furthermore, infant death rates differ dramatically by race and income level (Healthy People, 2014; OECD, 2013), and increases in health care spending do not consistently translate into fewer infant deaths (Kiely, Brett, Yu, & Rowley, 1995; OECD, 2013; Retzlaff-Roberts, Chang, & Rubin, 2004). Medical science has also failed to find effective ways to prevent prenatal risks, such as toxemia, or effective treatment for prenatal conditions, such as many neural tube defects (Maynard & Thadhani, 2009; Sahin, 2003). Moreover, health care is not easily tailored to the psychosocial needs of individual women with diverse backgrounds and cultural heritage (Sagrestano & Finerman, 2012).

Why has the United States made slower progress than other nations, and why have some risks actually increased for American women and children? We argue that the lure of medicalization introduces new opportunities for complications in otherwise normal pregnancies and births, particularly as interventions in the United States are not reserved exclusively for high-risk cases. Medicalization and technological advances are inextricably bound to shifts in place, person, and process in the birthing experience—from home to hospital, from individualized and relaxed to regimented and schedule-driven, and from female midwives to male physicians (although currently almost one-half of obstetricians and gynecologists are women) (ACOG, 2012).

THE RISE OF MEDICALIZED PREGNANCY AND BIRTH IN THE UNITED STATES

Before the 18th century, women gave birth at home, attended by midwives. If birth complications arose, colonial Americans would summon a barber-surgeon, even though such intervention was largely unsuccessful. These rare but vivid experiences began to build a culture of fear related to childbirth. This, coupled with the availability of professional male health practitioners, provided a rationale for displacing female midwives with "man-midwives" and surgeons. This transition was furthered by the exclusion of women from attending medical school and the use of new birthing techniques, such as pain-reduction medications and technologies, thus shifting the locus of childbirth expertise from women and lay midwives to professionally trained male physicians (Cheyney, 2011; Davis-Floyd, 2004). This reflected a paternalistic movement to control women's bodies and women's access to reproductive knowledge (Cahill, 2001; McCool & Simeone, 2002; Stone, 2009). In addition, the biomedical establishment made a conscious effort to discredit Black midwives as "witch doctors" and instead encouraged their would-be patients to seek care from hospital-sanctioned physicians, often aided by female nurses assigned to the wards, many of which were racially segregated until the 1960s (Wailoo, 2001).

Early hospital delivery attended by physicians did not yield anticipated improvements in maternal and child well-being. Rather, the frequency of complications rose among low-risk women; for instance, rates of deadly puerperal infection or "childbed fever" soared with hospitalization as compared to the lower rates with home birth and midwifery (Hallett, 2005; Wertz & Wertz, 1989). Despite the limitations of hospital-based birth, home births in the United States fell into disfavor. In 1940, nearly one-half of all births took place outside hospitals, and by 1970, this had declined to only 1%, where it remains today (CDC, 2012). Contemporary home and alternative birth movements are regarded with skepticism in the United States (Cheyney, 2008). For example, certified professional midwives are legally authorized to practice in just 28 states, some of which allow them to practice only within a hospital and under the supervision of a licensed physician (Certified Professional Midwives NOW, 2014).

MEDIA, FEAR, AND MEDICALIZATION

Information about pregnancy currently comes not only from medical professionals and social support networks, but also from popular media sources, such as television, magazines, and the Internet (Jordan, 1993). Today's increasingly connected and data-driven environment facilitates access to information on pregnancy, yet provokes uncertainty and anxiety.

Such diverse, readily available, and at times contradictory sources create information overload that can support or confound informed decisions. Media sources also foster two disparate impressions of pregnancy and motherhood: one an unrealistic ideal, the other an exaggerated danger. Both impressions feed into a culture of fear (Lagan, Sinclair, & Kernohan, 2010; Morris & McInerney, 2010).

Further, media sources promote medicalization by localizing authority for pregnancy care in the hands of physicians (Song, West, Lundy, & Dahmen, 2012). For instance, an analysis of reality-based birth television showed that birth is often portrayed as unpredictable and dangerous and that the optimal solution is a regimented labor process. Moreover, women who fail to conform to prescribed, time-sensitive benchmarks or who question interventions, such as pain management or episiotomy, are depicted as uncooperative (Morris & McInerney, 2010). Media portrayals can be key sources of information that allow parents to visualize the birthing process; yet, framing birth as both dangerous and idealized may create unnecessary fears and undermine a woman's confidence in her natural abilities. This heightened fear, compounded by anecdotal "war stories" from friends and family, can reinforce dependence on medicalized interventions (Fisher, Hauck, & Fenwick, 2006; Geissbuehler & Eberhard, 2002; Jordan, 1993; Morris & McInerney, 2010; Reiger & Dempsey, 2006).

MARKET-DRIVEN INSURANCE, LITIGATION, AND MEDICALIZATION

Medicalization in the United States is also propelled by the economic pressures of commercialization and litigation. Providers profit from the use of new and costly reproductive technologies, procedures, and products. These are advertised to create demand among consumers with the resources to insist on the highest level of care. Yet this consumer-patient population is shrinking as voluntary fertility rates decline, which has intensified competition among providers. At the same time, the growing number of procedures exhausts the ability of governing agencies to oversee quality and safety, which poses a potential for substandard care. When this occurs, the most affordable and efficient means for patients remains malpractice lawsuits (Sloan & Hsieh, 2012).

Historically, malpractice awards were limitless and often punitive (Budetti & Waters, 2005). High awards have the potential to spur increases in malpractice premiums, forcing providers to pass along costs to patients in order to stay in business (Hellinger & Encinosa, 2006). Many states have responded by instituting award caps (Fairchild, 2010), which has led to a reduction in malpractice premiums since the 1970s (Hellinger & Encinosa, 2006). However, providers' fear of litigation remains and fosters an atmosphere of defensive medicine. In this way, physicians have expanded testing that was initially indicated only for high-risk patients to a standard of care for all patients, regardless of their risk level (Fairchild, 2010). This is exemplified by a plethora of screening, testing, treatment, and other interventions in the reproductive domain, as discussed below.

THE MEDICALIZED PREGNANCY

In much of the world, pregnancy and birth are viewed as natural stages in the lifecycle and embedded within a more humanistic, holistic approach to health. Yet, U.S. health systems regard all aspects of reproduction as invariably risky medical conditions, which almost always require professional and technological intervention to ensure the well-being of mothers and infants (Lock & Nguyen, 2010; Stone, 2009; Unnithan-Kumar, 2004). In the United States, each phase of pregnancy is associated with different medical risks, which are subjected to tests and interventions that grow more numerous and complex each year (Browner & Press, 1995; Jordan, 1997). Moreover, the emphasis has shifted to prevent any possible risk, even among low-risk women. Activities that would otherwise appear innocuous, such as eating unpasteurized cheese, relaxing in a sauna or hot tub, tending a garden, or having an occasional glass of wine or cup of coffee, have been recast as perilous—and even illegal during pregnancy in select states. The only behaviors not subjected to distrust are prenatal visits, which create the impression that physicians can resolve all risks, a promise that remains unfulfilled.

Fear, the desire to control the unknown, and the quest for "perfect" babies (in terms of health, gender, or other desirable traits) underlie prenatal testing, interventions, and new reproductive technologies (Boardman, 2014; Buchbinder & Timmermans, 2011; Davis-Floyd & Dumit, 2013; Press, Browner, Tran, Morton, & LeMaster, 1998; Press, Wilfond, Murray, & Burke, 2011; Rapp, 1999, 2014). This fear drives the desire to detect pregnancy at the earliest possible stage, and the pregnancy test-kit industry exploits these fears. Multiple brands of at-home pregnancy tests bank on the profitable and persistent (albeit remote) fear of birth defects and complications, which are promoted as "common" outcomes of maternal missteps (e.g., smoking, use of alcohol) during the first three months of pregnancy (CDC, 2014c). In reality, at-home pregnancy test reliability varies, depending on the length of time since conception and the time of day when the test is conducted. Once pregnancy is positively "diagnosed," women are given an estimated due date (EDD), which is an estimate in every sense; the length of normal pregnancy differs from woman to woman and can vary by as much as 37 days (Jukic, Baird, Weinberg, McConnaughey, & Wilcox, 2013). As ultrasound technology grows more advanced, physicians seek to zero in on the EDD with greater precision. The EDD then serves as the benchmark for determining overdue and induction dates, despite the normal variation among women (Hunter, 2009; Jukic et al., 2013).

The positive pregnancy test initiates a regimen of personal and medical management of pregnancy, including the adoption of social norms that inform the "do's and don'ts" of pregnancy, as well as the seemingly endless repertoire of prenatal tests, which can reveal manageable health conditions. For example, gestational diabetes and hypertension might be controlled through a combination of behavior change and medical intervention. A comprehensive physical examination and a repertoire of blood, urine, and ultrasound tests are routinely conducted to detect everything from dietary and metabolic imbalances, Rh incompatibility, infections, and pregnancy complications to hereditary and congenital defects. Pregnant women are further instructed on "proper" diet, weight, and behavioral practices. These tests and practices reinforce a culture of fear, which has sometimes culminated in criminalization. Some states have passed legislation criminalizing drug use in pregnancy, even though few substance abuse programs reportedly accept patients who are pregnant (ACOG, 2001; Gregory, 2010; Nash, 2001; Steverson & Rieckmann, 2009).

More invasive tests accrue with each trimester, and each test poses both benefits and risks. Benefits include the ability to detect conditions that might be treated or that allow parents to anticipate and make informed choices about the viability of a pregnancy. Indicators of fetal abnormality (e.g., open neural tubal defects or lung immaturity) can allow both doctors and parents to prepare for specialized infant care, which might include surgery or treatment prior to or immediately after birth. In these situations, detecting an abnormality during the prenatal period can make the difference between life and death. However, prenatal testing also reinforces a cultural fear of disability; it "publicly implies that disabled people are an outcome to be avoided" (Landsman, 2009, p. 44). In addition, tests can be costly, invasive, or harmful to the fetus. Some tests also have a high false-positive rate, which poses the potential that parents might abort a healthy fetus based on inaccurate test results. Moreover, only a few fetal conditions can be treated, and intervention may be culturally or religiously unacceptable for some parents, which makes the testing irrelevant for them (Rapp, 1999, 2014; Root & Browner, 2011).

Early tests (e.g., chorionic villus sampling, first trimester screen, and maternal serum alpha-fetoprotein) are particularly susceptible to a false-positive diagnosis and thus require further testing. Others (e.g., amniocentesis, cordocentesis, and percutaneous umbilical cord sampling) may yield spontaneous miscarriage or other fetal damage (which indicates its own series of further tests). The American Congress of Obstetricians and Gynecologists' guidelines recommend that all pregnant women be offered prenatal screening, but that such testing should be reserved for women with elevated risk factors (ACOG, 2007). Nevertheless, these tests are increasingly becoming routine, independent of risk (Rapp, 2001; Root & Browner, 2011).

Screenings can also place disproportionate liability on mothers for fetal health. Parents, and especially mothers, may be held legally, socially, or personally responsible for fetal disability. Indeed, women who receive positive diagnoses of fetal abnormalities often feel pressured to prove to doctors that they are "doing everything right" (Landsman, 2009, p. 17). Women with a family history of disability are even more likely to voluntarily seek prenatal testing, despite the invasive nature of the tests and their associated risks (Cappelli et al., 2008). Furthermore, public policy legitimizes the sense of maternal responsibility, as women can be prosecuted for poor fetal health outcomes (Mills, 1998). Fear of judicial and social repercussions may foster a greater dependency on the medical system.

The Medicalized Labor

The onset of labor initiates a new cascade of medicalized interventions. Although many pregnant women create a birth plan that includes freedom of movement during labor, water birth, choice of attendants, or minimally invasive and medication-free childbirth, that plan is often abandoned soon after arrival at the hospital (Lothian, 2000). As a setting for birth, hospitals are foreign territory: The rules are obscure and complex, the staff unfamiliar, and the environment cold and clinical. Control over health care decisions is surrendered in the face of regimented policies and procedures that favor providers' authority over patients' wishes (Jordan, 1997). In high-risk births, this process saves lives. However, in routine labor and birthing, medicalization introduces unnecessary complications (Chen & Wang, 2006). This is especially the case for first-time mothers (Spong et al., 2012; Tracy et al., 2007).

Prior to admission, a woman in labor must pass the first litmus test: Her water must have broken, or her cervix must be at least three centimeters dilated. If neither benchmark is met, she will probably be sent home (and charged a fee for her visit). If at least one is met, hospital routine dictates how she is processed, admitted, and shown to a room. Alternatively, when the mother is believed to be well past her estimated due date or has had a prior cesarean section, intervention may be prescribed. In contrast, unnecessary intervention may be introduced merely for the convenience of scheduling labor and birth. Elective induction or scheduled cesarean section allows a woman to bypass the litmus test for admission (Glantz, 2005).

Once admitted, the labor regimen begins (McCourt, 2010). For some women, surrendering to the physician's care and a high-tech birth can be a reassuring and desirable experience, whereas others may prefer a less invasive process. Unlike a childbirth at home, hospital rooms feature limited privacy and are stocked with intimidating equipment (Jordan, 1993). Visitors are restricted, which leaves the woman to make many decisions alone or with only one family member or friend to advocate on her behalf. A parade of unfamiliar staff may feel her cervix every 30 minutes to check the speed of dilation; the number of staff and cervix checks varies by hospital, but tends to be highest in teaching institutions. Moreover, women in labor may not eat or drink in case cesarean section and anesthesia are indicated. In a prolonged labor, lack of sustenance might weaken a woman's resolve and lower her stamina for the rigors of childbirth, which increases the potential for medical intervention.

In many hospitals, standard procedures also include inserting an intravenous drip, urinary catheter, or an electronic fetal monitor (EFM), which evaluates the fetus's condition. Traditional EFM also requires stripping membranes (i.e., manually opening the amniotic sac), which might introduce a risk of infection. All of these procedures interfere with the woman's ability to stand and walk, which is a natural way to promote dilation; the result is a domino effect that increases a woman's risk for cesarean section (Chen & Wang, 2006; Spong et al., 2012). Women may also be shaved and given an enema, procedures that have no demonstrated medical benefit; their continued use appears to serve the convenience of the attending physicians (Chen & Wang, 2006). The cumulative effect of these medicalized interventions can slow the course of labor (Jordan 1997; Leggitt & Ringdahl, n.d.). If labor is slow, further intervention may be imposed, including medications such as oxytocin, which "ripens" or speeds up cervical dilation. However, this process can be painful for women, poses risks, and is not always effective. Studies have shown that over one-half of all women who receive these medications remain in the slow or "latent" stage of labor far longer than other women, which places them at greater risk for cesarean section (Spong et al., 2012; Tracy et al., 2007).

Pain management is another component of medicalized labor. A skillfully administered epidural can make labor a far more comfortable experience without diminishing the ability to push. However, epidurals are risky, and their effects vary from woman to woman. An epidural may prolong the latent phase of labor; can deaden the woman's muscle response and sensation, leaving her unable to bear down; and requires that she lie flat on her back, which poses further challenges at the point of crowning (Anim-Somuah, Smyth, & Jones, 2011; Jordan, 1993).

The Medicalized "Delivery"

By the time a woman is ready to give birth to her baby, the original birth plan is likely to have been overridden, her partner sidelined with secondary tasks, and the process subsumed so that the physician—rather than the mother—"delivers" the baby. Women may have little voice in the entire context of the birth. For example, rather than moving into a posture that feels most comfortable for vaginal birth, the typical U.S. birth position is supine, with the mother flat on her back, her legs elevated, and her feet in stirrups. This practice again benefits the attendant by providing an unrestricted view, but forces the mother to fight gravity while attempting to push (Blaz, 2011; Jordan, 1993). Studies also indicate that supine deliveries are more likely to result in tearing of the perineum, the tissue between the vagina and anus (Terry, Westcott, O'Shea, & Kelly, 2006).

During vaginal birth, physicians may also perform an episiotomy (i.e., cut the perineum) in the belief that the procedure facilitates the infant's passage. This may be deemed necessary because medication used to speed labor shortcuts the body's natural ability to stretch and accommodate the infant. Episiotomies pose further complications because the incision fails to heal as effectively as a natural tear (should one occur) and it both delays recovery and increases costs (Hartmann et al., 2005; Jordan, 1993). The final episiotomy suture is dubbed by some as the "husband's stitch" or the "love knot" as it tightens the vaginal opening. If these various interventions are not effective, the physician may apply forceps or use vacuum suction to pull the baby from the birth canal. All of this reflects regimented time constraints that are common in hospital births (Jordan, 1993; McCourt, 2010; Unzila & Norwitz, 2009).

Alternately, the physician may decide that a cesarean section is indicated. This intervention is justified in high-risk situations, such as fetal or maternal distress; however, its use may be inappropriate, and even counterproductive, in low-risk situations. Caesarean rates increased tenfold between 1970 and 1990 (Villar et al., 2006) and continue to rise worldwide (OECD, 2013). Today the United States has one of the world's highest rates of cesarean section, irrespective of risk level (34% in 2012; Meloni et al., 2012), despite recommendations by the ACOG and World Health Organization (WHO) to minimize its use (ACOG, 2014; Gibbons et al., 2010). Rate increases appear to be linked to defensive medicine and physicians' convenience rather than medical need. For example, rather than automatically resort to a cesarean for all breach presentations, providers can use techniques, such as external cephalic version, to move the baby into position for vaginal birth. Unfortunately, these techniques are no longer routinely included in the training of U.S. physicians, but they are a standard part of professional midwife certification (North American Registry of Midwives, 2014). Women may have little choice in cesarean decisions; indeed, physicians have been known to obtain a court order to perform the procedure against the wishes of their patient (Curran, 1990; Deshpande & Oxford, 2012; Irwin & Jordan, 1987). Cesarean section delays recovery and increases the risk of maternal and infant morbidity, maternal mortality, and complications in future births (OECD, 2013; Villar et al., 2006). It is also double the cost of vaginal birth (OECD, 2013), and the associated discomfort may interfere with mother–infant bonding and reduce the likelihood of breastfeeding (Zanardo et al., 2010). Moreover, few physicians support vaginal birth after cesarean because they fear possible uterine rupture and malpractice suits, even though the risk of rupture is less than 1%. This forces women into perpetual intervention in future births despite its risks (Agency for Healthcare Research and Quality, 2010; Romano, Gerber, & Andrews, 2010).

The Medicalized Recovery

Postpartum care is similarly managed and regimented both in the hospital and following discharge in the United States. In hospital settings, physicians tend to clamp and sever the umbilical cord immediately after birth as a part of time management, whereas birth attendants in other settings allow the cord to finish transferring blood to the newborn before it is tied and cut. Attendants must also wait for the mother to expel the placenta. In many cultures, the placenta and cord are treated with respect and may be used in a variety of postpartum rituals. In hospital delivery, the placenta is treated as medical waste; it is discarded and incinerated. Depending on prior planning, the cord may be incinerated, cryogenically frozen for future medical use, or donated for research (Lloyd, 2006; Stone, 2009).

The next step in medicalized postbirth care is to manage mother–infant interactions. Newborns in most societies are entrusted to the mother; in U.S. hospitals, the baby is cleaned, evaluated (the Apgar test of the newborn's condition is conducted at one minute and five minutes after birth), and then handed to the mother to hold. At some point, the baby undergoes routine postnatal procedures. Depending on the mother's condition, the newborn's condition, and the hospital's policy, babies may stay in the newborn nursery, which offers little time for bonding between mother and child. An increasing number of hospitals now allow a healthy newborn to room with the mother, a practice that makes it easier for a mother to bond and breastfeed while she is hospitalized (Kennell & McGrath, 2005; WHO & UNICEF, 2012b).

Exclusive breastfeeding for the first 6 to 12 months is recommended by numerous health organizations such as the WHO, the National Institutes of Health, and the American Medical Association. U.S. breastfeeding rates have increased in recent years but remain low relative to other industrialized nations (Bartick & Reinhold, 2010; CDC, 2013; Farrell, 2013). After a generation of primarily formula-fed babies, contemporary women may lack role models for breastfeeding. Although hospitals encourage mothers to breastfeed, they enable formula feeding by supplying parents with samples and resources for bottle feeding. Mothers who want to breastfeed exclusively may have to overcome the pressure to formula feed. Some hospitals provide breastfeeding educators, but they are few in number and their availability varies. Some mothers are discharged before they can connect with an educator, and those who have undergone a cesarean may not receive any guidance during recovery. At the same time, mothers may hold unrealistic expectations about the ease of breastfeeding, when the process can actually be challenging and even painful. Difficult or uncomfortable experiences may leave women unsure that they can successfully breastfeed a healthy baby. A number of cities in the United States have recently initiated campaigns to promote breastfeeding education, ban formula gifts in hospitals, and distribute free breast pumps; collectively, these actions hold promise for more informed feeding choices (Perrine et al., 2011; Raphael, 2012).

Following a routine birth, the mother is typically discharged within 24 hours. If her newborn is in distress, it will be admitted to a neonatal intensive care unit, where it may remain for some time. Such units greatly increase the chance for survival in infants with high-risk conditions (Lorch, Baiocchi, Ahlberg, & Small, 2012), although such care comes at a high cost (Muraskas & Parsi, 2008). However, pending doctor's orders, even healthy newborns may be held for a longer period of observation and assessment after the mother is discharged. For example, about 50% to 60% of newborns display neonatal jaundice; although a fraction of these cases require care, jaundice is usually normal and adaptive, and it does not need medicalized intervention (AAP, 2004; Brett & Niermeyer, 1999). Novice parents may also engage more fully in the medicalization process by seeking reassurance for natural yet potentially alarming characteristics of newborns. For instance, vaginally birthed newborns may exhibit a number of normal conditions that can provoke concern in new parents, such as blue skin tone (cyanosis), a misshapen skull (molding), and irregular breathing.

Novice parents may be further alarmed by a fresh round of fear-inducing information when they leave the hospital. Parents may be handed discharge orders with a litany of medicalized "do's and don'ts" related to diet, sexual behavior, secondhand smoke, and infant care and feeding. For instance, infants' sleep is flagged as life-threatening; parents are instructed to place infants to sleep on their back, avoid soft bedding, and never bed-share if they are to avoid suffocating their newborn. These guidelines are evidence based (AAP, 2011), but they invoke fear and insecurity. The taboo against bed-sharing also fails to accommodate both cultural tradition and pragmatics: it is likely that most mothers fall asleep with the baby in their bed at some point, which can induce feelings of guilt (Gettler & McKenna, 2011; McKenna & McDade, 2005). Indeed, first-time parents can grow so anxious that they may question their every action and decision. Yet, rather than turn to experienced family and friends, the medicalized process of pregnancy and birth leaves them dependent on health care networks and the media as default experts, which extends medicalization into childrearing.

CONCLUSION

Advances in medical diagnosis, treatment, and technology have demonstrated value to save the lives of women and infants at high risk. At the same time, the universal application of these tools, regardless of risk, leads to a growing tide of interventions and complications in what would otherwise be routine pregnancy and birth.

With each phase of pregnancy and birth, the market-driven medical model yields fresh opportunities for commodification and expensive and defensive techniques, all of which lead to overburdened patients with greater uncertainty about their decision-making abilities (Thomas & Zimmerman, 2007). Furthermore, the United States is exporting this invasive model around the world, replacing and marginalizing existing systems that can be safer and more effective for low-risk pregnancies (Cahill, 2001; Jordan, 1997; Selin & Stone, 2009). Controversy over this approach to "health" has sparked a growing movement in the United States to reverse medicalization and reinstate natural childbirth and a greater variety of potential birth attendants. Even so, the natural childbirth movement has exerted only minimal influence against the legitimacy of the medical model, and its impact varies by class, education, ethnicity, and state regulations (Davis-Floyd & Sargent, 1997).

An antidote to unwarranted medicalization is accessible, informed, and empowered decision making, as advocated by the reproductive justice movement (Chrisler, 2012; Sagrestano & Finerman, 2012). Accessible care requires the elimination of health disparities, universal health coverage, and the geographic availability of multiple and alternative reproductive care options, including fertility and family planning services, midwives and doulas, birthing clinics, and quality hospital care (Walker & Chesnut, 2010). Informed decision making hinges on the availability of medically accurate, balanced, and culturally appropriate educational resources that outline women's choices without provoking unnecessary fear and insecurity. Empowerment is contingent on social and legislative reforms that ensure reproductive health care choices for all women (Davis-Floyd & Sargent, 1997; Jordan, 1997; Machizawa & Hayashi, 2012; Sagrestano & Finerman, 2012). At present, these basic human rights remain unrealized for many women and their partners in the United States and worldwide. Accomplishing these aims will depend on collaboration, political will, and strategic action at all levels.

REFERENCES

Agency for Healthcare Research and Quality. (2010). *Vaginal birth after cesarean: New insights* (AHRQ Publication No. 10-E003). Retrieved from http://www.ahrq.gov/research/findings/evidence-based-reports/er191-abstract.html.

American Academy of Pediatrics [AAP] Subcommittee on Hyperbilirubinemia. (2004). Management of hyperbilirubinemia in the newborn infant 35 or more weeks of gestation. *Pediatrics, 114,* 297–316.

American Academy of Pediatrics [AAP] Task Force on Sudden Infant Death Syndrome. (2011). SIDS and other sleep-related infant deaths: Expansion of recommendations for a safe infant sleeping environment. *Pediatrics, 128,* 1030–1039.

American Congress of Obstetricians and Gynecologists [ACOG]. (2001). Substance abuse reporting and pregnancy: The role of the obstetrician-gynecologist. Retrieved from ACOG's Committee Opinion on Healthcare for Underserved Women website: http://www.acog.org/Resources_And _Publications/Committee_Opinions/Committee_on_Health_Care_for _Underserved_Women/Substance_Abuse_Reporting_and_Pregnancy _The_Role_of_the_Obstetrician_Gynecologist.

American Congress of Obstetricians and Gynecologists [ACOG]. (2007). ACOG's screening guidelines on chromosomal abnormalities: What they mean to patients and physicians. Retrieved from http://www.acog.org /About_ACOG/News_Room/News_Releases/2007/ACOGs Screening _Guidelines_on Chromosomal_Abnormalities.

American Congress of Obstetricians and Gynecologists [ACOG]. (2012). *2011 women's health stats & facts.* Retrieved from http://www.acog.org/~/media /NewsRoom/MediaKit.pdf.

American Congress of Obstetricians and Gynecologists [ACOG]. (2014). Obstetric care consensus: Safe prevention of the primary cesarean delivery. Retrieved from http://www.acog.org/Resources_And_Publications/Obstetric_Care _Consensus_Series/Safe_Prevention_of_the_Primary_Cesarean_Delivery.

Anim-Somuah, M., Smyth, R. M. D., & Jones, L. (2011). Epidural versus non-epidural or no analgesia in labour. *Cochrane Database of Systematic Reviews, 12,* CD000331.

Bartick, M., & Reinhold, A. (2010). The burden of suboptimal breastfeeding in the United States: A pediatric cost analysis. *Pediatrics, 125,* e1048–e1056.

Blaz, A. (2011, January 18). Dorsal lithotomy position vs. non-supine position during 2nd stage of labor: Quadriped. Retrieved from Lamaze International's website: http://www.scienceandsensibility.org/?p=1939.

Boardman, F. K. (2014). Knowledge is power? The role of experiential knowledge in genetically 'risky' reproductive decisions. *Sociology of Health & Illness, 36,* 137–150.

Brett, J., & Niermeyer, S. (1999). Is neonatal jaundice a disease or an adaptive process? In W. R. Trevathan (Ed.), *Evolutionary medicine* (pp. 75–100). New York: Oxford University Press.

Browner, C., & Press, N. (1995). The normalization of prenatal diagnostic screening. In F. Ginsburg & R. Rapp (Eds.), *Conceiving the new world order: The global politics of reproduction* (pp. 307–322). Berkeley, CA: University of California Press.

Buchbinder, M., & Timmermans, S. (2011). Medical technologies and the dream of the perfect newborn. *Medical Anthropology, 30*(1), 56–80.

Budetti, P., & Waters, T. M. (2005). Medical malpractice law in the United States. Retrieved from the Kaiser Family Foundation website: http://kff.org/health-costs/report/medical-malpractice-law-in-the-united-states/.

Cahill, H. A. (2001). Male appropriation and medicalization of childbirth: An historical analysis. *Journal of Advanced Nursing, 33*, 334–342.

Cappelli, M., Coyle, D., Etchegary, H., Graham, I., Howley, H., & Potter, B. (2008). The influence of experiential knowledge on prenatal screening and testing decisions. *Genetic Testing, 12*(1), 115–125.

Centers for Disease Control and Prevention [CDC]. (2012). *Home births in the United States, 1990–2009.* (NCHS Data Brief No. 84, January). Retrieved from http://www.cdc.gov/nchs/data/databriefs/db84.htm.

Centers for Disease Control and Prevention [CDC]. (2013). U.S. breastfeeding rates continue to rise. Retrieved from http://www.cdc.gov/media/releases/2013/p0731-breastfeeding-rates.html.

Centers for Disease Control and Prevention [CDC]. (2014a). Severe maternal morbidity in the United States. Retrieved from http://www.cdc.gov/reproductivehealth/MaternalInfantHealth/SevereMaternalMorbidity.html.

Centers for Disease Control and Prevention [CDC]. (2014b). Pregnancy complications. Retrieved from http://www.cdc.gov/reproductivehealth/maternalinfanthealth/pregcomplications.htm.

Centers for Disease Control and Prevention [CDC]. (2014c). Facts about birth defects. Retrieved from http://www.cdc.gov/ncbddd/birthdefects/facts.html.

Central Intelligence Agency [CIA]. (2013). *The world factbook 2013–14: Maternal mortality rate country comparison.* Retrieved from https://www.cia.gov/library/publications/the-world-factbook/rankorder/2223rank.html.

Certified Professional Midwives NOW. (2014). Big push for midwives: PushStates in action. Retrieved from http://pushformidwives.org/what-we-do/pushstates-in-action/.

Chen, C-Y., & Wang, K-G. (2006). Are routine interventions necessary in normal birth? *Taiwanese Journal of Obstetrics and Gynecology, 45*, 302–306.

Cheyney, M. J. (2008). Homebirth as systems-challenging praxis: Knowledge, power, and intimacy in the birthplace. *Qualitative Health Research, 18*, 254–267.

Cheyney, M. J. (2011). *Born at home: The biological, cultural, and political dimensions of maternity care in the United States.* Belmont, CA: Wadsworth.

Chrisler, J. C. (Ed.). (2012). *Reproductive justice: A global concern.* Santa Barbara, CA: Praeger.

Curran, W. J. (1990). Court-ordered cesarean sections receive judicial defeat. *New England Journal of Medicine, 323*, 489–492.

Davis-Floyd, R. E. (2004). *Birth as an American rite of passage.* Berkeley, CA: University of California Press.

Davis-Floyd, R. E., & Dumit, J. (Eds.). (2013). *Cyborg babies: From techno-sex to techno-tots.* New York: Routledge.

Davis-Floyd, R. E., & Sargent, C. F. (Eds.). (1997). *Childbirth and authoritative knowledge: Cross-cultural perspectives*. Berkeley, CA: University of California Press.

Deshpande, N. A., & Oxford, C. M. (2012). Management of pregnant patients who refuse medically indicated cesarean delivery. *Reviews in Obstetrics and Gynecology, 5*, e144–e150.

Fairchild, J. (2010). The defensive medicine debate: Driven by special interests. *Annals of Health Law Advance Directive, 19*, 297–305.

Farrell, J. (2013). We can't afford to ignore the benefits of breastfeeding. Retrieved from the Center for American Progress website: http://americanprogress.org/issues/women/news/2013/03/08/55769/we-cant-afford-to-ignore-the-benefits-of-breastfeeding/.

Fisher, C., Hauck, Y., & Fenwick, J. (2006). How social context impacts on women's fears of childbirth: A Western Australian example. *Social Science & Medicine, 63*, 64–75.

Geissbuehler, V., & Eberhard, J. (2002). Fear of childbirth during pregnancy: A study of more than 8000 pregnant women. *Journal of Psychosomatic Obstetrics & Gynecology, 23*, 229–235.

Gettler, L. T., & McKenna, J. J. (2011). Evolutionary perspectives on mother–infant sleep proximity and breastfeeding in a laboratory setting. *American Journal of Physical Anthropology, 144*, 454–462.

Gibbons, L., Belizan, J. M., Lauer, J. A., Betran, A. P., Merialdi, M., & Althabe, F. (2010). *The global numbers and costs of additionally needed and unnecessary cesarean sections performed per year: Overuse as a barrier to universal coverage* (World Health Report, Background Paper No. 30). Retrieved from the World Health Organization website: http://www.who.int/healthsystems/topics/financing/healthreport/30C-sectioncosts.pdf.

Glantz, J. C. (2005). Elective induction vs. spontaneous labor associations and outcomes. *Journal of Reproductive Medicine, 50*, 235–240.

Gregory, J. (2010). (M)Others in altered states: Prenatal drug-use, risk, choice, and responsible self-governance. *Social and Legal Studies, 19*, 49–66.

Hallett, C. (2005). The attempt to understand puerperal fever in the eighteenth and early nineteenth centuries: The influence of inflammation theory. *Medical History, 49*(1), 1–28.

Hartmann, K., Viswanathan, M., Palmieri, R., Gartlehner, G., Thorp, J., & Lohr, K. N. (2005). Outcomes of routine episiotomy: A systematic review. *Journal of American Medical Association, 293*, 2141–2148.

Healthy People. (2014). Leading health indicators: Maternal, infant, and child health. Retrieved from the U.S. Department of Health and Human Services, Healthy People website: http://www.healthypeople.gov/2020/LHI/micHealth.aspx?tab=overview.

Hellinger, F. J., & Encinosa, W. E. (2006). The impact of state laws limiting malpractice damage awards on health care expenditures. *American Journal of Public Health, 96*, 1375–1381.

Hogan, M. C., Foreman, K. J., Naghavi, M., Ahn, S. Y., Wang, M., Makela, S. M., . . . Murray, C. J. (2010). Maternal mortality for 181 countries, 1980–2008: A systematic analysis of progress towards millennium development goal 5. *Lancet, 375,* 1609–1623.

Hunter, L. A. (2009). Issues in pregnancy dating: Revisiting the evidence. *Journal of Midwifery & Women's Health, 54,* 184–190.

Irwin, S., & Jordan, B. (1987). Knowledge, practice, and power: Court-ordered cesarean sections. *Medical Anthropology Quarterly, 1,* 319–334.

Jordan, B. (1993). *Birth in four cultures* (4th ed.). Long Grove, IL: Waveland.

Jordan, B. (1997). Authoritative knowledge and its construction. In R. Davis-Floyd & C. Sargent (Eds.), *Childbirth and authoritative knowledge* (pp. 55–79). Berkeley: University of California Press.

Jukic, A. M., Baird, D. D., Weinberg, C. R., McConnaughey, D. R., & Wilcox, A. J. (2013). Length of human pregnancy and contributors to its natural variation. *Human Reproduction, 28,* 2848–2855.

Kennell, J., & McGrath, S. (2005). Starting the process of mother-infant bonding. *Acta Paediatrica, 94,* 775–777.

Kiely, J., Brett, K., Yu, S., & Rowley, D. (1995). Low birth weight and intrauterine growth retardation. In L. Wilcox & J. Marks (Eds.), *From data to action: CDC's public health surveillance for women, infants, and children* (pp. 185–202). Atlanta, GA: Centers for Disease Control and Prevention.

Lagan, B. M., Sinclair, M., & Kernohan, W. G. (2010). Internet use in pregnancy informs women's decision making: A web-based survey. *Birth, 37,* 106–115.

Landsman, G. H. (2009). *Reconstructing disability and motherhood in the age of "perfect" babies.* New York: Routledge.

Leggitt, K., & Ringdahl, D. (n.d.). What factors influence the progression of childbirth? Retrieved from the University of Minnesota's Center for Spirituality and Healing website: http://www.takingcharge.csh.umn.edu/explore-healing-practices/holistic-pregnancy-childbirth/what-factors-influence-progression-childbirt.

Lloyd, E. (2006, April 6). Umbilical cord research: The future of stem cell research? *National Geographic News.* Retrieved from http://news.nationalgeographic.com/news/2006/04/0406_060406_cord_blood.html.

Lock, M., & Nguyen, V.K. (2010). *An anthropology of biomedicine.* Chichester, UK: Wiley-Blackwell.

Lorch, S. A., Baiocchi, M., Ahlberg, C. E., & Small, D. S. (2012). The differential impact of delivery hospital on the outcomes of premature infants. *Pediatrics, 130,* 270–278.

Lothian, J. A. (2000). The birth plan revisited. *Journal of Perinatal Education, 9*(2), viii–xi.

Loudon, I. (1991). On maternal and infant mortality 1900–1960. *Social History of Medicine, 4*(1), 29–73.

Machizawa, S., & Hayashi, K. (2012). Birthing across cultures: Toward the humanization of childbirth. In J. C. Chrisler (Ed.), *Reproductive justice: A global concern* (pp. 231–251). Santa Barbara, CA: Praeger.

Maynard, S., & Thadhani, R. (2009). Pregnancy and the kidney. *Journal of the American Society of Nephrology, 20,* 14–22.

McCool, W. F., & Simeone, S. A. (2002). Birth in the United States: An overview of trends past and present. *Nursing Clinics of North America, 37,* 735–746.

McCourt, C. (Ed.). (2010). *Childbirth, midwifery and concepts of time.* New York: Berghahn Books.

McKenna, J. J., & McDade, T. (2005). Why babies should never sleep alone: A review of the co-sleeping controversy in relation to SIDS, bedsharing and breast feeding. *Paediatric Respiratory Reviews, 6*(2), 134–152.

Meloni, A., Loddo, A., Martsidis, K., Deiana, S. F., Porru, D., Antonelli, A., & Melis, G. B. (2012). The role of caesarean section in modern obstetrics. *Journal of Pediatric and Neonatal Individualized Medicine, 1*(1), 53–58.

Mills, M. D. (1998). Fetal abuse prosecutions: The triumph of reaction over reason. *DePaul Law Review, 47,* 989–1040.

Morris, T., & McInerney, K. (2010). Media representations of pregnancy and childbirth: An analysis of reality television programs in the United States. *Birth, 37,* 134–140.

Muraskas, J., & Parsi, K. (2008). The cost of saving the tiniest lives: NICUs versus prevention. *Virtual Mentor, 10,* 655–658.

Nash, E. (2001). High court invalidates involuntary drug tests on pregnant women. *Guttmacher Report on Public Policy, 4*(2). Retrieved from http://www.guttmacher.org/pubs/tgr/04/2/gr040213a.html.

North American Registry of Midwives. (2014). *Certification: The CPM credential.* Retrieved from http://narm.org/certification.

Omran, A. R. (1977). A century of epidemiologic transition in the United States. *Preventive Medicine, 6,* 30–51.

Organization for Economic Cooperation and Development [OECD]. (2013). Health at a glance 2013: OECD indicators. Retrieved from http://www.oecd.org/health/health-systems/health-at-a-glance.htm.

Perrine, C. G., Shealy, K. R., Scanlon, K. S., Grummer-Strawn, L. M., Galuska, D. A., Dee, D. L., & Cohen, J. H. (2011). Vital signs: Hospital practices to support breastfeeding—United States, 2007 and 2009. *Morbidity and Mortality Weekly Report, 60,* 1020–1025.

Press, N., Browner, C. H., Tran, D., Morton, C., & Le Master, B. (1998). Provisional normalcy and "perfect babies": Pregnant women's attitudes toward disability in the context of prenatal testing. In S. Franklin & H. Ragone (Eds.), *Reproducing reproduction: Kinship, power, and technological innovation* (pp. 46–65). Philadelphia: University of Pennsylvania Press.

Press, N., Wilfond, B. S., Murray, M., & Burke, W. (2011). The power of knowledge: How carrier and prenatal screening altered the clinical goals of genetic testing. In W. Burke, K. A. Edwards, S. Goering, S. Holland, & S. B. Trinidad (Eds.), *Achieving justice in genomic translation: Re-thinking the pathway to benefit* (pp. 95–108). New York: Oxford University Press.

Raphael, D. (Ed.). (2012). *Breastfeeding and food policy in a hungry world.* Waltham, MA: Elsevier.

Rapp, R. (1999). *Testing women, testing the fetus: The social impact of amniocentesis in America* (vol. 1). New York, NY: Psychology Press.

Rapp, R. (2001). Gender, body, biomedicine: How some feminist concerns dragged reproduction to the center of social theory. *Medical Anthropology Quarterly, 15*, 466–477.

Rapp, R. (2014). Constructing amniocentesis: Maternal and medical discourses. In L. Lamphere, H. Ragone, & P. Zavella L. (Eds.), *Situated lives: Gender and culture in everyday life* (pp. 128–141). New York: Routledge.

Reiger, K., & Dempsey, R. (2006). Performing birth in a culture of fear: An embodied crisis of late modernity. *Health Sociology Review, 15*, 364–373.

Retzlaff-Roberts, D., Chang, C., & Rubin, R. (2004). Technical efficiency in the use of health care resources: A comparison of OECD countries. *Health Policy, 69*, 55–72.

Romano, A. M., Gerber, H., & Andrews, D. (2010). Social media, power, and the future of VBAC. *Journal of Perinatal Education, 19*(3), 43–52.

Root, R., & Browner, C. H. (2011). Cultural context of reproductive health. In P. Van Look, K. Heggenhougen, & S. Quah (Eds.), *Sexual and reproductive health: A public health perspective* (pp. 314–319). San Diego, CA: Academic Press.

Sagrestano, L. M., & Finerman, R. (2012). Pregnancy and prenatal care: A reproductive justice perspective. In J. C. Chrisler (Ed.), *Reproductive justice: A global concern* (pp. 203–230). Santa Barbara, CA: Praeger.

Sahin, G. (2003, March). *Incidence, morbidity and mortality of preeclampsia and eclampsia.* Paper presented at the Twelfth Postgraduate Course in Reproductive Medicine and Biology, Geneva, Switzerland. Retrieved from http://www.gfmer.ch/Endo/Course2003/Eclampsia.htm.

Selin, H., & Stone, P. (Eds.). (2009). *Childbirth across cultures: Ideas and practices of pregnancy, childbirth, and the postpartum.* New York: Springer.

Sloan, F. A., & Hsieh, C. R. (2012). *Health economics.* Cambridge, MA: MIT Press.

Song, F. W., West, J. E., Lundy, L., & Dahmen, N. S. (2012). Women, pregnancy, and health information online: The making of informed patients and ideal mothers. *Gender & Society, 26*, 773–798.

Spong, C. Y., Berghella, V., Wenstrom, K. D., Mercer, B. M., & Saade, G. R. (2012). Preventing the first Cesarean delivery. *Obstetrics and Gynecology, 120*, 1181–1193.

Steverson, J., & Rieckmann, W. (2009). Legislating for the provision of comprehensive substance abuse treatment programs for pregnant and mothering women. *Duke Journal of Gender Law and Policy, 1*, 315–346.

Stone, H. (2009). A history of Western medicine, labor, and birth. In H. Selin & P. Stone (Eds.), *Childbirth across cultures: Ideas and practices of pregnancy, childbirth, and the postpartum* (pp. 41–54). New York: Springer.

Terry, R. R., Westcott, J., O'Shea, L., & Kelly, F. (2006). Postpartum outcomes in supine delivery by physicians vs. nonsupine delivery by midwives. *Journal of the American Osteopathic Association, 106,* 199–202.

Thomas, J. E., & Zimmerman, M. K. (2007). Feminism and profit in American hospitals: The corporate construction of women's health centers. *Gender & Society, 21,* 359–383.

Tracy, S. K., Sullivan, E., Wang, Y. A., Black, D., & Tracy, M. (2007). Birth outcomes associated with interventions in labour amongst low risk women: A population-based study. *Women and Birth, 20*(2), 41–48.

Unnithan-Kumar, M. (2004). Introduction: Reproductive agency, medicine and the state. In M. Unnithan-Kumar (Ed.), *Reproductive agency, medicine, and the state: Cultural transformations in childbearing* (pp. 1–23). New York: Berghahn.

Unzila, A. A., & Norwitz, E. R. (2009). Vacuum-assisted vaginal delivery. *Reviews in Obstetrics and Gynecology, 2*(1), 5–17.

Villar, J., Valladares, E., Wojdyla, D., Zavaleta, N., Carroli, G., Velazco, A., . . . Acosta, A. (2006). Caesarean delivery rates and pregnancy outcomes: The 2005 WHO global survey on maternal and perinatal health in Latin America. *Lancet, 367,* 1819–1829.

Wailoo, K. (2001). *Dying in the city of the blues: Sickle cell anemia and the politics of race and health.* Chapel Hill: University of North Carolina Press.

Walker, L. O., & Chesnut, L. W. (2010). Identifying health disparities and social inequities affecting childbearing women and infants. *Journal of Obstetric, Gynecologic, & Neonatal Nursing, 39,* 328–338.

Wertz, R. W., & Wertz, D. C. (1989). *Lying-in: A history of childbirth in America.* New Haven, CT: Yale University Press.

World Health Organization, & UNICEF. (2012a). Trends in maternal mortality, 1990 to 2010: WHO, UNICEF, UNFPA and the World Bank estimates. Retrieved from http://www.who.int/reproductivehealth/publications/monitoring/9789241503631/en/.

World Health Organization, & UNICEF. (2012b). Baby-friendly hospital initiative. Retrieved from http://www.babyfriendlyusa.org/about-us/baby-friendly -hospital-initiative.

Zanardo, V., Svegliado, G., Cavallin, F., Giustardi, A., Cosmi, E., Litta, P., & Trevisanuto, D. (2010). Elective cesarean delivery: Does it have a negative effect on breastfeeding? *Birth, 37,* 275–279.

Chapter 2

(Re)Productive Disorders: The Expanding Marketplace of Infertility Medicine

Emily Breitkopf and Lisa R. Rubin

In September 2014, the story of the Gardner couple emerged in national media outlets; after eight years of infertility, they were pregnant with quadruplets. The story first caught media attention when the couple posted photos on their private Facebook account, showing the face of a shocked 27-year-old Ashley Gardner and her husband just after learning she was pregnant with multiples. The photos went viral on Facebook, were quickly picked up by national entertainment and news outlets (CNN, *The Today Show*), where the couple gave various interviews and brought significant media attention to the topic of infertility and to the couple themselves. In an interview with Babycenter.com, Gardner said, "I was so close to giving up right before we did IVF, but I got up and dusted myself off one more time —and look what happened" (McGinnis, 2014). They shared a 13-minute video documenting their "fertility journey" on YouTube, culminating in what was deemed (by the media, the couple themselves, and their doctors) as a "successful" pregnancy, and they invited others to follow their story by way of their public Facebook page titled "A Miracle Unfolding." According to Gardner, her "'whole goal in opening up about this [was] to promote infertility awareness. . . . It's not something that's talked about a lot and it's a really hard trial that people go through'" (Pawlowski, 2014).

Infertility and impaired fecundity are surprisingly common health issues with implications for individual, relational, and social well-being. Population-based studies suggest that 6% of reproductive-age married women are infertile, and 12% experience impaired fecundity (Chandra, Copen, & Stephen, 2013).[1] Infertility is *not* a uniquely contemporary issue, and, despite popular representations, rates of infertility and impaired fecundity are *not* on the rise in the United States. In fact, evidence suggests that infertility may even be on the decline (Stephen & Chandra, 2006). Nonetheless, in the United States, the past few decades have been marked by growing awareness and concern with infertility and assisted reproductive technologies (ARTs). Although ARTs have been the subject of considerable media attention and popular fascination, infertility continues to be, for many, a stigmatized condition endured with shame and in silence. Online spaces have emerged as an alternative to these dichotomous realities—the silence of stigmatization on one hand and the explosion of media coverage on the other—as individuals, such as Ashley Gardner, turn to blogs and social media networks for advice, knowledge, and support regarding infertility.

In the United States, infertility and ARTs have increasingly been positioned at the nexus of a wide range of social issues, such as gender politics; lesbian, gay, bisexual, transgender, and queer (LGBTQ) rights; economic inequality; the goals of medicine; and the meaning of personhood and life itself. Sandelowski and de Lacy (2002) suggested that social and technological issues related to infertility and its treatment "offer something for everyone" to debate. This chapter contextualizes contemporary debates and dilemmas surrounding infertility and reproductive technologies through the lens of biomedicalization theory (Clarke, Shim, Mamo, Fosket, & Fishman, 2003), highlighting in particular the role of social media and online engagement in the promotion of, and resistance to, the marketplace of reproductive medicine.

BIOMEDICALIZATION THEORY

Biomedicalization theory was introduced by a group of feminist scholars (Clarke, Shim, Mamo, Fosket, & Fishman, 2003) working to update and expand the scope of scholarship on medicalization. Clarke and colleagues (2003, 2010) suggested that earlier approaches to medicalization may have overly emphasized the top-down processes by which the patriarchal institution of medicine objectifies, controls, and surveils the body, particularly the female body. They developed a biomedicalization theory to capture a more nuanced power dynamic and suggested that institutions, identities, and technologies of medicalization are not only *imposed* on the (gendered) body, but that individuals are also agents of power who *engage* with medical technologies in complex ways and for a variety of different reasons. They discussed these ever-changing medicalization processes in relation to a biomedical field that is defined by its use of technology.

Biomedicalization theory provides a framework that helps us to understand how reproductive medicine, particularly ARTs, can further bind women to the mandates of traditional motherhood by producing new boundaries of desire and deviance, but without dismissing what these technologies may make possible for individual users (Sawicki, 1991). For example, access to ARTs can open up new possibilities of parenthood for LGBTQ individuals and couples (Mamo, 2007). For lesbians marginalized by heterosexist ideologies of motherhood, ARTs can serve as an important site of resistance that can be used to challenge the status quo of motherhood and traditional familial gender arrangements.

However, the logic of medicalization "link[s] up with the logic of consumerism and commodification by inciting the desire for 'better babies' and by creating a market in reproductive body parts" (Sawicki, 1999, p. 194). As health itself becomes a commodity, the medical patient, framed as a consumer, is seemingly offered a "vast array of possibilities" purchasable through the medical marketplace. In the marketplace of reproductive medicine, or what Mamo (2010, p. 173) has described as "Fertility, Inc.," reproductive technologies are marketed as lifestyle technologies whereby the family a person has always wanted is made available for purchase.

Biomedicalization theory also takes into account "new social [identities and relationships] constructed around and through" processes of medicalization, what feminist scholars call "biosocialities" (Clarke et al., 2003, p. 165). In the context of infertility and reproductive technologies, the Internet has been an important arena for the development, organization, and elaboration of biosocialities, which underscore the ways that technologies (i.e., information, computer, reproductive) converge through processes of biomedicalization. As Mamo suggested, "Internet technologies point the way enabling new forms of communication, information exchange, expression and visibilities . . . [which] are part of biomedical expansions [by] . . . enabling parents-in-waiting, poised to self-enterprise and become biomedical users of Fertility Inc." (2013, p. 237). For example, Ashley Gardner's public Facebook page became a site where other women dealing with infertility converged to post on her page, share their experiences, and seek support and knowledge from others about how to navigate Fertility, Inc.

Furthermore, biomedicalization theory underscores the increasingly stratified nature of medicalization. Medicalization is rarely enacted evenly across patient groups, and this is particularly evident in the context of infertility and ARTs, a field of medicine often considered elective within the U.S. health care system. Thus, the provision of treatment is characterized by what Clarke et al. (2003, p. 168) described as "dual tendencies of selective medicalization and selective exclusion from care, based on [one's] ability to pay." These stratifications are further exacerbated by new population-dividing practices and emerging biosocialities and technoscientific identities, the latter of which are often formed and reinforced through social media networks. Thus, some patients are presented with a dramatic expansion of technologies available to diagnose and treat fertility issues, whereas others are excluded from knowing about and accessing even the most basic of care.

Throughout this chapter we use the framework of biomedicalization theory to examine the construction of infertility and the marketplace for in vitro fertilization (IVF), and we discuss three rising reproductive technologies that illustrate many of the dimensions of biomedicalization theory: third-party reproduction, preimplantation genetic diagnosis (PGD), and oocyte cryopreservation. We highlight key feminist positions and debates about infertility, ARTs, and medicalization within an era defined by the increased dependence on technology and online spaces, and we consider the ways each form of treatment has both transformed and been transformed by this contemporary landscape.

DEFINING INFERTILITY

What does it mean to be infertile? Definitions vary across settings. For example, the World Health Organization defined infertility as a "disease of the reproductive system defined by the failure to achieve a clinical pregnancy after 12 months or more of regular unprotected sexual intercourse" (Zegers-Hochschild et al., 2009, p. 1523). The Practice Committee of the American Society for Reproductive Medicine (ASRM, 2013a, p. 63) defined infertility as "the failure to achieve a successful pregnancy after 12 months or more of appropriate, timed unprotected intercourse or therapeutic donor insemination." As the subtle differences in these definitions suggest, when it comes to defining infertility, the devil is in the details. As Thompson (2005, p. 55) noted, and the above definitions make clear, "contemporary infertility and its treatment are conceptualized and structured around a strong, coupled, heterosexual, consumer-oriented, normative nuclear-family scenography."

Medical technologies play an important role in contemporary constructions of sickness and health, normality and deviance. As such, feminist and critical health scholars have noted the ways in which contemporary notions of infertility emerged as a medical condition alongside the development of ARTs (Clarke et al., 2010; Sandelowski & de Lacy, 2002; van Balen & Inhorn, 2002). Denoting infertility as a *disease* suggests that its manifestation represents a deviation from the "normal" structure or function of the body. However, whereas "normal" fertility declines for both women and men over time, the above definition provides little guidance to distinguish "normal" age-related fertility decline from "non-normative" biological impairment. Rather, turning logic on its head, for individuals over the age of 35, when fertile decline is "normal" and expected, individuals are encouraged to pursue an expedited path to diagnosis, with infertility evaluation and diagnosis recommended after only six months of unprotected intercourse to prevent treatment delay. Although earlier use of reproductive technologies among those over 35 may, in fact, increase the chances of "successful" treatment, defining illness categories in relation to treatment options is a hallmark of medicalization. Indeed, many (Ashley Gardner included) frame reproductive medicine both as a first place to turn and as a last hope for achieving a pregnancy. By constructing infertility as a medical issue, "medical science offers sufferers a logical cause for [an] unwanted condition, and often holds out the possibility of controlling or eliminating it through concrete medical interventions" (Heitman, 1999, p. 24). Yet, even when men are diagnosed with infertility, it is largely women whose bodies are the sites of intervention, and thus women bear the brunt of treatment, regardless of the source of the infertility (Rothman, 2000).

Through the processes of biomedicalization, the definition of *infertility* is in constant transformation and obscures the social context in which women are "compelled to try" in the first place (Sandelowski, 1991). Many women carry a long-held desire to have a child, a desire rooted in early gender-role socialization (Larkin, 2006). Nancy Felipe Russo (1976, p. 143) introduced the term "the motherhood mandate" to describe how motherhood is socially constructed as integral to one's identity as a woman. This social imperative is commonly transformed throughout mainstream U.S. cultural discourse into a biological imperative, such that some believe that women have a natural desire to reproduce that emerges as a "baby itch" driven by an innate "biological clock" (Friese, Becker, & Nachtigall, 2006). Feminists and queer theorists have critiqued these discourses extensively by outlining the essentialist assumptions about reproductivity and gender that underlie them (Chodorow, 1999; Edelman, 2004; Friese et al., 2006; Rothman, 2000).

The concept and imagery of the biological clock has offered a useful selling point for reproductive medicine, which depends on these assumptions and has enforced a logic that frames women as inadequate if they are unable to "overcome" infertility by reproducing a child (Gentile, 2013). This "logic" contributes to the trend of seeking repeated infertility treatments (Sandelowski, 1991), and it considers women without children as *not yet pregnant* (Greil, 1991). Gentile (2013, p. 265) framed this situation as an "ongoing crisis state" whereby women's hopes of reproducing are hinged upon the efficacy of their biomedical treatment and their ability to fulfill (what is perceived as) a biologically rooted reproductive mandate.

In this sense, biological motherhood is normalized alongside a technological imperative that claims, with regard to infertility, "if something *can* be done, then it *ought* to be done" (Rubin & Phillips, 2012, p. 175). Despite the potential for failure, and despite the impact of ARTs on the reproductive body, women are still "compelled to try" (Sandelowski, 1991, p. 29).

It stands to reason that, in this context, the inability to fulfill this "innate," "biological" role can provoke intense feelings of psychological loss (Horowitz, Galst, & Elster, 2010). The struggle and loss often occur behind closed doors, as infertility remains highly stigmatized in the United States. Like Ashley Gardner, many women turn to blogs and social media sites to share their stories and seek support to cope with their experience of infertility. Social media also contribute to the definition of infertility, as new social networks form around collective experience. Thus, through processes of biomedicalization, technologies (both reproductive and personal) and gendered desire have a direct impact on how infertility is defined, experienced, and navigated in the United States. New options for responding to these "shortcomings" of the reproductive body become available for purchase via Fertility, Inc., which extends one's reproductive potential and hope to fulfill it in new technological ways. However, many women are unable to gain access to infertility treatment. Stereotypical representations of infertility offer a vision of White middle- or upper-class heterosexual couples or single women seeking, at any cost, the ability to bear a genetically related child. In reality, in the United States, it is poor and working-class women of color who face the highest rates of infertility and who regularly lack the socioeconomic resources to seek biomedical treatment (Greil, McQuillan, Shreffler, Johnson, & Slauson-Blevins, 2011). The Centers for Disease Control and Prevention (2013) frame infertility as a "public health issue," but there are no structural policies in place to increase women's access to these services. Thus, the ability to treat infertility using biomedical tools has become stratified along boundaries of race, ethnicity, sexual identity, and class, which suggests that the government's concern about infertility as a "public health issue" applies largely to White, heterosexual, cisgender[2] women who can afford these services (Myers, 2014; Roberts, 2014).

Infertility must be considered within the context of these intertwining social structures, which illuminate who is taken into account and who is left out, by its definition. As we have discussed, the meanings of infertility are not static; they are constantly impacting, and impacted by, processes of biomedicalization. Yet, in the field of reproductive medicine, infertility is defined by an imperative to treat, control, and eliminate it, increasingly through the use of ARTs. This has culminated in a multibillion-dollar fertility industry in the United States that both expands and restricts possibilities for women (Mamo, 2010). At the center of this industry lies one key technology: in vitro fertilization.

IN VITRO FERTILIZATION IN AN ERA OF ONLINE ENGAGEMENT

IVF first entered the larger public imagination in 1978 with the birth of Louise Brown in the United Kingdom. Over 35 years later, its use has grown tremendously in the United States (van Balen & Inhorn, 2002), doubling over the past decade (CDC, 2013). In 2012 alone, over 170,000 IVF cycles were performed (CDC, 2013). IVF is a foundational technology in the treatment of infertility, and it is used in a variety of contexts (e.g., third-party reproduction, oocyte cryopreservation, PGD). During a cycle of IVF, eggs are extracted from a woman's body and fertilized, and the resulting embryos are then implanted into a woman's uterus.

IVF is a technology that interfaces with various other technologies and media that affect how it is used in the field of reproductive medicine. For instance, IVF has inspired the production of smartphone applications and online tools meant to be used during an IVF cycle (e.g., iVitro, My Fertility Diary). As IVF and computer and information technologies converge, we see the proliferation of certain types of information about IVF via blogs and social media sites (which are often sponsored by private biomedical corporations) and new ways of marketing motherhood online through the promotion of IVF. Gentile (2013) pointed out that IVF is highly researched by its clients; even a brief search on Google leads to thousands of sites offering information about the technology, the majority of which perpetuate the framework of biomedicalization. Online advocacy concerning infertility, an initiative taken up by Ashley Gardner through her Facebook page, often focuses on promoting awareness about IVF as a viable option for those facing infertility and calling for expanded mandates for insurance coverage, which in the United States is variable across states and generally quite limited, if it is available at all.

Framed as a technological "fix" to infertility, IVF is the primary technology used in the treatment of infertility, and it contributes strongly to the multibillion-dollar industry of Fertility, Inc. (Mamo, 2010). Heitman (1999, p. 25) noted the power held by physicians who are part of Fertility, Inc., "not only in terms of wealth and prestige, but also in the less tangible power that they hold over the creation of life and the control that they wield in the lives of their patients."

Gentile (2013, p. 264) pointed out that IVF "is the most profitable procedure for clinics," which is undoubtedly connected to the fact that individuals are compelled to carry out multiple cycles with the hopes of finding success. Women with the economic resources to do so are often willing to pay for multiple cycles (others may seek loans to finance IVF), despite the toll it takes on their bodies. In the United States, multiple embryo transfer is common, despite the increased likelihood of a twin, or higher order, pregnancy. Women and couples may prefer multiple embryo transfers in the belief that it will save time and money by decreasing the number of necessary cycles to achieve a pregnancy. Clinics often prefer multiple embryo transfers to promote higher pregnancy success rates, which is important to their marketing efforts. These preferences and practices exist despite research that indicates no impact on the cumulative birth rate when legislative restrictions limit the number of embryos that can be transferred (Peeraer et al., 2014). The story of Nadya Suleman (known as "Octomom") brought some public scrutiny to the practice of multiple embryo transfers (Rao, 2011). This sensationalized media story merely reinforced the extant bifurcated view of reproductive medicine and its medical practitioners as *either* miracle workers (Gentile, 2013) or vigilante quacks, but did little to upend routine practices that increase risks to women and babies in order to accommodate the medical marketplace.

Furthermore, Spar (2006, p. 57) contended that fertility clinics are compelled to "put the most positive spin they can on their technologies and data, touting procedures that frequently have a low probability of success and an unknown potential to do harm." Because IVF is carried out through women's bodies, it is often women (and not the technologies themselves) who are blamed for a failed cycle (Heitman, 1999), which echoes old narratives that fault women for their own infertility (van Balen & Inhorn, 2002). As Throsby (2004, p. 59) contended, "success goes to the clinic, failure to the woman."

Because of the booming industry of Fertility, Inc., many seeking IVF travel to the United States from countries where ARTs are more strictly regulated (Martin, 2014). However, many in the United States remain unable to access this technology because IVF costs are as high as $15,000 to $20,000 per cycle (Bell, 2010). There are no government subsidies to increase access to IVF for poor and working-class women of color, who face the highest rates of infertility in the United States (Greil et al., 2011).

The prioritizing of contraceptives by the federal government suggests that old eugenic threads (regarding who should reproduce and who should not) are still current and continue to define access to medical services according to racist and classist imperatives. Alongside this restricted access, the privatization and commodification of IVF further enhances the status of Fertility, Inc., and the biomedicalization of infertility itself as a largely White and upper-class matter.

Another way IVF access is restricted is through health insurance guidelines. Insurance companies that cover IVF treatment often require doctors to prove medical necessity in order to gain coverage, or the policies contain caveats that support the heterosexist definition of infertility (Conrad & Leiter, 2004; Johnson, 2012). For example, a policy might only cover IVF for the treatment of infertility due to biological causes, such as blocked or damaged fallopian tubes, or "only when a woman's egg is fertilized by her spouse's sperm" (Johnson, 2012, p. 396). Thus, single individuals and lesbian couples seeking IVF coverage are sometimes excluded from it. Even if they have access to health insurance and their insurance policy covers IVF, they may not be covered because their experience of infertility does not meet the insurance company's guidelines. Furthermore, the medicalization of infertility means that, whereas IVF may be covered by health insurance, nonbiomedical strategies for family building are not. Thus, individuals may be compelled toward reproductive technologies because they are financially more feasible and thus more accessible and preferable than other options, such as adoption (Gentile, 2013). Thus, with regard to IVF, boundaries of restriction and possibility, privilege and access, are drawn along lines that perpetuate inequities through the mechanisms of biomedicalization, an issue that becomes more complex as we situate IVF within the different biomedical responses to infertility.

THIRD-PARTY REPRODUCTION

Despite extensive media coverage of reproductive technologies and the promises they hold, considerably less attention has been devoted to their high failure rates. According to the CDC (2012), the average per-cycle success rate of ARTs is less than 30%. When IVF fails, many individuals and couples turn to "third-party reproduction" to increase their chances of becoming a parent. *Third-party reproduction* is a term used to describe reproductive arrangements that involve the body or bodily products of a "third" person—an oocyte (egg) or sperm donor,[3] or surrogate—to achieve parenthood.[4] There is a significant body of work on the ethical, social, and legal issues involved in third-party reproduction. Thus, a comprehensive review of these issues is beyond the scope of this chapter. Rather, we focus our attention specifically on the ways in which medicalization and market forces come together within current practices in third-party reproduction, particularly commercial egg donation and surrogacy.[5]

Third-party reproduction, particularly commercial surrogacy and egg donation, epitomizes contemporary practices of biomedicalization. These technologies require medical professionals to subject healthy individuals (usually women) to medical treatments and concomitant medical risks in order to help others to meet their reproductive goals. Women's health advocates have noted the dearth of safety data available regarding the long- and short-term effects of infertility treatments for women without fertility problems (Beeson & Lippman, 2006). Indeed, fertility clinics have nothing to gain from studying possible risks. Thus, there has been considerable critique of third-party reproduction as dangerous and exploitive of vulnerable women (e.g., Dickenson, 2002; Papadimos & Papadimos, 2004). In contrast, others have challenged exploitation concerns and emphasized that the vast majority of third-party providers of reproductive matter *choose* to exchange their "body bits" for compensation (Chavkin & Maher, 2010). The emphasis on choice and agency is consistent with shifts from a medicalization to a biomedicalization framework of health, illness, and contemporary medical practice. Thus, more recent scholarship tends to bypass questions of exploitation versus agency and instead examines broader social and contextual issues at stake in the buying and selling of reproductive matter.

The United States has been described as the "Wild West" of procreative possibilities due to the lack of a meaningful regulatory agency and the free-market approach to reproductive technologies (Spar, 2011). Indeed, the lack of restrictions governing reproductive technologies has made the United States an ideal marketplace, particularly for those seeking reproductive resources (i.e., gametes, wombs) from others (Martin, 2014). Throughout most of the developed world, commercial surrogacy (i.e., surrogacy for pay) is outlawed, and the selling of gametes is prohibited or highly regulated. In the United States, the field of reproductive medicine is governed primarily through professional self-regulation, as professional associations set forth guidelines but lack enforcement authority. For example, the ASRM's (2007) Ethics Committee considers that payment in excess of $10,000 to oocyte donors is inappropriate compensation and advises against different compensation according to the donor's racial, ethnic, or personal characteristics. However, as a quick perusal of many elite college and university newspapers' advertisements will quickly demonstrate, egg brokers, fertility clinics, and intended parents often offer tens of thousands of dollars for egg donors with particular racial or ethnic backgrounds, physical characteristics, or talents or abilities (e.g., academic achievement).

Infertility clinics, even those housed within academic medical centers, engage in aggressive marketing to recruit patients in this highly profitable branch of reproductive medicine (Kolata, 2002). Clinics that offer third-party reproductive technologies (e.g., donor gametes) may use the donors' profiles to market and retain intended parents as clinic patients. Almeling's (2011) ethnography of the egg and sperm market in the United States revealed the gendered organization of the market for "sex cells." For example, men providing sperm are encouraged to think about their payment as compensation for doing a "job," whereas women are encouraged to think of egg donation as a "gift" and to construct their profiles to convey their desire to give, rather than to receive compensation.

Third-party reproduction, which involves the costs of IVF as well as third-party (and often a brokering agency's) payment, is expensive and cost prohibitive for many. The United States is a destination for individuals and couples, particularly from Western Europe and the Middle East, seeking to use reproductive technologies that are prohibited in their home countries, but it is also a point of departure for many Americans, who seek less expensive treatments available abroad. The Internet has contributed to a globalized marketplace for reproductive technologies, where direct advertising as well as infertility blogs and chat rooms help individuals to find clinics across the globe that offer less restrictive and less expensive options for buying gametes and contracting with surrogates, a practice described alternatively as "fertility tourism" or "cross-border reproductive care." Here, the specter of exploitation of women providing reproductive matter rises. Women who serve as third-party providers may ultimately be seeking to "gain a sense of dignity within global capitalism," as Nahman (2008, p. 76) concluded in her study of Romanian egg providers, but there may also be fewer protections if medical procedures or contractual arrangements go awry. For example, the widely publicized account of surrogate baby Gammy, who was left with his surrogate in Thailand by his Australian commissioning parents after he was born with Down syndrome and a congenital heart defect, has raised awareness of the need for regulation and global oversight over third-party reproductive practices (Howard, 2014).

As noted earlier, biomedicalization theory emphasizes biosocialities, or new social forms and arrangements fueled by emerging medical knowledge and shifting medical practices. Third-party providers, whose anonymity had previously eluded organization, are beginning to connect around their new identity (e.g., as egg donors or surrogates) and to add their voice as meaningful stakeholders in the marketplace of reproductive medicine. For example, the grassroots group We Are Egg Donors (2015) has created a web-based community open exclusively to egg providers that aims to "offer a safe space where women can connect about aspects of being an egg donor—the highs and the lows and even the TMIs [too much information]." The group provides support, resources for education, and advocacy in support of donors' health, without taking a position in support or opposition to the practice of providing eggs for others.

PREIMPLANTATION GENETIC DIAGNOSIS

PGD entails an additional testing phase in the IVF cycle that involves the removal and genetic testing of one or two cells from an embryo, and the transfer of selected embryos to the uterus, with the hope of establishing a pregnancy (Baruch, Kaufman, & Hudson, 2006). When PGD first entered public discourse in the early 1990s, there was fear that dystopian tales of "designer babies" had finally come true (Spar, 2006). By 2002, approximately 1,000 babies had been born after PGD, and the number of such babies born each year has increased since then (Preimplantation Genetic Diagnosis International Society, 2008). Indeed, the practice of PGD expands genetic choices in ways previously thought impossible, thus enabling the selection of preferred embryos during a cycle of IVF, based on genetic criteria. It adds an estimated monetary cost of at least $3,500 (Spar, 2006) to the price of IVF in the United States, and it is generally not covered by health insurance. Franklin and Roberts (2006, p. 130) contended that it is "difficult to say in any simple sense what PGD 'is,' since there are many 'PGDs'."

PGD was first used as an alternative to prenatal diagnosis for known carriers of serious hereditary conditions who wish to have a genetically related child without that particular condition (Franklin & Roberts, 2006). It is also technology that has enabled controversial "savior siblings" (an embryo selected in the hopes of bearing a child who is genetically compatible with an already existing ill child). In this potentially lifesaving procedure, the child born through PGD will then provide an organ or cell transplant for an ill sibling, an intervention dramatized and sensationalized in Jodi Picoult's (2005) novel-turned-movie *My Sister's Keeper*. More recently, PGD has begun to be utilized to avoid conditions that confer increased *risk* of disease, such as hereditary breast, ovarian, or colon cancer risk (Offit et al., 2006). Perhaps most controversially, it is also used for sex selection. Although discouraged, sex selection is not prohibited in the United States, and it is even marketed for purposes of "family balancing," a practice rooted in gender assumptions of personhood that perpetuates gender stereotypes (ASRM, 1999, 2001).

With little federal regulation, the United States has become a global destination for sex selection (Darnovsky, 2009). PGD use was once rare, but, over the past decade, reproductive medicine has begun to strengthen the relation between PGD and infertility and framed it as a potentially more effective option for treating infertility than IVF alone, specifically for women who are deemed "at risk" for "nonsuccess" (Chang et al., 2012; Colls et al., 2007; Lathi, Westphall, & Milki, 2008). Because PGD is carried out during an IVF cycle, the relation between PGD and infertility has always been complicated, and sometimes it brings often-fertile couples into the domain of infertility care. However, as PGD begins to be more regularly used to treat infertility, the fields of infertility care and clinical genetics will further intertwine.

One central use of PGD is to select embryos without aneuploidy[6] and chromosomal defects, which might impact infertility. Research suggests that the risk for such issues increases significantly for women over age 35 (Marquard, Westphal, Milki, & Lathi, 2010). According to the ASRM's Practice Committee for Assisted Reproductive Technology (2008):

> Aneuploidy is the most common cause for early pregnancy failure. The prevalence of oocyte [egg] and embryo aneuploidy increases with maternal age and also may be increased in chromosomally normal couples with recurrent early pregnancy loss or repeated failed IVF cycles despite the transfer of high-quality embryos. (p. S139)

During pregnancy, it is common to screen for aneuploidy conditions (such as trisomy 21 and Turner's syndrome) using prenatal diagnosis (PND). If these conditions are detected, it may lead one to terminate the pregnancy, which can be costly in many ways, particularly for an individual undergoing IVF with its high costs and low success rates. PGD is marketed as an alternative to PND for the screening of aneuploidy as a way to mitigate some of these potential costs. Thus, PGD is cited as a way to increase the likelihood of "selecting embryos that will reach term" (Colls et al., 2007, p. 53), whether by selecting out conditions that might lead to pregnancy termination or by choosing the embryos that are not at risk for those conditions. Franklin and Roberts (2006) noted that, for those already struggling to conceive through IVF, the risk of having to terminate a pregnancy that is so costly and unlikely in the first place will convince them to seek PGD in order to ensure that their transferred embryo is free of genetic risk.

Although these practices have been used in reproductive medicine over the past decade (Franklin & Roberts, 2007), the increased focus in biomedical research on the contribution of PGD to the efficacy of infertility treatment is telling, perhaps alluding to a further merging of PGD and ARTs (Mamo, 2010). As PGD is used more regularly to "treat risk" for women facing the possibility of infertility, its technological possibilities shift into the domain of Fertility, Inc., ushering in new options of genetic selection during the treatment of infertility and bringing old ethical questions into new light.

Issues of access and availability invariably come into play. As with IVF, access to PGD is highly stratified due to its significant expense and the dearth of insurance coverage. Thus, the option of genetic choice is only available to those who can afford it. In the context of biomedicalization, PGD risks becoming yet another way to commodify health and bring it into the realm of Fertility, Inc., as it allows individuals seeking treatment for infertility simultaneously to increase their chances for a successful pregnancy and to be a responsible parent by choosing the "healthiest" genes (Mamo, 2013). Thus, once it is fully routinized into IVF practices, it may be difficult to opt out. When PGD is framed as a parental responsibility (Rubin, 2011), as a way of doing everything that can be done to benefit prospective children (Zeiler, 2004), parents may feel obliged to choose this option, particularly in a social context where services for persons with disabilities and their caretakers are limited.

Disability rights activists have suggested that such genetic choice distracts from initiatives that address existing social stratification and sources of oppression that eschew biological difference and diversity (Shakespeare, 1999). Instead of focusing on important changes to the social environment and improving resources for disabled individuals, biomedicalized tools, such as PGD and PND, offer the possibility of eliminating disability in the first place. This devalues the lives of individuals with genetic differences and disabilities (Galpern, 2007) by deploying PGD to enforce problematic norms regarding the human body and boundaries of identity (Mamo, 2013). Thus, the allure of technological innovation further removes the focus from nonbiomedicalized responses to disability and infertility.

EGG FREEZING

Few medical procedures illustrate processes of biomedicalization as explicitly as fertility preservation technologies, particularly oocyte cryopreservation (popularly known as egg freezing). Oocyte cryopreservation is a newer reproductive technology that involves stimulation of a woman's ovaries with fertility medications to promote maturation of multiple eggs, rather than the typical single egg released during a menstrual cycle; the release is followed by an oocyte harvesting procedure. Oocytes are then cooled and stored at subzero temperatures. Costs can range from $9,000 to $15,000 per cycle, with additional storage fees (Martin, 2010).

Due to its invasiveness and relatively low success rates, the medical use of oocyte cryopreservation has been, until recently, generally limited to reproductive-age women prior to undergoing medical treatments, such as chemotherapy, that can cause infertility. However, consistent with processes of medicalization, the boundaries of use have expanded rapidly over the years, such that the current target population includes virtually all healthy reproductive-age women with ovaries and, of course, the financial means to pay for treatment.

The ASRM recently issued new guidelines on oocyte cryopreservation; they removed the "experimental" label that had previously been applied to the procedure (ASRM, 2013b). Although certainly a victory for cancer patients, as insurance often does not cover experimental procedures, the real beneficiary was Fertility, Inc. With more women delaying childbearing, the fertility industry had already been marketing oocyte cryopreservation to healthy women as a way to "beat" or "freeze" their "biological clock" (Friese et al., 2006). ASRM has explicitly discouraged the use and marketing of oocyte cryopreservation to delay childbearing; they described the data on safety, efficacy, cost-effectiveness, and emotional risks as "insufficient" and warned: "Marketing this technology for the purpose of deferring childbearing may give women false hope" (ASRM, 2013b, p. 41). This statement was lost amid the media and commercial hype that touted ASRM's *endorsement* of egg freezing.[7]

Martin (2010) proposed the term *anticipated infertility* as a descriptor for the "condition" of young women who anticipate delayed childbearing and, thus, are viewed as "at risk" for age-related fertility decline. Although not (yet) considered a medical diagnosis, women who anticipate the possibility of infertility are encouraged to manage this risk by taking preventive action, which can include medical procedures, such as ovarian reserve screening (Kushnir, Barad, & Gleicher, 2014) and the invasive procedures involved in oocyte cryopreservation years in advance of intended childbearing, ironically using the same treatment to prevent infertility as they might utilize if they were actually diagnosed as infertile in the future. This is consistent with contemporary transformations in Western medicine, and particularly in the U.S. context, in which, "individuals are increasingly *obligated* to formulate life strategies, to seek to maximize their life chances" (Novas & Rose, 2000, p. 487, emphasis added), and in which "the categories of health and illness have become vehicles for self-production" (Greco, 1993, p. 358, as cited in Novas & Rose, 2000).

As with other reproductive technologies, egg freezing has been celebrated by its practitioners and consumers as a procedure that elevates the status of women by freeing women from the dilemmas and constraints of biology and leveling the playing field at work and in heterosexual relationships. Although cautious about appearing to advocate limits on women's reproductive autonomy, feminist scholars and activists have raised particular concern with egg freezing as a solution to these contemporary dilemmas. Whereas feminist perspectives were previously obscured within mainstream media representations of infertility treatments, a recent announcement that Apple and Facebook, trendsetting employers in the tech industry, would provide insurance coverage to women for oocyte cryopreservation (Sydell, 2014) served as a tipping point that moved feminist concerns from margin to center.

As the ASRM did, feminist scholars and activists raised concerns about the safety and efficacy of these procedures, but feminists also highlighted the procedures' downstream consequences. Specifically, oocyte cryopreservation offers an individual solution to the societal dilemma of balanced work/life policies by maintaining (or even exacerbating) the status quo. Indeed, as Almeling, Radin, and Richardson (2014, para. 9) contended, "the structural organization of work has proved more inflexible than women's ovaries." Use of these technologies further exacerbates stratified reproduction (Colen, 1995). As these technologies take pressure off political advocacy for actual workplace reform, women unable to afford access to them may be especially disadvantaged. The scores of entrepreneurial businesses that have arisen to support Fertility, Inc., market the "treatments" as "lifestyle" technologies and define their preferred clientele as women of economic means.

Manufacturing women's anxieties about their fertility is a profitable enterprise; it results in scores of entrepreneurs who carve out niche businesses to support Fertility, Inc. For example, businesses that offer "financing options" (i.e., interest-bearing loans) and related "concierge services" are now emerging.[8] Their target audience is young "career-minded" women, as exemplified by their marketing efforts, which highlight the cost of egg freezing as "cheaper than a cold juice press a day!"[9] The company hosts "egg freezing cocktail parties" across the country that are heavily advertised through Twitter, Facebook, and other forms of social media, with hash tags such as #letschill. Their events, held in major cities across the country, "bring together fertility doctors, first person testimonials, Q&A sessions, financing information and cocktails."[10] On their site, EggBanxx claims: "The empowering movement, of educating women on how they can be proactive with their fertility options, has been selling out and silencing those ticking biological clocks." This discourse co-opts feminist ideas about choice and empowerment and transforms them into a marketing tool.

Egg freezing and related enterprises claim to offer a "solution" to the competing desires of full-time employment and reproduction. However, instead of advocating for access to egg freezing for poor and working-class women, addressing oppressive systems that compel women to experience these roles (work and motherhood) as mutually exclusive, or advocating for family-friendly workplaces and universal childcare, women are directed to loans and "financing options" as the ultimate solution. In true biomedicalized fashion, egg freezing becomes the answer to social problems.

CONCLUSION

Despite tremendous media attention and increased online engagement, infertility continues to be a stigmatized issue for many. The framework of biomedicalization theory allows us to consider the social and psychological weight of infertility for those facing it, yet it also looks critically at the larger social, technological, political, and economic trends that shape how infertility is understood and experienced and the possibilities for responding to it. Throughout this chapter, we have illustrated the gendered and socioeconomically stratified nature of the contemporary marketplace of U.S. infertility and reproductive technologies. We have highlighted the rapid expansion of this marketplace, as new technologies mutate in their uses, initially developed to treat rare health conditions and concerns, but later refashioned for mass appeal, and produce a shift in ideas about "normative" and "deviant" reproduction. Sometimes these technologies democratize reproductive technologies and expand notions of kinship by providing access where there were once restrictions. Yet, they also further stratify populations, first creating a *possible* means of fulfilling one's reproductive desires, but then providing it only to those who can afford access.

The same online spaces and ARTs that perpetuate biomedicalization can help foster supportive communities for women dealing with fertility concerns (as we saw with Ashley Gardner) and also offer important possibilities to resist the very narratives upheld by Fertility, Inc. Critical feminist media scholars have pointed out that online spaces can offer sites for social and political resistance to oppressive power structures (Koerber, 2001; Orgad, 2005) and support and encourage advocacy and alternatives, including voluntary childfree living, adoption, and other alternative family arrangements that challenge the hegemony of reproductive technologies. As women continue to discuss and challenge the biomedicalization of infertility, perhaps online spaces will serve as an important site to expand the discussion of infertility beyond the boundaries of Fertility, Inc.

Although the proliferation of social media use has certainly widened the global(ized) network of Fertility, Inc., it has also served as a useful platform to create new alliances to counter these trends. Increased restriction of ARTs has the potential to drive seekers underground or overseas, but an improved oversight of Fertility, Inc., could help to support those parties who are particularly vulnerable in this marketplace. Social media networks and community blogs also can be used to advocate for a disability rights movement that focuses on support for those living with disability, rather than on preventing the birth of people with disabilities. As domains of reproductive technologies and information and computer technologies continue to intertwine, we must attend to the changing meanings of infertility that are produced through processes of biomedicalization and continue to reimagine these technologies as tools to expand the scope of reproductive justice.

NOTES

1. According to the U.S. National Health Statistics Reports, if a woman and her consistent male partner have not become pregnant despite regular unprotected intercourse over 12 months, the woman is identified as infertile in their methodology, regardless of whether the infertility stems from the man or the woman (Chandra et al., 2013). Among infertile couples, the male partner is a sole or contributing cause of infertility in approximately 40% of cases (ASRM, 2014).

2. Cisgender refers to individuals whose gender identity is consistent with the sex assigned to them at birth.

3. The term *donor* suggests generosity and gift giving, which illustrates the ways in which language regarding third-party reproduction is euphemized to avoid discomfort within a marketplace model of reproduction, despite the fact that the majority of gamete transfers involve monetary exchange (Shanley, 2002).

4. Although the reference to a *third* party assumes a couple, or two persons who are in need of reproductive resources from another, single adults may also use so-called third-party interventions to become parents, including single women through donor sperm and single men who contract with a surrogate to become a parent.

5. We focus in this chapter on egg donation and surrogacy because of their higher cost and the greater extent of biomedical involvement.

6. A condition caused by an extra or a missing chromosome.

7. See, for example, Texas Fertility Center (http://txfertility.com/pressrelease/tfc-austin-egg-freezing-program), Pacific Fertility Center (http://www.pacific fertilitycenter.com/blog/asrm-endorses-egg-freezing).

8. For example, FertilityFunds.com, EggBanxx.com.

9. From http://www.fertilityfunds.com/how-it-works.

10. From http://wwww.eggbanxx.com/events.

REFERENCES

Almeling, R. (2011). *Sex cells: The medical market for eggs and sperm*. Berkeley: University of California Press.

Almeling, R., Radin, R., & Richardson, S. (2014, October 20). Egg-freezing a better deal for companies than for women. Retrieved from http://www.cnn.com/2014/10/20/opinion/almeling-radin-richardson-egg-freezing/.

American Society of Reproductive Medicine [ASRM]. (1999). Sex selection and preimplantation genetic diagnosis. *Fertility and Sterility, 72*, 595–598.

American Society of Reproductive Medicine [ASRM]. (2001). Preconception gender selection for nonmedical reasons. *Fertility and Sterility, 75*, 861–864.

American Society of Reproductive Medicine [ASRM]. (2007). Financial compensation of oocyte donors. *Fertility and Sterility, 88*, 305–309.

American Society for Reproductive Medicine [ASRM]. (2008). Preimplantation genetic testing: A practice committee opinion. *Fertility and Sterility, 90*, S136–S143.

American Society for Reproductive Medicine [ASRM]. (2013a). Definitions of infertility and recurrent pregnancy loss. *Fertility and Sterility, 90*, 63.

American Society for Reproductive Medicine [ASRM]. (2013b). Mature oocyte cryopreservation: A guideline. *Fertility and Sterility, 99*, 37–43.

American Society for Reproductive Medicine [ASRM]. (2014). Quick facts about infertility. Retrieved from http://www.asrm.org/detail.aspx?id=2322.

Baruch, S., Kaufman, D., & Hudson, K. L. (2006). Genetic testing of embryos: Practices and perspectives of U.S. IVF clinics. *Fertility and Sterility, 83*, 1708–1716.

Beeson, D., & Lippman, A. (2006). Egg harvesting for stem cell research: Medical risks and ethical problems. *Reproductive BioMedicine Online, 13*, 573–579.

Bell, A. V. (2010). Beyond (financial) accessibility: Inequalities within the medicalisation of infertility. *Sociology of Health & Illness, 32*, 631–646.

Centers for Disease Control and Prevention [CDC]. (2012). *Assisted reproductive technology fertility clinic success rates report*. Retrieved from http://www.cdc.gov/art/ART2 012/PDF/ART_2012_Clinic_Report-Full.pdf.

Centers for Disease Control and Prevention [CDC]. (2013). *Infertility*. Retrieved from http://www.cdc.gov/reproductivehealth/Infertility.

Chandra, A., Copen, C. E., & Stephen, E. H. (2013). Infertility and impaired fecundity in the United States, 1982–2010: Data from the National Survey of Family Growth. *National Health Statistics Reports, 67*, 1–18.

Chang, E. M., Han, J. E., Kwak, I. P., Lee, W. S., Yoon, T. K., & Shim, S. H. (2012). Preimplantation genetic diagnosis for couples with a Robertsonian translocation: Practical information for genetic counseling. *Journal of Assisted Reproduction and Genetics, 29*, 67–75.

Chavkin, W., & Maher, J. (Eds.). (2010). *The globalization of motherhood: Deconstructions and reconstructions of biology and care.* New York: Routledge.

Chodorow, N. J. (1999). *The reproduction of mothering: Psychoanalysis and the sociology of gender.* Berkeley: University of California Press.

Clarke, A. E., Shim, J., Mamo, L., Fosket, J. R., & Fishman, J. R. (2003). Biomedicalization: Theorizing techno-scientific transformations of health, illness, and US biomedicine. *American Sociological Review, 68*, 161–194.

Clarke, A. E., Shim, J. K., Mamo, L., Fosket, J. R., & Fishman, J. R. (2010). Biomedicalization: A theoretical and substantive introduction. In A. E. Clarke, L. Mamo, J. R. Foscket, J. R. Fishman, & J. K. Shim (Eds.), *Biomedicalization: Technoscience, health, and illness in the U.S.* (pp. 1–44). Durham, NC: Duke University Press.

Colen, S. (1995). "Like a mother to them": Stratified reproduction and West Indian childcare workers and employers in New York. In F. D. Ginsburg & R. Rapp (Eds.), *Conceiving the new world order: The global politics of reproduction* (pp. 78–102). Berkeley: University of California Press.

Colls, P., Escudero, T., Cekleniak, N., Sadowy, S., Cohen, J., & Munné, S. (2007). Increased efficiency of preimplantation genetic diagnosis for infertility using "no result rescue." *Fertility and Sterility, 88*, 53–61.

Conrad, P., & Leiter, V. (2004). Medicalization, markets and consumers. *Journal of Health and Social Behavior, 45*, 158–176.

Darnovsky, M. (2009). *Countries with laws or policies on sex selection.* A memo prepared for the April 2009 New York City sex selection meeting. Retrieved from http://www.geneticsandsociety.org/downloads/200904_sex_selection_memo.pdf.

Dickenson, D. (2002). Commodification of human tissue: Implications for feminist and development ethics. *Developing World Bioethics, 2*, 55–63.

Edelman, L. (2004). *No future: Queer theory and the death drive.* Durham, NC: Duke University Press.

EggBanxx. (2015). Egg freezing informational events & egg freezing cocktail parties. Retrieved from https://www.eggbanxx.com/events.

Fertility Funds. (2014). How it works. Retrieved from http://www.fertilityfunds.com/how-it-works.

Franklin, S., & Roberts, C. (2006). *Born and made: An ethnography of preimplantation genetic diagnosis.* Princeton, NJ: Princeton University Press.

Friese, C., Becker, G., & Nachtigall, R. D. (2006). Rethinking the biological clock: Eleventh-hour moms, miracle moms and meanings of age-related infertility. *Social Science & Medicine, 63*, 1550–1560.

Galpern, E. (2007). *Assisted reproductive technologies: Overview and perspective using a reproductive justice framework.* Retrieved from http://www.geneticsand society.org/downloads/ART.pdf.

Gentile, K. (2013). The business of being made: Exploring the production of temporalities in assisted reproductive technologies. *Studies in Gender and Sexuality, 14,* 255–276.

Greil, A. L. (1991). *Not yet pregnant: Infertile couples in contemporary America.* New Brunswick, NJ: Rutgers University Press.

Greil, A. L., McQuillan, J., Shreffler, K. M., Johnson, K. M., & Slauson-Blevins, K. S. (2011). Race-ethnicity and medical services for infertility stratified reproduction in a population-based sample of US women. *Journal of Health and Social Behavior, 52,* 493–509.

Heitman, E. (1999). Social and ethical aspects of in vitro fertilization. *International Journal of Technology Assessment in Health Care, 15,* 22–35.

Horowitz, J. E., Galst, J. P., & Elster, N. (2010). *Ethical dilemmas in fertility counseling.* Washington, DC: American Psychological Association.

Howard, S. (2014). Taming the international commercial surrogacy industry. *British Medical Journal, 349,* g6334.

Johnson, K. M. (2012). Excluding lesbian and single women? An analysis of U.S. fertility clinic websites. *Women's Studies International Forum, 35,* 394–402.

Koerber, A. (2001). Postmodernism, resistance, and cyberspace: Making rhetorical spaces for feminist mothers on the web. *Women's Studies in Communication, 24,* 218–240.

Kolata, G. (2002, January 1). Fertility, Inc.: Clinics rate to lure clients. *New York Times.* Retrieved from http://www.nytimes.com/2002/01/01/science /fertility-inc-clinics-race-to-lure-clients.html.

Kushnir, V. A., Barad, D. H., & Gleicher, N. (2014). Ovarian reserve screening before contraception? *Reproductive Biomedicine Online, 29,* 527–529.

Larkin, L. (2006). Authentic mothers, authentic daughters and sons: Ultrasound imaging and the construction of fetal sex and gender. *Canadian Review of American Studies, 36,* 273–292.

Lathi, R. B., Westphal, L. M., & Milki, A. A. (2008). Aneuploidy in the miscarriages of infertile women and the potential benefit of preimplanation genetic diagnosis. *Fertility and Sterility, 89,* 353–357.

Mamo, L. (2007). *Queering reproduction: Achieving pregnancy in the age of technoscience.* Durham, NC: Duke University Press.

Mamo, L. (2010). Fertility Inc.: Consumption and subjectification in lesbian reproductive practices. In A. E. Clarke, L. Mamo, J. R. Foscket, J. R. Fishman, & J. K. Shim (Eds.), *Biomedicalization: Technoscience, health, and illness in the U.S.* (pp. 173–196). Durham, NC: Duke University Press.

Mamo, L. (2013). Queering the fertility clinic. *Journal of Medical Humanities, 34,* 227–239.

Marquard, K., Westphal, L. M., Milki, A. A., & Lathi, R. B. (2010). Etiology of recurrent pregnancy loss in women over the age of 35 years. *Fertility and Sterility, 94,* 1473–1477.

Martin, L. J. (2010). Anticipating infertility: Egg freezing, genetic preservation, and risk. *Gender & Society, 24,* 526–545.

Martin, L. J. (2014). The world's not ready for this: Globalizing selective technologies. *Science, Technology & Human Values, 39,* 432–455.

McGinnis, S. (2014, October 2). Gardner quadruplets: Inside one couple's infertility and IVF journey. [Blog post]. Retrieved from http://blogs.babycenter.com/mom_stories/gardner-quadruplets-ivf-10022014-infertility-story-video.

Myers, C. E. (2014). Colonizing the (reproductive) future: The discursive construction of ARTS as technologies of self. *Frontiers, 35,* 73–106.

Nahman, M. (2008). Nodes of desire: Romanian egg sellers, dignity and feminist alliances in transnational ova exchanges. *European Journal of Women's Studies, 15,* 65–82.

Novas, C., & Rose, N. (2000). Genetic risk and the birth of the somatic individual. *Economy and Society, 29,* 485–513.

Offit, K., Kohut, K., Clagett, B., Wadsworth, E. A., Lafaro, K. J., Cummings, S., . . . Davis, J. G. (2006). Cancer genetic testing and assisted reproduction. *Journal of Clinical Oncology, 24,* 4775–4782.

Orgad, S. (2005). The transformative potential of online communication: The case of breast cancer patients' Internet spaces. *Feminist Media Studies, 5,* 141–161.

Papadimos, T. J., & Papadimos, A. T. (2004). The student and the ovum: The lack of autonomy and informed consent in trading genes for tuition. *Reproductive Biology and Endocrinology, 2*(1), 56.

Pawlowski, A. (2014, October 6). After 8 years of infertility, parents' shocked reactions to quadruplet pregnancy go viral. [Blog post]. Retrieved from http://www.today.com/parents/parents-shocked-reactions-quadruplet-pregnancy-go-viral-2D80195978.

Peeraer, K., Debrock, S., Laenen, A., De Loecker, P., Spiessens, C., De Neubourg, D., & D'Hooghe, T. M. (2014). The impact of legally restricted embryo transfer and reimbursement policy on cumulative delivery rate after treatment with assisted reproduction technology. *Human Reproduction, 29,* 267–275.

Picoult, J. (2005). *My sister's keeper.* New York: Washington Square Press.

Preimplantation Genetic Diagnosis International Society. (2008). History of preimplantation genetic diagnosis (PGD). Retrieved from http://www.pgdis.org/history.html.

Rao, R. (2011). How (not) to regulate ARTs: Lessons from Octomom. *Albany Law Journal of Science & Techology, 21,* 313.

Roberts, D. (2014). *Killing the black body: Race, reproduction, and the meaning of liberty.* New York: Random House.

Rothman, B. K. (2000). *Recreating motherhood*. New Brunswick, NJ: Rutgers University Press.

Rubin, L. (2011, March). *Family risk and parental responsibility: Repro-genetic testing for inherited breast/ovarian risk among BR(east)CA(ncer) mutation carriers*. Invited presentation to the doctoral program in Social Personality Psychology, the Graduate Center, City University of New York.

Rubin, L. R., & Phillips, A. (2012). Infertility and assisted reproductive technologies: Matters of reproductive justice. In J. C. Chrisler (Ed.), *Reproductive justice: A global concern* (pp. 173–199). Santa Barbara, CA: Praeger.

Russo, N. F. (1976). The motherhood mandate. *Journal of Social Issues, 32*(3), 143–153.

Sandelowski, M. (1991). Compelled to try: The never-enough quality of conceptive technology. *Medical Anthropology Quarterly, 5*, 29–47.

Sandelowski, M., & de Lacy, S. (2002). The uses of a "disease": Infertility as rhetorical vehicle. In M. C. Inhorn & F. van Balen (Eds.), *Infertility around the globe: New thinking on childlessness, gender, and reproductive technologies* (pp. 33–51). Berkeley: University of California Press.

Sawicki, J. (1991). *Disciplining Foucault: Feminism, power, and the body*. New York: Routledge.

Sawicki, J. (1999). Disciplining mothers: Feminism and the new reproductive technologies. In J. Price & M. Shildrick (Eds.), *Feminist theory and the body: A reader* (pp. 190–202). New York: Routledge.

Shanley, M. L. (2002). Collaboration and commodification in assisted procreation: Reflections on an open market and anonymous donation in human sperm and eggs. *Law & Society Review, 36*, 257–284.

Shakespeare, T. (1999). "Losing the plot"? Medical and activist discourses of contemporary genetics and disability. *Sociology of Health & Illness, 21*, 669–688.

Spar, D. (2006). *The baby business: How money, science, and politics drive the commerce of conception*. Boston: Harvard Business School Press.

Spar, D. (2011, September 13). Fertility industry is a Wild West. *New York Times*. Retrieved from http://www.nytimes.com/roomfordebate/2011/09/13/making-laws-about-making-babies/fertility-industry-is-a-wild-west.

Stephen, E. H., & Chandra, A. (2006). Declining estimates of infertility in the United States: 1982–2002. *Fertility and Sterility, 86*, 516–523.

Sydell, L. (2014, October 17). Silicon Valley companies add new benefit for women: Egg-freezing. Retrieved from http://www.npr.org/blogs/alltechconsidered/2014/10/17/356765423/silicon-valley-companies-add-new-benefit-for-women-egg-freezing.

Thompson, C. (2005). *Making parents: The ontological choreography of reproductive technologies*. Cambridge, MA: MIT Press.

Throsby, K. (2004). *When IVF fails: Feminism, infertility and the negotiation of normality*. New York: Palgrave Macmillan.

van Balen, F., & Inhorn, M. C. (2002). Interpreting infertility: A view from the social sciences. In M. C. Inhorn & F. van Balen (Eds.), *Infertility around the globe:*

New thinking on childlessness, gender, and reproductive technologies (pp. 3–32). Berkeley: University of California Press.

We Are Egg Donors. (2015). About us. Retrieved from http://weareeggdonors.com/about-us/.

Zegers-Hochschild, F., Adamson, G.D., de Mouzon, J., Ishihara, O., Mansour, R., Nygren, K., ... Vanderpoel, S. (2009). International Committee for Monitoring Assisted Reproductive Technology (ICMART) and the World Health Organization's (WHO) revised glossary of ART terminology. *Fertility and Sterility, 95,* 1520–1524.

Zeiler, K. (2004). Reproductive autonomous choice—A cherished illusion? Reproductive autonomy examined in the context of preimplantation genetic diagnosis. *Medicine, Heath Care, and Philosophy, 7,* 175–183.

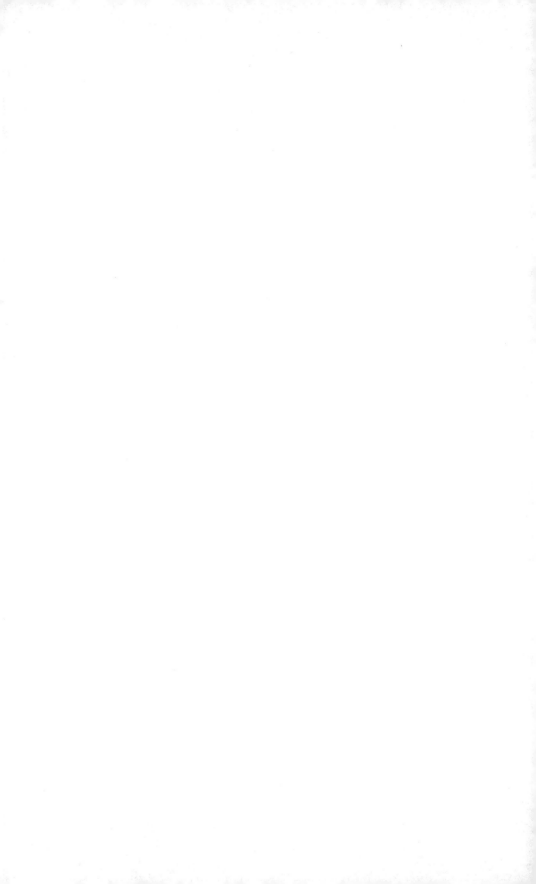

Chapter 3

The Medicalization of the Menstrual Cycle: Menstruation as a Disorder

Jessica Barnack-Tavlaris

Choice is an important word with significant meaning when it comes to reproductive health. Whether or not to menstruate has become a choice for some, as medical technology has advanced to develop ways of suppressing menstruation. In a sense, women can now have menstruation "treated" as if it were a medical disease with the potential to harm their health. As a result, people have come to question the purpose and necessity of menstruation, an already stigmatized reproductive event. This chapter discusses the different perspectives about whether menstruation is necessary, the details of menstrual suppression and the arguments for and against it, how the media portray menstrual suppression and how pharmaceutical companies stand to profit, and women's attitudes toward menstruation and menstrual suppression. Finally, I provide some conclusions and recommendations to consider.

IS MENSTRUATION NECESSARY? BIOMEDICAL VERSUS BIOPSYCHOSOCIAL PERSPECTIVES

According to the American Congress of Obstetricians and Gynecologists (ACOG), the average age of menarche (a girl's first menstrual period) in the United States is about 12 years old (range of 8 to 15 years) (ACOG, 2006). The ACOG defined a normal menstrual cycle for adolescent and young adult women as ranging between 21 and 45 days (mean of 32.2 days), menstrual flow of seven or fewer days, and normal use of three to six pads or tampons per day while bleeding. The ACOG has called menarche an important developmental milestone of adolescence and recommended that physicians use their assessment of an adolescent's menstrual cycle as a vital sign, just as they would blood pressure or heart rate. In other words, normal menstrual cycles are a sign of good health status. In their report on the importance of the menstrual cycle as a vital sign, the ACOG also stressed the need for physicians to educate girls and young women about the menstrual cycle because those who have more accurate information about menstruation will have better emotional development (i.e., less anxiety). In other words, this medical organization, whose members have expertise on reproductive health issues, acknowledges the value and importance of the menstrual cycle and views menarche as a normal, healthy developmental event. So does the Society for Menstrual Cycle Research, which has endorsed the vital sign campaign and promoted body literacy education for adolescents (Stubbs, 2008).

Today, women in industrialized societies menstruate far more often than they did hundreds of years ago. This is because contemporary women have earlier menarche, reproduce later in life, have fewer children, spend less time breastfeeding (which means women begin to menstruate sooner postpartum), and experience menopause later in life than their ancestors did. Age at menarche in the United States decreased from the 1800s to the mid-1950s; however, the mean age at menarche has remained relatively stable since then (ACOG, 2006). Some proposed reasons for earlier age at menarche include girls' higher body mass index and environmental factors, such as nutrition and better access to preventive care (ACOG, 2006). There is debate across the fields of medicine and the social sciences about what the increase in number of lifetime menstrual cycles means for women's health and what, if anything, should be done about it. Those who view menstruation as unnecessary reference these changes as unnatural and argue that women can and should return to a state of having fewer periods. On the other hand, those who challenge the claims of menstruation as unnecessary highlight the positive aspects of menstruation and argue that there are many aspects of modern life that differ from hundreds of years ago that we do nothing to reinstate. For example, giving birth to 10 or more children may have been the norm in the early 1800s, but we do not consider that normal today, nor do we encourage women to return to that lifestyle.

Scientists and health professionals who believe menstruation to be unnecessary tend to view menstruation from a biomedical perspective and often express their views by discussing the negative aspects some women may experience during menstruation (e.g., headaches, cramps, bloating). From this view, menstruation appears to be a bodily process with symptoms and risks, thus medical management is deemed necessary. Most of the studies that support the claim that menstruation is harmful and in need of treatment have been conducted by researchers who have been involved in clinical trials of drugs that treat or suppress menstruation or those whose work has been funded by various pharmaceutical companies (e.g., Bitzer, Serrani, & Lahav, 2013; Lin & Barnhart, 2007) that manufacture drugs to treat menstrual symptoms and "manage" the menstrual cycle (e.g., to produce cycles of a predictable length, to produce shorter and lighter menstrual flows, or to treat severe cramps).

In the 1990s, Elsimar Coutinho, a Brazilian gynecologist, and his colleague Sheldon Segal, a researcher who has worked on the design of contraceptives, wrote a book titled *Is Menstruation Obsolete?* They argued that "menstruation is unnecessary and can be harmful to the health of women. It is a needless loss of blood" (Coutinho & Segal, 1999, p. 159). They supported their argument that menstruation is harmful by referring to the disorders related to menstruation (e.g., endometriosis, anemia, premenstrual syndrome) and the negative impact those disorders can have on women's physical and psychological well-being. The media enthusiastically publicized the book and promoted Coutinho and Segal's campaign to educate *all* women (who were not trying to get pregnant) that menstruation is unnecessary (Johnston-Robledo, Barnack, & Wares, 2006). Of course, their campaign aimed to educate women about ways to suppress menstruation, which include the continuous use of oral contraceptives and injectable progestins (e.g., Depo Provera). The media rarely noted that Coutinho was involved in the creation of Depo Provera and Segal was involved in the discovery of Norplant (both suppress the menstrual cycle); thus they stood to benefit significantly from convincing women of the uselessness of menstruation (Hitchcock & Prior, 2004a).

Not everyone agrees with Coutinho and Segal's claim that menstruation is obsolete or unnecessary. Feminist researchers have provided evidence that challenges the legitimacy of this claim (e.g., Gunson, 2010; Hitchcock, 2008). Researchers who reject Coutinho and Segal's claims view menstruation from a biopsychosocial perspective and acknowledge it as a bodily process that is experienced within psychological and sociocultural contexts. From this model, negative experiences with menstruation have the potential to be alleviated by examining and addressing psychological and sociocultural factors such as attitudes and stigma.

Johnston-Robledo and Chrisler (2013) argued that menstruation is stigmatized in North American societies and that this stigma has negative implications for women's physical and emotional well-being. Some women experience shame associated with menstruation, and those with negative attitudes toward menstruation are more likely than other women to self-objectify (e.g., to have high levels of body shame and self-surveillance; Johnston-Robledo, Sheffield, Voight, & Wilcox-Constantine, 2007). As a result of this stigma and shame, women often go to great lengths to conceal their menstrual status (e.g., hide tampons or pads, wear loose and dark clothing, avoid sexual contact during menstruation, keep their menstrual status secret); thus, women limit their behavior during menstruation. Negative attitudes and beliefs may also lead women to choose medical regimens to manage or suppress their cycles, which can affect their physical health. In fact, in an early study (Johnston-Robledo, Ball, Lauta, & Zekoll, 2003), college-aged women who were more interested in and supportive of menstrual suppression were also those who viewed menstruation as shameful and as a disability. Treating menstruation as a normal healthy process should have positive psychological effects on women's experiences with menstruation. For example, in one study, college women who were high in optimism reported less pain and negative behavior change during menstruation than women who were low in optimism (Chrisler, Rose, Dutch, Sklarsky, & Grant, 2006).

WHAT IS MENSTRUAL SUPPRESSION?

Menstrual suppression is becoming an easily prescribed medical management of menstruation. Currently, there are various birth control methods that women can use to regulate or suppress their menstrual cycles. Some of the common and more effective regimens include traditional oral contraceptive pills or "the ring" used continuously, specific types of oral contraceptive pills created specifically to suppress menstruation (e.g., Seasonale), and hormonal contraceptive injections (e.g., Depo Provera). The number of "periods" a woman will experience depends on the exact contraceptive regimen.

When women take a traditional oral contraceptive pill, they are given 21 days of hormones (i.e., estrogen and progestin), then seven days of placebo pills that do not contain any hormones. The week the women take the placebo pills is the week that they bleed. The bleeding is actually withdrawal bleeding from the lack of hormones (Jacobson, Likis, & Murphy, 2012) rather than a normal menstrual period. The oral contraceptive pill was developed in this way to mimic the natural 28-day menstrual cycle. When women take oral contraceptive pills to suppress menstruation, they are instructed to skip the seven days of placebo pills and continue directly to a new pack of active pills that contains hormones (Jacobson et al., 2012). In this way, women experience no hormone withdrawal because there is no placebo week, and, therefore, they do not experience the bleeding they would have had with the traditional oral contraceptive regimen. However, women who use continuous oral contraceptives may experience unpredictable spotting, which is more likely to happen when they first begin taking the pill continuously; the spotting usually subsides with time. Yet, women who wish to avoid all bleeding or to know when to expect bleeding find the unpredictable spotting to be disappointing and disconcerting. In 2003, the U.S. Food and Drug Administration (FDA) approved the first oral contraceptive pill (Seasonale) that was created specifically to reduce the number of periods women have in a year from about 12 to 4. Some women who have used Seasonale have also reported some breakthrough bleeding, especially in the beginning stages of the regimen (Anderson & Hait, 2003).

Oral contraceptives have been commonly prescribed to "regulate" women's menstrual cycles, and studies have shown that women who use oral contraceptives report fewer premenstrual symptoms than women who do not use them (e.g., Adrist, Hoyt, Weinstein, & McGibbon, 2004). In one study, 91% of providers reported that they had prescribed oral contraceptives to women for reasons other than pregnancy prevention (Andrist, Arias et al., 2004). The extended or continued use of oral contraceptive pills to suppress menstruation is prescribed for both lifestyle (e.g., travel, military deployment) and therapeutic reasons (Andrist, Arias et al. 2004; Jacobson et al., 2012). Some therapeutic reasons for prescribing the regimen include menstruation-related disorders, such as migraines, endometriosis, and disorders that cause abnormal or heavy uterine bleeding (Jacobson et al., 2012).

In a recent study by Lakehomer, Kaplan, Wozniak, and Minson (2013), 1,719 college women were surveyed about their use of hormonal contraceptives to control menstruation. Almost 80% of women had currently or recently used hormonal contraceptives, and about 17% (n = 228) of them had used the contraceptives specifically to suppress menstruation. The most common reason women reported for modifying their cycles was "convenience or social scheduling" (51.3%), followed by "personal preference" (28.9%), to "reduce menstrual symptoms" (16.7%), and for "sports or athletic reasons" (3.1%) (Lakehomer et al., 2013, p. 429). What is perhaps most interesting about the findings of this study is that when women were asked how they learned to modify their cycles with their contraceptives, 47% reported they learned from medical professionals, 30% from family or friends, 9% from the Internet, and 2% from other media (Lakehomer et al., 2013). This means that many women were not necessarily suppressing their cycles under the recommendation or supervision of their physicians. Rather, they were choosing and implementing this method on their own. Physicians should ask their patients who use oral contraceptives if they are taking them as prescribed, and, if not, physicians should inform women about what we do and do not know about the long-term effects of menstrual suppression.

Proponents of menstrual suppression have argued that the regimen is safe and effective in alleviating the discomfort some women experience during menstruation. On the other hand, opponents have argued that more long-term studies on the effects of menstrual suppression on the woman's whole body are needed before its safety can be assured. For instance, menstrual suppression with continuous oral contraceptive use can expose women to 25% to 33% more estrogen than traditional oral contraceptive use, and there is no convincing evidence that such increased exposure will not negatively impact women's health in the long term (Prior & Hitchcock, 2007). The regular use of oral contraceptives (i.e., not continuous) has been found to slightly increase breast cancer risk (National Cancer Institute, n.d.); it is unknown whether the increased amount of hormones from the continuous use would further increase that risk. At the same time, however, it should also be pointed out that regular use of oral contraceptives (i.e., not continuous) has been found to reduce ovarian and endometrial cancer risk (National Cancer Institute, n.d.).

Hitchcock and Prior (2004b) conducted a systematic review of the scientific literature on the continuous use of oral contraceptives. They found that, although women who used continuous oral contraceptives had less bleeding than women who used traditional oral contraceptives, those women who used the continuous regimen had more random bleeding and spotting. Sporadic and unexpected bleeding is a common reason women give for discontinuing the continuous oral contraceptive regimen. In their review, Hitchcock and Prior (2004b) also found a paucity of research regarding the physiological effects of continuous oral contraceptive use. For example, it is unknown how the regimen impacts reproductive development, as well as how soon women's reproductive functioning returns to normal after discontinuing the regimen (Hitchcock & Prior, 2004b). These questions are particularly important because developing girls and young women are suppressing their cycles. Furthermore, evidence is needed to determine whether or not suppressing menstruation is actually safer than normal monthly menstruation (Hitchcock, 2008). Finally, we also need to consider the psychological consequences of women's decision to suppress menstruation. If more and more women choose to "manage" or suppress their cycles, the stigma and shame of menstruation could be exacerbated for women who choose to menstruate regularly (Johnston-Robledo & Chrisler, 2013).

MENSTRUAL SUPPRESSION IN THE MEDIA AND WHAT PHARMACEUTICAL COMPANIES HAVE TO GAIN

It is important to examine the representation of menstrual suppression in the media because some studies have shown that women report the media as their primary source of information about menstrual suppression, much more so than physicians and other sources (Gorman, Chrisler, & Couture, 2008; Johnston-Robledo et al., 2003). The media's portrayal of menstrual suppression through advertisements and articles in the popular press has been biased in favor of suppression and reinforces the stigma of menstruation, which can ultimately have an impact on women's attitudes and experiences with menstruation. Although there may be medical reasons for some women to choose menstrual suppression, the vast majority of media coverage and marketing strategies do not advertise the regimen as a way to alleviate symptoms of menstrual cycle–related disorders. Rather, menstrual suppression is presented as a way for *all* women to have a more convenient life that is free from the negative aspects of menstruation.

Prior to the FDA approval of Seasonale, researchers (Johnston-Robledo et al., 2006) examined articles in the U.S. and Canadian media about menstrual suppression. The articles explicitly instructed readers about how to suppress menstruation (by skipping placebo pills), but fewer than one-half (40.9%) of them encouraged women to seek information from their doctors before trying such a regimen. The majority of articles recommended suppression for women with endometriosis, premenstrual syndrome, severe cramps, and anemia; however, 50% suggested menstrual suppression for any woman taking oral contraceptives or any woman with vague or general "menstrual problems." The information provided in the articles was also biased in that 90% of them quoted proponents of suppression, but only 45% quoted its opponents. Of particular concern is how little information there was in the articles about the need for long-term studies on the effects of menstrual suppression.

Following the FDA approval of Seasonale, Mamo and Fosket (2009) analyzed the content of Seasonale advertisements between 2003 and 2004. They concluded that, although menstrual suppression can be used to alleviate symptoms of disorders related to the menstrual cycle (e.g., endometriosis), it has not necessarily been marketed in that way. Rather, it is marketed to women as a way to reduce the inconvenience of menstruation, which is indeed a larger (and thus more profitable) audience than women who have menstrual cycle–related disorders. Mamo and Fosket (2009, p. 928) argued that "Seasonale® produces the nonmenstrual woman as both embodiment and subjectivity." Thus, the nonmenstruating woman is positioned as the feminine ideal, an easy sell in a society that shames menstruation. Not only is the ideal woman free of stigmatized leaks and odors, but, because she no longer needs to observe the sex taboo, she is sexually available to her partner at any time (Johnston-Robledo & Chrisler, 2013).

Some articles and advertisements that promote menstrual suppression have specifically targeted adolescent girls. For example, a recent article on a website geared toward girls provides step-by-step instructions on how to suppress the menstrual cycle using traditional oral contraceptive pills

(Booth, 2013). The article also gives many reasons (e.g., mood swings, cramps, and convenience) why girls would want to suppress menstruation. The tone of the article suggests that menstrual suppression is easy and safe, which, of course, would make it appealing to young girls who are already being exposed to negative messages about menstruation and who may be using oral contraceptives for a variety of off-label reasons (e.g., acne). The Affordable Care Act will increase the number of U.S. women who have access to free birth control, which indeed is important in terms of family planning options, but this also means an even greater incentive for pharmaceutical companies to market their brands and the "benefits" of menstrual suppression.

In 2012, the profits of the top 11 pharmaceutical companies reached an astonishing $83.9 billion (Rome, 2013). Although the companies claim that the high prices of their products are needed for research and development, spending for marketing is 19 times that of research and development (Rome, 2013). Pharmaceutical company media campaigns have created a profitable market for oral contraceptive use in general and for menstrual suppression more specifically. Findings from the National Survey of Family Growth (2006 to 2008) revealed that 11.2 million women and girls aged 15 to 44 use oral contraceptives; about 1.5 million of them reported that they use the pills for noncontraceptive reasons (Jones, 2011). About 9% of pill users are not even sexually active, and most of those are adolescents (Jones, 2011). In fact, 59% of the girls or women aged 15 to 19 who were using contraceptives had never had sex or had not had sex in the past three months (Jones, 2011). In other words, the financial benefit from contraceptives extends well beyond family planning.

In order to further their agenda in making menstrual suppression seem beneficial and even necessary, pharmaceutical companies have also provided funding support for studies and articles written in support of the regimen. For example, the Association for Reproductive Health Professionals (AHRP) receives funding from pharmaceutical companies; thus, it is no surprise that AHRP has published supportive and "how to" articles about menstrual suppression (Hitchcock, 2008).

In their marketing campaigns, some pharmaceutical companies have capitalized on messages about reproductive choice, empowerment, and convenience to create the desire for their products (Mamo & Fosket, 2009). In her study of television commercials for menstrual suppression products, Kissling (2012) reported that the dialogue that takes place in these commercials reflects postfeminist and neoliberal values, such as questioning authority, taking control over one's own body, and self-definition. Proponents of menstrual suppression also incorporate this rhetoric in pushing their agenda. For example, in their book about the uselessness of menstruation, Coutinho and Segal (1999) even quoted feminist Margaret Sanger as saying that "No woman is completely free unless she has control over her own reproductive system." They followed that quote with these words: "Let this new freedom begin" (p. 164).

Some of the television commercials for oral contraceptives that can be used to suppress menstruation can be persuasive, especially to adolescents and young women who have already received many negative messages about menstruation. For example, Loestrin 24Fe is an oral contraceptive that reduces menstrual periods to three days, and its commercial suggests that five to seven days of menstruating is much too long. Furthermore, the commercials instruct women to "call your doctor and ask for the pill with the short period" (Gee, 2013). A television advertisement for Seasonique asks women: "Did you know that when you're on the pill there is no medical need to have a period? . . . Who says that time of the month needs to be every month? . . . Repunctuate your life" (MLCip, 2009). Kissling (2012) pointed out that that commercial in particular plays on the idea that menstruation is not natural (and that pill periods are "fake periods"); thus, by suppressing menstruation, women are taking control over their lives.

WOMEN'S ATTITUDES TOWARD MENSTRUATION AND MENSTRUAL SUPPRESSION

In response to its growing popularity, researchers have sought to examine what women know about menstrual suppression and how they feel about it. Some of this research has been reassuring in that many women view menstruation as a normal, healthy process. Women who are not trying to conceive also appreciate menstruation as a sign that reassures them that they are not pregnant and that they have a normally functioning reproductive system capable of conceiving when or if they choose to do so. However, there are also studies that reveal women's negative attitudes toward menstruation and these attitudes' association with a desire to suppress or manage menstruation. Such findings illustrate the impact negative cultural views of menstruation can have on women's attitudes and experiences.

Andrist, Hoyt, and colleagues (2014) conducted a survey to examine women's (aged 18 to 40) attitudes toward menstruation and menstrual suppression. They found that women with negative attitudes toward menstruation reported more interest in suppressing menstruation than did women with positive attitudes. Women who did not use oral contraceptives were more interested in menstrual suppression than women who did use them. Not all women in the study were in favor of menstrual suppression. In fact, women who were uninterested in menstrual suppression reported that *not* menstruating seemed abnormal to them and would cause them anxiety and that having a period reassured them that they were not pregnant. Forty-four percent of participants believed that having a monthly period is necessary, and those who believed it is necessary were less likely to be interested in menstrual suppression.

In another survey study, researchers examined women's and health care providers' attitudes toward using continuous oral contraceptives to suppress the menstrual cycle (Andrist, Arias, et al., 2004). Most women in the sample had never heard of (73%) or had never tried (78%) menstrual suppression. One-half of the participants believed that it is necessary for women to menstruate monthly. With regard to women's attitudes toward menstruation, 59% reported they would be interested in not menstruating monthly, and 30% would prefer never to menstruate, but 54% thought the argument that menstruation is unhealthy was strange. Most physicians (91%) reported that they had prescribed oral contraceptives to women for reasons other than pregnancy prevention, such as menstrual suppression and menstrual cycle regulation. Reasons for prescribing menstrual suppression were patient request, lifestyle, menorrhagia (i.e., abnormally heavy bleeding), dysmenorrhea (i.e., severe menstrual cramps), and endometriosis. Few health care providers (7%) believed monthly menstruation is physically necessary, and only 11% thought monthly menstruation is important to women; however, 69% of physicians disagreed that menstruation is harmful to a woman's health. Both the women and the physicians expressed concerns about the possible long-term health effects of menstrual suppression (Andrist, Arias, et al., 2004).

Although many women who show an interest in menstrual suppression are women who experience disorders related to the menstrual cycle, there are also some women without severe symptoms who show interest in menstrual suppression. For example, Ferrero and colleagues (2006) surveyed a sample of Italian women without menstrual cycle–related symptoms about their attitudes toward menstruation and their desire for fewer periods. The areas in which women reported the most interference from menstruation were sexual life and sports activities; fewer women found menstruation to interfere with their work or choice of clothes. About 28% of women reported an interest in reducing the number of menstrual periods they had, and another 28% reported an interest in never menstruating (Ferrero et al., 2006). It should be noted that the survey questions about whether menstruation interfered with women's lives and whether the women desired fewer periods were all posed to women in the "negative" direction, which could have influenced the negativity of women's responses (e.g., "Menstrual periods interfere with my sexual life," "Menstrual periods interfere with my work"; p. 538).

Gorman and her colleagues (2008) tested the idea that women's attitudes and willingness to suppress the menstrual cycle could be influenced by the types of questions (positive vs. negative) women are asked beforehand. In their study, U.S. college women completed questionnaires about menstrual distress, menstrual joy (i.e., positive aspects related to the menstrual cycle), beliefs about and attitudes toward menstruation, and willingness to suppress menstruation; however, the order in which the women completed these questionnaires differed. One group completed the Menstrual Joy Questionnaire before answering questions about their willingness to suppress menstruation (positive priming group), and the other group completed the Menstrual Distress Questionnaire before the willingness to suppress menstruation questions (negative priming group). After the willingness to suppress menstruation questions, all participants responded to the Beliefs about and Attitudes toward Menstruation questionnaire, then either the Menstrual Distress Questionnaire (first group) or the Menstrual Joy Questionnaire (second group). Thirty-three percent of participants reported a willingness to suppress menstruation, and that willingness increased to 68% if there were no negative side effects; in fact, concerns about safety were most commonly referenced when participants were asked about factors that affected their willingness to suppress their cycles. Women in the positive priming group were less likely to endorse myths about women's limited abilities during menstruation. However, there were no priming effects on women's willingness to suppress menstruation. Women with more positive attitudes toward menstrual suppression and women who used oral contraceptives were more willing to suppress menstruation than women with negative attitudes or those who did not use oral contraceptives.

In a more recent study, 12 Canadian women were interviewed about their attitudes toward menstrual suppression; one-half of the sample had suppressed their periods and the other one-half had never tried menstrual suppression (Repta & Clarke, 2013). All of the women who had suppressed their cycles viewed menstrual suppression as convenient. Additional motivations for their menstrual suppression included managing pain and not having to experience the body dissatisfaction that they felt while menstruating. On the other hand, women who had never suppressed their menstrual cycles viewed menstrual suppression as unhealthy, expressed distrust of pharmaceutical products in general, and mentioned the importance of natural menstruation. One woman who had never suppressed her cycle said: "It [your menstrual cycle] is not something that should be suppressed. It's something natural. The whole idea of suppressing menstruation gives the idea that menstruation is some kind of disease" (Repta & Clarke, 2013, p. 101). In sum, women who suppressed their cycles largely cited convenience as a factor, and women who did not suppress cited "natural" menstruation as important. It should not be surprising, then, that media campaigns that promote menstrual suppression incorporate messages about menstruation as unnecessary and incredibly inconvenient, as women may be especially susceptible to such messages.

Women's displeasure with menstruation has been well documented; however, it would be unwise not to question whether negative attitudes toward menstruation are at least in part related to the stigma and shame associated with menstruation in our society. If we lived in a society that celebrated menstruation as a healthy and empowering experience, would there be so much discomfort and disdain? As a woman who has coped with endometriosis and uterine fibroids for many years, I want to be careful not to minimize the severity of symptoms that can accompany disorders related to menstruation and the extent to which they can interfere with one's life. However, I argue that it is not menstruation *itself* that is a disorder. Furthermore, I believe that women's ability to cope with disorders related to menstruation would improve if there were less shame associated with menstruation.

CONCLUSION

Menstruation is a normal, healthy, bodily experience that has been stigmatized for a long time in many cultures and societies. The stigmatization of menstruation has serious implications for how women view their bodies and themselves. Women who have more positive attitudes toward menstruation also have more positive menstrual experiences. Pharmaceutical companies have billions of dollars to gain through the perpetuation of beliefs that menstruation is a disorder in need of treatment or a cure. Such beliefs are advertised and reinforced in the media in an effort to sell products that will make the "problem" of menstruation go away. These messages have the potential to negatively impact the extent to which teens and young women are able to connect with and maintain a healthy relationship with their bodies.

What we need are more media messages that embrace menstruation specifically and women's natural bodily experiences more generally. Such messages should incorporate the same feminist ideals that have been used by the pharmaceutical companies to make menstruation seem irrelevant and inconvenient. Perhaps it could be pointed out that surrendering one's body to synthetic hormones and pharmaceutical profit is not gaining control over one's body; it really is the opposite.

The Society for Menstrual Cycle Research (SMCR) is an international, interdisciplinary organization that has worked hard to challenge the stigma of menstruation and continues to play an important role in educating and challenging negative and inaccurate beliefs about women's reproductive health and well-being. On their website (www.menstruationresearch.org) one can find various resources, such as access to research, teaching materials, and information about activism. As more and more women choose to suppress their cycles, menstruation is at risk of becoming even more stigmatized, which will make the work of organizations such as SMCR even more necessary.

There are critical questions we need to ask and information we need to evaluate if we want women to embrace their bodies and resist the medicalization of normal reproductive experiences. For example, we need to think about how we can reconcile telling young girls that menstruation is normal if, one day, the majority of women are taking contraceptives to suppress it. Even more, we need answers about how the long-term continuous use of contraceptives (beginning in adolescence) affects girls' and women's reproductive well-being. Finally, we need to think about how menstrual suppression will further the stigma associated with menstruation. Who will choose to menstruate, and how will those women be viewed by a society that has deemed menstruation unnecessary and unhealthy?

REFERENCES

American Congress of Obstetricians and Gynecologists [ACOG]. (2006). Menstruation in girls and adolescents: Using the menstrual cycle as a vital sign. Retrieved from http://www.acog.org/~/media/Committee%20 Opinions/Committee%20on%20Adolescent%20Health%20Care/co349.pdf ?dmc=1&ts=20140416T1431026190.

Anderson, F. D., & Hait, H. (2003). A multicenter, randomized study of an extended-cycle oral contraceptive. *Contraception, 68*, 89–96.

Andrist, L. C., Arias, R. D., Nucatola, D., Kaunitz, A. M., Musselman, B. L., Reiter, S., . . . Emmert, S. (2004). Women's and providers' attitudes toward menstrual suppression with extended use of oral contraceptives. *Contraception, 70*, 359–363.

Andrist, L. C., Hoyt, A., Weinstein, D., & McGibbon, C. (2004). The need to bleed: Women's attitudes and beliefs about menstrual suppression. *Journal of the American Academy of Nurse Practitioners, 16*(1), 31–37.

Bitzer, J., Serrani, M., & Lahav., A. (2013). Women's attitudes towards heavy menstrual bleeding, and their impact on quality of life. *Open Access Journal of Contraception, 4*, 21–28.

Booth, J. (2013, May). Want to skip your period? Here's how to do it. Retrieved from http://www.gurl.com/2013/05/07/how-to-skip-your-period/.

Chrisler, J. C., Rose, J. G., Dutch, S. E., Sklarsky, K. G., & Grant, M. C. (2006). The PMS illusion: Social cognition maintains social construction. *Sex Roles, 54*, 371–376.

Coutinho, E. M., & Segal, S. J. (1999). *Is menstruation obsolete?* New York: Oxford University Press.

Ferrero, S., Abbamonte, L. H., Giordano, M., Alessandri, F., Anserini, P., Remorgida, V., & Ragni, N. (2006). What is the desired menstrual frequency of women without menstruation-related symptoms? *Contraception, 73*, 537–541.

Gee, J. (2013, September 21). Loestrin 24Fe commercial. May 23, 2006. Retrieved from http://www.youtube.com/watch?v=zCx_Ncz6p_0.

Gorman, G. R., Chrisler, J. C., & Couture, S. (2008). Young women's attitudes toward continuous use of oral contraceptives: The effect of priming positive attitudes toward menstruation on women's willingness to suppress menstruation. *Health Care for Women International, 29*, 688–701.

Gunson, J. S. (2010). "More natural but less normal": Reconsidering medicalization and agency through women's accounts of menstrual suppression. *Social Science & Medicine, 71*, 1324–1331.

Hitchcock, C. (2008). Elements of the menstrual suppression debate. *Health Care for Women International, 29*, 702–719.

Hitchcock, C. L., & Prior, J. C. (2004a). Review [*Is menstruation obsolete?*]. *Women & Therapy, 27*(3–4), 195–203.

Hitchcock, C. L., & Prior, J. C. (2004b). Evidence about extending the duration of oral contraceptive use to suppress menstruation. *Women's Health Issues, 14*, 201–211.

Jacobson, J. C., Likis, F. E., & Murphy, P. A. (2012). Extended and continuous combined contraceptive regimens for menstrual suppression. *Journal of Midwifery & Women's Health, 57*, 585–592.

Johnston-Robledo, I., Ball, M., Lauta, K., & Zekoll, A. (2003). To bleed or not to bleed: Young women's attitudes toward menstrual suppression. *Women & Health, 38*(3), 59–75.

Johnston-Robledo, I., Barnack, J., & Wares, S. (2006). "Kiss your period good-bye": Menstrual suppression in the popular press. *Sex Roles, 54*, 353–360.

Johnston-Robledo, I., & Chrisler, J. C. (2013). The menstrual mark: Menstruation as social stigma. *Sex Roles, 68*, 9–18.

Johnston-Robledo, I., Sheffield, K., Voight, J., & Wilcox-Constantine, J. (2007). Reproductive shame: Self-objectification and young women's attitudes toward their reproductive functioning. *Women & Health, 46*(1), 25–39.

Jones, R. K. (2011). Beyond birth control: The overlooked benefits of oral contraceptive pills. Guttmacher Institute. Retrieved from http://www.guttmacher.org/pubs/Beyond-Birth-Control.pdf.

Kissling, E. A. (2012). Pills, periods, and postfeminism. The new politics of marketing birth control. *Feminist Media Studies, 13*, 490–504.

Lakehomer, H., Kaplan, P. F., Wozniak, D. G., & Minson, C. T. (2013). Characteristics of scheduled bleeding manipulation with combined hormonal contraception in university students. *Contraception, 88*, 426–430.

Lin, K., & Barnhart, K. (2007). The clinical rationale for menses-free contraception. *Journal of Women's Health, 16*, 1171–1180.

Mamo, L., & Fosket, J. R. (2009). Scripting the body: Pharmaceuticals and the (re)making of menstruation. *Signs: Journal of Women in Culture and Society, 34*, 925–949.

MLCip. (2009, May 1). Seasonique "Repunctuate your life" commercial. Retrieved from: http://www.youtube.com/watch?v=6xsnKcNgZW8.

National Cancer Institute. (n.d.). Oral contraceptives and cancer risk. Retrieved from http://www.cancer.gov/cancertopics/factsheet/Risk/oral-contraceptives.

Prior, J. C., & Hitchcock, C. L. (2007). Manipulating menstruation with hormonal contraception—what does the science say? Retrieved from http://www.cemcor.ubc.ca/help_yourself/articles/manipulating_menstruation.

Repta, R., & Clarke, L. H. (2013). "Am I going to be natural or am I not?" Canadian women's perceptions and experiences of menstrual suppression. *Sex Roles, 68*, 91–106.

Rome, E. (2013, April 8). Big pharma pockets $711 billion in profits by robbing seniors, taxpayers. *Huffington Post*. Retrieved from http://www.huffingtonpost .com/ethan-rome/big-pharma-pockets-711-bi_b_3034525.html.

Stubbs, M. L. (2008). Cultural perceptions and practices around menarche and adolescent menstruation in the United States. *Annals of the New York Academy of Sciences, 1135*, 58–66.

Chapter 4

The Medicalization of Women's Moods: Premenstrual Syndrome and Premenstrual Dysphoric Disorder

Joan C. Chrisler and Jennifer A. Gorman

It may be difficult to believe, but there was once a time (only a few decades ago) when few people had ever heard of premenstrual syndrome, when women's occasional irritability, bloating, and pimple outbreaks were normal experiences, part of the ups and downs of everyday life. In those days (before 1980), people thought that women were angry when there was something to be angry about, irritable because something was irritating, and tearful because there was reason to be sad. Today, however, an angry, irritable, or tearful woman is almost automatically assumed to be premenstrual, her mood caused by her hormones, at the mercy of her menstrual cycle. She is also assumed to need medical treatment to "balance" her hormones and return her to the serene comportment (Cosgrove & Riddle, 2003) that the feminine gender role stereotype teaches us to expect. But is it normal to be calm and placid all the time? When did mood and emotion become "symptoms" of a disorder?

WHAT ARE PMS AND PMDD?

Premenstrual syndrome (PMS) refers to the cyclic recurrence of certain physical, psychological, and behavioral changes that begin during the week prior to menstruation and disappear soon after menstruation has begun. The most commonly reported premenstrual change is fluid retention, especially in the breasts and abdomen (Chang, Holroyd, & Chau, 1995; Johnson, McChesney, & Bean, 1988). Other changes that women often report include acne, cravings for sweet or salty foods, aches and pains in the muscles or joints, fatigue, irritability, tension, anxiety, sadness, moodiness, constipation or diarrhea, feeling out of control, insomnia, and changes in sex drive. Some self-help books and magazine articles suggest that there are 100 or more possible "symptoms" of PMS, including some that are so gendered that they would never be considered a problem if men reported them (e.g., food cravings, increased sex drive, anger, arguments with family or friends; Chrisler & Levy, 1990, Figert, 1996; Taylor & Colino, 2002) and others that are more typical of the menstrual than the premenstrual phase (e.g., uterine or pelvic cramps; Chrisler & Johnston-Robledo, 2002). Some women also report positive premenstrual changes that they welcome and appreciate, such as bursts of energy or activity, increased creativity, increased sex drive, and feelings of affection (Chrisler, Johnston, Champagne, & Preston, 1994; Lee, 2002; Nichols, 1995), but these are rarely mentioned in the professional or popular literature because they do not fit the conceptualization of the premenstrual phase as a time of illness and disorder. Other changes (e.g., difficulty concentrating, poor judgment, decreased efficiency, worse work or school performance) that are often associated with the premenstrual phase are not supported by research; no cognitive deficits are reliably associated with any phase of the cycle, although some women may think they are (see Epting & Overman, 1998, or Gordon & Lee, 1993, for a review of the literature).

The prevalence of PMS is unknown because there is little agreement among researchers and health care providers about the criteria that should be used to diagnose it. There are at least 65 different questionnaires to assess premenstrual symptoms (Budeiri, LiWanPo, & Dornan, 1994), and no laboratory test or hormone assay has ever been shown to discriminate reliably between women who report premenstrual complaints and those who do not (Freeman, 2003). Researchers often differentiate between normal experience and PMS by restricting PMS to reports of symptoms that are severe enough to interfere with a woman's daily life. If it is relatively easy to cope with premenstrual changes through self-care (e.g., rest, aspirin, planning, problem solving), then the woman does not have PMS. Yet, the World Health Organization (1996) has suggested that women and girls can be diagnosed with PMS if they experience one or more physical or mood symptoms during the premenstrual phase, a criterion that includes almost every woman, especially given that the severity does not seem to matter. The American Congress of Gynecologists (2011) has estimated that 85% of women experience at least one symptom during most cycles, but only 5% to 10% of those women have symptoms severe enough to interfere with their daily functioning.

Premenstrual dysphoric disorder (PMDD) is classified as a depressive disorder. Diagnosis requires the presence of five or more symptoms during most premenstrual phases, and those symptoms must diminish within a few days of the beginning of menstruation. At least one of the symptoms must be related to mood. The diagnostic criteria (i.e., symptoms) are "marked" affective lability (e.g., suddenly sad or tearful, mood swings, increased sensitivity to rejection); "marked" irritability or anger or increased interpersonal conflicts; "marked" depressed mood, feelings of hopelessness, or self-deprecating thoughts; "marked" anxiety, tension, or feeling "on edge"; decreased interest in usual activities; subjective difficulty concentrating; lethargy, fatigue, or "marked" lack of energy; "marked" change in appetite; hypersomnia or insomnia; sense of being overwhelmed or out of control; physical symptoms (e.g., bloating, joint or muscle pain, breast swelling, weight gain) (American Psychiatric Association, 2013). The symptoms must be severe enough to interfere with women's daily functioning or with their relationships.

The American Psychiatric Association (2013) has recommended that daily symptom ratings be collected over the course of two menstrual cycles in order to confirm the diagnosis, although it seems unlikely that most clinicians would insist on this. Researchers (Pearlstein & Steiner, 2008) who have used this method have found that fewer than 5% of women with severe premenstrual complaints actually meet the criteria for PMDD. Many women (30% to 76%) who have been diagnosed with PMDD have a history of depression, which suggests that PMDD may be an instance of what Woods, Mitchell, and Lentz (1999) referred to as premenstrual magnification of an existing disorder (or PMM). PMM describes cases in which menstrual cycle–related biochemical changes aggravate an existing condition (e.g., depression) or trigger a flare-up of a chronic illness (e.g., migraine headaches, epilepsy).

Risk factors for PMDD include stress, interpersonal trauma, and sociocultural aspects of women's gender role (American Psychiatric Association, 2013), which critics (Caplan, 2004, 2008) have noted means that most women of reproductive age are at risk. The diagnostic criteria themselves have been criticized (Caplan, 2004), as it is not easy to agree on what a "marked" change would be. The criteria also make it possible to be diagnosed with a depressive disorder without reporting depressed mood. Thus, both PMS and PMDD remain controversial diagnoses among experts, even though the general public has come to accept them.

A BRIEF HISTORY OF PMS AND PMDD

During the Great Depression, the American gynecologist Robert Frank (1931) published an article in which he described some of his patients as being tense and irritable, crying more easily than usual, and engaging in "foolish and ill considered actions" just prior to menstruation (p. 1054). He coined the term *premenstrual tension* (PMT) to explain changes in their mood and behavior. Frank did not suggest that the premenstrual phase of the menstrual cycle caused problems for all women; however, some feminist critics (Chrisler & Caplan, 2002; Martin, 1988) have suggested that his article about this new "condition" came at an appropriate moment. It suggested a reason why women should stay out of the workforce and leave any jobs that were available in those dire economic times to men.

In the 1950s, the British endocrinologist Katharina Dalton began to study behavior changes associated with the menstrual cycle. As Martin (1988) noted, many women entered the workforce during the 1940s to participate in the war effort, and postwar governments encouraged them to vacate their jobs and leave them available for recently demobilized or rehabilitated soldiers and sailors. Although Dalton may not have intended to provide a reason why women's activities in public life should be limited, her work has had that effect. She greatly expanded the list of signs and symptoms associated with the premenstrual phase of the cycle and coined the term *premenstrual syndrome* (Dalton, 1964). The term PMS itself was a major marker in the medicalization of women's reproductive processes. Whereas PMT might seem simply to be a label for a phenomenon, once a set of "symptoms" is labeled a "syndrome," it is taken more seriously and seen as needing medical attention (Chrisler & Caplan, 2002). Dalton published several studies in medical journals in which she intended to demonstrate that girls perform worse on their examinations and women are more likely to commit crimes when they are premenstrual; the methodology she used in her studies and the statistical analyses she did have been soundly criticized (e.g., Parlee, 1973), and her results have not been verified by other researchers. Nevertheless, because she wrote about these studies in a book for the general public (Dalton, 1979) and spoke of them to journalists who interviewed her for various media outlets, many people believe that all women are incapacitated to some extent during the premenstrual phase.

Like Frank, Dalton did not believe that all women have PMS. She saw it as a medical condition caused by a hormonal imbalance, and she treated her patients with progesterone injections. She reported that many of her patients improved and were no longer subject to mood and behavioral changes premenstrually, but double-blind scientific studies have never shown progesterone to have these effects. Perhaps having their frustrations taken seriously by a famous physician and being offered a treatment of any sort were enough to cause a placebo effect. However, Dalton trumpeted her cure in the press, and she even suggested to reporters that women owe it to their families to seek treatment for their premenstrual symptoms (Rome, 1986).

PMS did not become well known to the general public until 1980, when two sensational murder trials in the United Kingdom received media coverage around the world. In both cases, the women who had been charged with a violent crime were visited in jail by Dalton, who decided that they had been premenstrual at the time of their crimes, diagnosed them with PMS, and began progesterone treatment. She testified at their trials, and, as a result, the courts accepted a plea of diminished responsibility, and the women did not receive prison sentences. One of the women, who had stabbed a coworker during an argument, had a history of mental illness and a criminal record. The other, who was a victim of domestic violence, killed her lover by hitting him with her car after they had been drinking heavily and arguing. The media coverage of the trials introduced people to the term PMS and reported the attorneys' argument that premenstrual hormonal fluctuations could change normally calm and peaceful women into angry and violent criminals. What the media did not report is that the stress associated with committing the crime and being jailed might be the reason why the women were menstruating when Dalton interviewed them (i.e., stress can delay menstruation or bring it on earlier than expected, as many women know from personal experience); there was never any proof that they were premenstrual at the time of their criminal acts. (See Boorse, 1987, or Chrisler, 2002, for more details about the crimes and trials.) Yet, the idea that women commonly suffer from PMS became firmly entrenched in many Western cultures as a result of the trial publicity and Dalton's many interviews with the press.

Feminist scholars (Chrisler & Caplan, 2002; Martin, 1988; Ussher, 2013) have also pointed out that the time was right for a renewed emphasis on ways that women's biology makes them unfit for certain roles in public life. A backlash against feminism had begun in the late 1970s (Faludi, 1991), and conservative activists were already engaged in attempts to erode the gains made by the Women's Liberation Movement of the 1960s and 1970s. Accusations of PMS proved to be a useful tool against women whom antifeminists considered "too" powerful (e.g., Hillary Clinton, U.S. Supreme Court Justice Sonia Sotomayor [Chrisler, 2011]; Canadian Prime Minister Kim Campbell [Chrisler & Caplan, 2002]).

Soon after the publicity about the trials ended, a committee of psychiatrists in the United States met to discuss the possibility of adding a new diagnosis for extreme cases of PMS to the forthcoming edition of the *Diagnostic and Statistical Manual of Mental Disorders* (DSM-IIIR; American Psychiatric Association, 1987). They coined the term *late luteal phase dysphoric disorder* (LLPPD), a term that reflects the committee's bio-medical emphasis, but it proved to be confusing to the general public, who did not realize that the late luteal phase of the menstrual cycle is commonly known as the premenstrual phase and that dysphoria means depression. The diagnostic criteria were a mix of physical (e.g., bloating, water retention, backaches) and emotional (e.g., anxiety, depression, crying) symptoms, and the variability among the symptoms (and the need to exhibit only a few of them) meant that a large number of women were at risk of being diagnosed with LLPPD. A coalition of both lay and professional women's groups (e.g., Association for Women in Psychology, Association of Women Psychiatrists, National Organization for Women, Feminist Therapy Institute) protested the inclusion of the new diagnosis in the *DSM* because they believed there was no evidence that such a disorder existed as such and because they feared that the diagnostic label would be used against women (e.g., in child custody cases or employment decisions). The activists achieved only a partial victory. The American Psychiatric Association voted to include the diagnosis in an appendix under "conditions that require further study" and said that they would not encourage their members to assign the diagnosis until strong evidence to support it had been produced by researchers. Although that strong evidence has never been produced (Chrisler & Caplan, 2002; Cosgrove & Caplan, 2004), the disorder—with its new name, premenstrual dysphoric disorder (PMDD)—was published in both the main text and the appendix of the *DSM-IV* (1994) and in the main text of the *DSM-5* (2013).

An important reason why PMDD was accepted as a legitimate disorder by professionals and the public alike is the approval in 1999 by the FDA of a medication to treat it. The patent on Prozac (fluoxetine), Eli Lilly and Company's[1] best-selling antidepressant, was due to expire shortly, which would make it possible for other pharmaceutical companies to manufacture and sell a generic equivalent. If another use could be found for fluoxetine, the patent could be renewed, which would mean significant profit for Lilly. Could fluoxetine help to alleviate symptoms of PMDD? Lilly convened an "expert panel" of psychiatrists to discuss the possibility. The psychiatrists discussed studies of PMDD treatments and their own experience with their patients, and they concluded that there was evidence that fluoxetine (and also calcium) were effective. They then published an article about their discussion in a medical journal, in which they highly recommended fluoxetine (but not calcium). The FDA relied on that article in their determination to renew Lilly's patent (Chrisler & Caplan, 2002; Cosgrove & Caplan, 2004). Lilly doubted that women would be willing to take Prozac for premenstrual moodiness, so they repackaged and renamed it (as Sarafem) and embarked on an extensive advertising campaign (e.g., "You may think you have PMS when you really have PMDD.") The FDA later chastised Lilly for misleading advertisements that did not differentiate PMS from PMDD, but, by then, the damage had already been done. Millions of American women blamed their menstrual cycles for their bad or sad moods and wanted to seek medical treatment for what used to be considered the normal ups and downs of life. (See Chrisler & Caplan, 2002, and Cosgrove & Riddle, 2003, for more details about the development of PMDD and Lilly's advertising campaign.)

A BIOPSYCHOSOCIAL APPROACH TO PREMENSTRUAL SYMPTOMS

Both PMS and PMDD are typically framed biomedically (i.e., something is "wrong" with the body that needs to be "fixed" by some form of medical treatment). Perhaps because the menstrual cycle is regulated by the activity of four hormones (estrogen, progesterone, follicle-stimulating hormone, luteinizing hormone), any physical, emotional, or behavioral changes that are associated with the cycle are assumed to be "hormonal" in nature. The biomedical approach is dominant in both the professional and popular literature, where premenstrual women's hormones are often described as "raging" or "unbalanced." In fact, hormone assays have never shown any difference between women with and without PMS complaints, and women's hormones are actually in balance, doing what they are designed to do, to prepare the uterus for a possible pregnancy. Researchers have also suggested that PMS symptoms are caused by neurotransmitter malfunction, nutritional deficits, low blood sugar, or sleep disturbances, but those studies have not been replicated successfully and are rarely discussed today. PMDD is theorized to result from low levels of the neurotransmitter serotonin, but that is because antidepressants that increase serotonin levels seem to elevate the mood of dysphoric women, a circular explanation.

We are not suggesting that physiology and biochemistry have nothing to do with women's premenstrual experience, only that they are not the *only* things that do. For example, high levels of progesterone (which are normal during the premenstrual phase and during pregnancy) cause water retention (i.e., the swelling of breasts, abdomen, and ankles) and weight gain. Water retention makes people uncomfortable and irritable; both irritability and swelling or bloating are key components of PMS. Changes in biochemistry can produce changes in women's experience, but it is how we feel and think about those changes (psychological) and what they mean to us (sociocultural) that turn "changes" into "symptoms." Therefore, a biopsychosocial model better explains why some women suffer from PMS.

Many of the common symptoms of PMS overlap with the signs of stress (e.g., tension, irritability, headaches, backaches, crying, fatigue), and a number of researchers (Beck, Gevirtz, & Mortola, 1990; Kuczmierczyk, Labrum, & Johnson, 1992; Ussher & Perz, 2013; Warner & Bancroft, 1990) have found that women who report that they suffer from PMS also tend to report that they experience high levels of stress in their lives (e.g., financial strain, marital dissatisfaction, heavy workload, work monotony, family conflict, hectic schedules). Women with PMS have also been shown to be more likely to use less effective methods of coping with their stress (e.g., avoidance, wishful thinking, appeasement, withdrawal, and focusing on or venting emotions) and less likely to use more effective methods (e.g., seeking social support, problem-focused coping, direct action, self-care) (Genther, Chrisler, & Johnston-Robledo, 1999; Ornitz & Brown, 1993; Ussher & Perz, 2013). Studies have also shown that women with PMS or PMDD exhibit higher than usual levels of trait anxiety (i.e., as a regular personality feature, not just during the premenstrual phase; Giannini, Price, Loiselle, & Giannini, 1985; Picone & Kirby, 1990), higher than average lifetime incidence of sexual assault and abuse (Taylor, Golding, Menard, & King, 2001), a higher than usual previous experience of depression (Dennerstein, Morse, & Varnanides, 1988; Warner, Bancroft, Dixson, & Hampson, 1991), a negative or pessimistic explanatory style (Chrisler, Rose, Dutch, Sklarsky, & Grant, 2006), negative attitudes toward menstruation (Marván & Cortés-Iniestra, 2001; Marván & Escobedo, 1999), a tendency to silence themselves rather than express their anger and frustration with others (Chrisler, Gorman, & Streckfuss, 2014; Ussher & Perz, 2010), and a tendency to adhere to the feminine gender role (e.g., to try to be an ideal wife and mother; Freeman, Sondheimer, & Rickels, 1987; Stout & Steege, 1985). It is easy to see how the psychological and biological factors can interact. A woman who tends to "swallow" her anger and frustration might be less willing or able to do so when she is premenstrual, but her angry outbursts might seem inexplicable to others who are unaware of why she is angry and see her as usually calm and serene (Cosgrove & Riddle, 2003; Swann & Ussher, 1995). A woman with negative attitudes toward menstruation and a pessimistic or anxious personality may expect to experience severe premenstrual symptoms; when she does notice changes, she might focus intensely on them, making herself feel worse, rather than seeking social support, resting, or telling herself that the symptoms will end soon. It is also possible that symptoms of stress are categorized as PMS when they occur premenstrually, but recognized as stress when they occur at other times.

Cultural beliefs and social interactions are important reasons why women might expect to experience PMS or attribute symptoms to it that could be the result of some other problem (e.g., depression, lack of social support) or circumstances (e.g., financial or relationship stress). Women who know other women who complain about PMS and women who frequently see jokes about PMS and illustrations of out-of-control premenstrual women in popular culture may be more likely to notice menstrual cycle–related changes and label them as PMS or PMDD.

Until recently, PMS was little known outside of Western industrialized countries, and it has been theorized to be a culture-bound syndrome (Chrisler, 1996; Johnson, 1987). To say that illness or dis-ease is culture bound does not mean that it is imaginary or illegitimate. Women around the world may experience water retention, irritability, tension, sadness, acne, or constipation prior to menstruation, but not everyone thinks of these premenstrual changes as abnormal or as a syndrome that needs treatment. Surveys conducted by the World Health Organization show that menstrual cycle–related complaints (except for cramps, which are universal) are most often reported by women who live in North America, Western Europe, and Australia. Data collected from women in Hong Kong (Chang et al., 1995) and mainland China (Yu, Zhu, Li, Oakley, & Reame, 1996) indicate that the most commonly reported premenstrual symptoms are water retention, fatigue, pain, and increased sensitivity to cold. American women do not report cold sensitivity, and Chinese women rarely report bad moods. The results of those studies provide support for the idea that culture shapes which symptoms are noticed and what they mean. As Watters (2010, p. 2) noted, "how a people in a culture think about mental illnesses—how they categorize and prioritize the symptoms, attempt to heal them, and set expectations for their course and outcome—influences the diseases themselves." Publicity by drug companies selling "cures" for PMDD is likely to play a large role in the medicalization of women's moods in countries that have never before seen everyday emotions and behavioral variability as problems.

Industrialization has contributed to a belief in modern societies that conformity is better than variability, that people should exercise self-control at all times, and that it is good to feel and behave the same way everyday (like well-oiled machines, rather than like seasonal and other rhythms related to nature; Koeske, 1983; Martin, 1988). Furthermore, mainstream American culture encourages people to believe that they have more control over themselves and their bodies than is actually possible (Brownell, 1991; Chrisler, 2008), and women are especially encouraged to control themselves by blocking their emotional, sexual, or appetitive impulses and by always putting other people's needs ahead of their own (Baumeister, Heatherton, & Tice, 1994; Chrisler, 2008). The feminine gender role emphasizes self-discipline; good women, especially good mothers, are assumed to be soft-spoken, receptive, nurturing, kind, and patient. Any woman who is turned inward or seen as unapproachable because she is irritable, angry, or exhausted is thought to be ill or "not herself" (Chrisler & Johnston-Robledo, 2002) or is judged harshly because of ruptures in self-discipline (Ussher, 2004). If self-control is indeed "the quintessential feminine virtue" (Baumeister et al., 1994, p. 10), then it is no wonder that so many women are afraid that PMS will make them lose control (Chrisler, 2008; Ritenbaugh, 1982).

Gender roles, the gendered division of household labor, and the rise in the frequency of nuclear families may also play a role in the increasing acceptance of the medicalization of women's moods. In preindustrial societies, where men and women worked together on a farm, or on their craft, or in their shop, children were always nearby where both parents could watch out for them and teach them to work in the household and family business. In extended families, the work was shared, even if the labor was divided by gender. If a child's mother was tired, irritable, in pain, or otherwise unwell, someone else (e.g., grandmother, aunt, cousin, elder sibling) was always nearby to take over child care duties.

Contemporary arrangements, where many women are employed outside the home, yet still responsible for most of the housework and child care, are stressful and provide less social support or time for women to rest and engage in other forms of self-care. Many desire to be "superwomen," who can effortlessly juggle their multiple roles and remain calm and serene all month (Chrisler, 2008). This desire (unlikely to be fulfilled) leaves women stressed, ashamed, and feeling unable to keep up with their many responsibilities for household management, child care, and maintenance of family harmony (Ussher & Perz, 2013). Lesbian couples, who tend to share household duties more equitably than heterosexual couples and who both experience menstrual cycle–related changes, cope better with premenstrual symptoms because they are supportive and encourage each other to engage in self-care (Ussher & Perz, 2013).

MEDIA MESSAGES ABOUT PMS AND PMDD

The media are major sources of information about health issues, and the information they convey shapes perceptions and attitudes (Parlee, 1987). For example, movies such as *Carrie* and *My Girl* and episodes of television shows such as *King of the Hill* and *South Park* contain strong, stigmatizing messages about menstruation (Kissling, 2002; Rosewarne, 2012) that contribute to the development of negative attitudes toward menstruation and support the medicalization of women's moods. As noted above, PMS was relatively unknown prior to 1980 when the media's sensationalized coverage of the criminal trials in the United Kingdom brought it to worldwide attention, and advertisements for Sarafem and press coverage of the addition of PMDD (and its precursor, LLPPD) to the *DSM* convinced women that their menstrual cycles could make them mentally, as well as physically, ill.

Content analyses of articles in the popular press have shown that the information about PMS is often inaccurate, menstruation is almost always negatively portrayed, and both women and men are warned to be careful of behavioral changes caused by women's "raging hormones" (Chrisler & Levy, 1990; Markens, 1996). An analysis (Chrisler & Levy, 1990) of 78 magazine articles that were published between 1980 and 1987 included coverage of premenstrual symptoms, behaviors, and treatments of PMS. The authors noticed that the titles of articles about PMS were often negative and misleading: "Premenstrual Misery," "How to Beat the Pre-period Uglies," "The Taming of the Shrew Inside of You," and "PMS: The Return of the Raging Hormones" (p. 97). They found that the information about PMS in the articles was confusing and unclear. For example, there was little agreement about the percentage of women who experience PMS; estimates ranged from 5% to 90%. The symptoms of PMS also varied, and some authors mentioned that there are over 100 different symptoms or behavioral criteria. The majority of articles mentioned negative symptoms and behaviors related to pain, water retention, eating changes, negative affect, and impaired concentration. Furthermore, the symptoms that were emphasized support "the stereotype of the maladjusted woman" (p. 97), and many articles quoted (without attribution) the attorneys who defended the women on trial in the United Kingdom in 1980, who described their clients as a "raging beast" or "Jekyll and Hyde" (Chrisler, 2002). Most individuals do not question the accuracy of material presented in newspapers and magazines, and if readers are confused or curious, menstruation is not a topic most people feel comfortable about discussing with others (Delaney, Lupton, & Toth, 1976; Houppert, 1999).

There is a communication taboo about menstruation: It is socially unacceptable to talk about menstruation, especially in mixed company (Houppert, 1999; Kissling, 1996). Therefore, many individuals turn to the Internet, where they can anonymously search for information. What do they find? A recent Google search of "PMS" yielded the following first three images: (a) a woman holding a gun that is pointed toward the camera with the phrase "PMS: Nature's way of leveling the playing field. Much in the same way that an earthquake would level it";[2] (b) an image of a stern-faced woman that states "PMS: Be afraid! Be very afraid!";[3] and (c) an image of a distressed woman with a word bubble that reads "I'm fine. I hate you. I love you. I want ice cream. Come here. Get away. Oranges?"[4] Similar images can be easily found online, such as a Yahoo! image that states "Your lady got PMS? What to do: Pray to God. Move out of the way. Sleep on the sofa. A Message from the Ministry of Homeland Security."[5] Thus, Internet messages about PMS are primarily negative and heavily influenced by the coverage of the criminal trials, despite the fact that women commit only a small percentage of violent crimes. The media create pictures of women who are out of control, violent, indecisive, and should be feared and avoided at all costs. The stereotype of the premenstrual woman in popular culture is a "frenzied, raging beast, a menstrual monster, prone to rapid mood swings and crying spells, bloated and swollen from water retention, out of control, craving chocolate, and likely at any moment to turn violent" (Chrisler et al., 2006, p. 371).

There are many Internet sources where information (and misinformation) about PMS is communicated. Twitter is an uncensored social network where users create accounts, post short tweets (no more than 140 characters), and follow other Twitter users or groups. Researchers are starting to use Twitter to collect data and examine social phenomena. For example, in a qualitative analysis of 2,211 tweets that referenced menstruation ("time of the month"), Thornton (2013) identified four themes: anger and frustration; physical and emotional change; deceit, decorum, and disdain; and validation and bonding. Tweets perpetuated stereotypes that "menstrual women are to be regarded as whores; as unclean and disgusting; and as appropriate victims of retaliation" (p. 47). The communication taboo was also expressed: "Sorry ladies, but you talkn abt THAT time of the month on twitter and specially in my timeline can gross me out" (pp. 47–48). The second most popular re-tweet was a quote from the comedian Roseanne Barr: "Women complain about premenstrual syndrome, but I think of it as the only time of the month that I can be myself" (p. 48). Rather than using proper terms, many tweets contained acronyms, euphemisms, and slang to describe, discuss, and make fun of women and menstrual cycle–related experiences.

Urban Dictionary is an online dictionary of over 7 million slang words and phrases. It is quite popular, with over 15 million visitors per month, mostly people younger than age 25 (Heffernan, 2009), and it has publicized its own definitions of PMS, which also promote the stereotype of an irrational, angry premenstrual woman. *Urban Dictionary*'s definitions are written by Internet users and ranked according to popularity. The current number one definition of PMS (with 17,664 votes) is "a powerful spell that women are put under about once every month, which gives them the strength of an ox, the stability of a Window's OS, and the scream of a banshee. Basically, man's worst nightmare." The number two definition (with 5,796 votes) correctly states that "PMS = Premenstrual Syndrome." However, it then incorrectly states that PMS is "the woman's 'time of the month' when her uterus sheds its lining because her monthly egg isn't fertilized and dies" (this refers to *menstruation*, not PMS). The definition further indicates that PMS is "the worst time to be around a woman, because she becomes an irrational psycho bitch which froths at the mouth with rage and seeks to destroy anything which stands in her way." These "definitions" are inaccurate, they are not from credible sources, and the popularity of the definitions depends heavily on how humorous or outlandish they are. However, *Urban Dictionary* does reveal current proscriptions, euphemisms, and cultural beliefs about PMS and premenstrual women.

Men do not often discuss menstruation with women, and men's discussions with other men usually involve jokes about menstruating or premenstrual women (Laws, 1990). Men's written accounts of women's premenstrual changes were recently examined by King, Ussher, and Perz (2014), who analyzed posts on PMSBuddy.com, an online forum targeted toward men and partners of menstruating women. The website offers tips for coping with PMS, a discussion page ("PMS stories"), and a free reminder notice of when men's partners are likely to be in their premenstrual phases. Although some men posted positive comments about premenstrual women and the importance of being supportive husbands (7%), the majority of the posts were negative. The most common themes were posts about "premenstrual women as mad, bad, and dangerous" (31%) and "men as victims of premenstrual women" (22%; p. 7). One man joked: "When my wife hits PMS she goes into search and destroy mode. She'll hunt me down and scream at me for something I did or did not do. I always know it's PMS because it's so illogical that I almost laugh—but dare I DO NOT!" (p. 11). Both men and women tell jokes about menstruation and PMS. Kissling (2006) suggested that, because of menstrual taboos, the only acceptable way to discuss menstruation publicly is by "complaining about menstrual symptoms, mocking menstruating women, or helping to sell something related to menstruation" (p. 1).

It can be a bonding experience to joke and complain about premenstrual symptoms (Chrisler et al., 2006). Even though very few women (less than 10%) experience premenstrual symptoms that are severe enough to interfere with normal functioning, "many women embrace the PMS label for themselves and also apply it to other women" (Chrisler et al., 2006, p. 371), sometimes as a way to excuse things they wish they had not said or done. Perhaps because of media messages, most people now believe that PMS is universal (Houppert, 1999), and even women who themselves have few negative premenstrual experiences believe that most women experience PMS (Chrisler et al., 2006; Sveinsdottir, Lundman, & Norberg, 2002). Self-fulfilling biases may account for why so many women strongly believe that PMS is widespread. Expectations about what to expect during the premenstrual phase affects the symptoms women report (Marván & Cortés-Iniestra, 2001; Marván & Escobedo, 1999; Ruble, 1977). Furthermore, women who experience severe premenstrual symptoms may believe that other women share their experience, whereas women who do not suffer premenstrually probably think that they are unique (Chrisler et al., 2006).

TREATMENT AND SELF-CARE

As mentioned above, Dalton (1964, 1979) recommended progesterone for women with PMS. In the 1980s, clinics opened up in the United States to offer progesterone treatment, and they were popular for a time. However, no double-blind studies ever demonstrated progesterone's effectiveness, and the clinics went out of business.

Prozac, which was renamed Sarafem, repackaged in pink and purple capsules, and remarketed to treat PMDD, has also been promoted as a cure for all premenstrual sufferers. Only Sarafem (fluoxetine) and Zoloft (sertraline), two antidepressants, have been approved by the FDA to treat premenstrual symptoms. However, "the European Union's equivalent of the FDA concluded that the research showed PMDD was not a well-established disease entity and criticized pertinent drug-company-sponsored research" (Caplan, 2008, p. 64); no drug has been approved there for treatment of premenstrual symptoms.

Is PMDD really a form of depression, as its name (dysphoric disorder) suggests? In order for someone to be diagnosed with depression, she or he must have symptoms for a minimum of two weeks. PMDD sufferers may only experience symptoms for a few days each month. Furthermore, approval of a medication to treat a disorder is not a guarantee that the medication will work or that it is safe. The negative side effects of fluoxetine are well documented (e.g., suicidal ideation, loss of libido, weight gain), and women should consider whether it is worth the risk of these negative effects if they experience depressive symptoms for only a few days per month. Women's experiences with Sarafem are not well documented in the medical literature, and more research is needed. Health care providers should talk to their patients "about what has been helpful to other people, including not only drugs but also self-help groups, cognitive behavior therapy, and changes to diet and nutrition" (Caplan, 2004, p. 65).

As noted above, there is no definitive cause for premenstrual symptoms. The etiology has been linked to a number of factors, such as calcium deficiency, hormonal imbalance, brain chemistry (increases in gamma-aminobutyric acid), adrenal gland dysfunction, hypoglycemia, and deficiencies in essential fatty acids and vitamin B_6. Thus, there are also a plethora of treatment recommendations. Antidepressants and oral contraceptives are effective for some women; other women have reported that diet and lifestyle changes help to alleviate premenstrual symptoms. A common medical approach is to identify and treat individual symptoms. For example, pain relievers can be taken for headaches, and bloating can be relieved by water pills. Other suggestions have included psychotherapy, physical therapy, acupuncture, hydrotherapy, light therapy, a change in diet (e.g., avoid salt, chocolate, and coffee; eat more fatty acids, fish, whole grains, olive oil; eat a vegetarian or vegan diet; take vitamin and nutritional supplements, such as B complex and calcium); herbal remedies (e.g., black cohosh, dong quai, vitex, ginkgo biloba, oil of evening primrose),[6] Chinese medicine; lifestyle changes (e.g., increase exercise, sleep), seek social support; develop a range of coping techniques (e.g., sense of humor, problem solving, assertiveness about one's needs); and other forms of self-care (e.g., meditate, get massages, take warm baths, read, relax, and do pleasurable activities).

In general, regardless of the severity of premenstrual symptoms, *all* women could benefit from engaging in more self-care. For example, getting adequate rest and sleep, maintaining a healthy diet, exercising, and managing stress on a regular basis are beneficial for overall health and wellness. Expanding social support networks and communicating with others during stressful life events are also good ways to cope. Although some women may think it is selfish to engage in self-care, they should remember that they cannot take care of others who need them if they have not taken care of themselves. Taking time for themselves is also a way to show children that women's needs are important, too. Life is full of daily hassles, stressors, and cyclic changes. The way that we perceive them and react to them can positively or negatively affect our physical and psychological well-being.

CONSEQUENCES OF THE MEDICALIZATION OF WOMEN'S MOODS

As Cosgrove and Riddle (2003, p. 39) noted, "Women are inundated with information in the popular media about how to assess for and manage their 'premenstrual moods.' As a result, women are increasingly encouraged to overlook the context in which their emotions are manifest, and instead see their affective experiences as simple by-products of (premenstrual) hormones." In the first television commercial for Sarafem, a woman was shown ferociously pulling a shopping cart from a line of carts that were stuck together. She was visibly aggravated and losing patience. As she fought with the cart, a voice declared: "It's that week before your period . . . the irritability, mood swings, bloating. Think it's PMS? Think again! It could be PMDD." Do only premenstrual women become frustrated when carts are difficult to dislodge? Do only premenstrual women ever feel bloated, irritable, or moody? Aren't those normal experiences that *all people* (women, men, and children) occasionally experience? Yes, they are; yet, the medicalization of women's moods suggests that when women have those normal experiences, their hormones are to blame.

The medicalization of women's moods makes it seem as though women are ill and in need of treatment whenever they experience an emotion that is considered negative (e.g., sadness, anxiety) or unfeminine (e.g., anger, irritability). Dalton once told a reporter that women who live alone do not complain of PMS (Rome, 1986). That is not surprising if we consider that our emotions are often a result of interactions with other people (especially intimate others with whom we share our personal lives) that make us happy, proud, sad, angry, frustrated, irritable, guilty, or tense. If women assume that their sadness or anger needs medical treatment, they might never address with their family and friends the issues that led to those emotions. They might even think it is their fault when others frustrate them or make them anxious. Even worse, others often see women's anger and irritability as unwarranted and illegitimate. It is easier to say or think "you're hormonal" or "she must be PMSing" than to apologize or ask what can be done to make her feel better.

Women's tendency to medicalize their moods by attributing them to PMS also causes them to distance themselves from their bodies (Ussher, 2004). This distancing, and negative attitudes toward menstruation, can contribute to self-objectification (a tendency to see oneself as an object on display for others; Fredrickson & Roberts, 1997) and self-sexualization (a tendency to distance oneself from parts of the body deemed sexual, e.g., breasts and buttocks; Bartky, 1990). Women who tend to self-objectify have been found to have a sense of shame related to normal reproductive events (e.g., menstruation, birthing, breastfeeding; Johnson-Robledo, Sheffield, Voigt, & Wilcox-Constantine, 2007). That shame is psychologically damaging and appears to contribute to decisions that can be harmful to women's physical health (e.g., menstrual suppression, elective cesarean sections, risky sexual behavior; Johnston-Robledo & Chrisler, 2013).

The medicalization of women's moods is a problem for all women in the public sphere, whether or not they experience premenstrual symptoms. Jokes about menstruation and premenstrual women and the dismissal of women's emotions as hormonal are forms of microaggression. Microaggressions are everyday remarks or behaviors, either subtle or overt, that communicate negative attitudes toward members of particular social groups. These remarks and behaviors are experienced by their targets as demeaning and marginalizing (i.e., a way to set the individual apart from the rest of the group). Jokes about premenstrual women make women feel like they are in a spotlight (i.e., as if others are constantly observing their behavior for evidence of PMS). If others laugh at the joke, women may feel embarrassed or ashamed. The mere mention of menstruation in a group setting can also be a form of stereotype threat (Wister, Stubbs, & Shipman, 2013). Stereotype threat makes women become aware of their gender and menstrual status, and they may try very hard to avoid doing or saying anything that might confirm the stereotype of the premenstrual woman (e.g., seem tense or irritable, eat too many snacks, lose concentration).

Thus, we encourage women to resist the medicalization of their moods—unless their premenstrual symptoms are severe enough to interfere with daily functioning. If not, they should engage in self-care, treat symptoms as needed (e.g., water pills, aspirin), and not refer to themselves as having

PMS. We should all try to develop more positive attitudes toward menstruation and our bodies in general (see Johnston-Robledo & Chrisler, 2013, and Sobczak, 2014, for suggestions about how to do that), and we should never let anyone dismiss a woman's feelings as merely "hormonal." We are all entitled to experience and express a full range of emotions.

NOTES

1. In 2004, Eli Lilly sold the rights to Sarafem to Warner-Chilcott for $295 million (Wilson, 2004).

2. From http://www.jucoolimages.com.

3. From http://www.psychologytoday.com.

4. From http://www.pcosaintpretty.com.

5. From http://www.naturopathnsw.com.au.

6. Keep in mind that research on herbal treatments, like research on drug treatments, is usually funded by the companies who manufacture and market them.

REFERENCES

American Congress of Obstetricians and Gynecologists. (2011). Women's health stats and facts. Retrieved from http://www.acog.org/-/media/NewsRoom/MediaKit.pdf.

American Psychiatric Association. (1987). *Diagnostic and statistical manual of mental disorders* (3rd ed., rev.). Washington, DC: Author.

American Psychiatric Association. (1994). *Diagnostic and statistical manual of mental disorders* (4th ed.). Washington, DC: Author.

American Psychiatric Association. (2013). *Diagnostic and statistical manual of mental disorders* (5th ed.). Washington, DC: Author.

Bartky, S. L. (1990). *Femininity and domination: Studies in the phenomenology of oppression*. New York: Routledge.

Baumeister, R. F., Heatherton, T. F., & Tice, D. M. (1994). *Losing control: How and why people fail at self-regulation*. San Diego, CA: Academic Press.

Beck, L. E., Gevirtz, R., & Mortola, J. F. (1990). The predictive role of psychosocial stress on symptoms severity in premenstrual syndrome. *Psychosomatic Medicine, 52*, 536–543.

Boorse, C. (1987). Premenstrual syndrome and criminal responsibility. In B. F. Ginsburg & B. F. Carter (Eds.), *Premenstrual syndrome: Ethical and legal implications in a biomedical perspective* (pp. 81–124). New York, NY: Plenum.

Brownell, K. (1991). Personal responsibility and control over our bodies: When expectation exceeds reality. *Health Psychology, 10*, 303–310.

Budeiri, D. J., LiWanPo, A., & Dornan, J. C. (1994). Clinical trials of treatment of premenstrual syndrome: Entry criteria and scales for measuring treatment outcomes. *British Journal of Obstetrics and Gynaecology, 101*, 689–695.

Caplan, P. (2004). The debate about PMDD and Sarafem: Suggestions for therapists. *Women & Therapy, 27*(3–4), 55–67.

Caplan, P. (2008, June). Pathologizing your period. *Ms, 63–64*.

Chang, A. M., Holroyd, E., & Chau, J. P. C. (1995). Premenstrual syndrome in employed Chinese women in Hong Kong. *Health Care for Women International, 16*, 551–561.

Chrisler, J. C. (1996). PMS as a culture-bound syndrome. In J. C. Chrisler, C. Golden, & P. D. Rozee (Eds.), *Lectures on the psychology of women* (pp. 106–121). New York: McGraw-Hill.

Chrisler, J. C. (2002). Hormone hostages: The cultural legacy of PMS as a legal defense. In L. H. Collins, M. R. Dunlap, & J. C. Chrisler (Eds.), *Charting a new course for feminist psychology* (pp. 238–252). Westport, CT: Praeger.

Chrisler, J. C. (2008). Fear of losing control: Power, perfectionism, and the psychology of women. *Psychology of Women Quarterly, 32*, 1–12.

Chrisler, J. C. (2011). Leaks, lumps, and lines: Stigma and women's bodies. *Psychology of Women Quarterly, 35*, 202–214.

Chrisler, J. C., & Caplan, P. (2002). The strange case of Dr. Jekyll and Ms. Hyde: How PMS became a cultural phenomenon and a psychiatric disorder. *Annual Review of Sex Research, 13*, 274–306.

Chrisler, J. C., Gorman, J. A., & Streckfuss, L. (2014). Self-silencing, perfectionism, loss of control, dualistic discourse, and the experience of premenstrual syndrome. *Women's Reproductive Health, 1*(2), 138–152.

Chrisler, J. C., Johnston, I. K., Champagne, N. M., & Preston, K. E. (1994). Menstrual joy: The construct and its consequences. *Psychology of Women Quarterly, 18*, 375–387.

Chrisler, J. C., & Johnston-Robledo, I. (2002). Raging hormones? Feminist perspectives on premenstrual syndrome and postpartum depression. In M. Ballou & L. S. Brown (Eds.), *Rethinking mental health and disorder* (pp. 174–197). New York, NY: Guilford.

Chrisler, J. C., & Levy, K. B. (1990). The media construct a menstrual monster: A content analysis of PMS articles in the popular press. *Women & Health, 16*(2), 89–104.

Chrisler, J. C., Rose, J. G., Sklarsky, K. E., & Grant, M. (2006). The PMS illusion: Social cognition maintains social construction. *Sex Roles, 54*, 371–376.

Cosgrove, L., & Caplan, P. J. (2004). Medicalizing menstrual distress. In P. J. Caplan & L. Cosgrove (Eds.), *Bias in psychiatric diagnosis* (pp. 221–230). Lanham, MD: Jason Aronson.

Cosgrove, L., & Riddle, B. (2003). Constructions of femininity and experiences of menstrual distress. *Women & Health, 38*(3), 37–58.

Dalton, K. (1964). *The premenstrual syndrome*. Springfield, IL: Charles C. Thomas.

Dalton, K. (1979). *Once a month*. Pomona, CA: Hunter House.

Delaney, J., Lupton, M. J., & Toth, E. (1976). *The curse: A cultural history of menstruation*. New York: Dutton.

Dennerstein, L., Morse, C. A., & Varanides, K. (1988). Premenstrual tension and depression: Is there a relationship? *Journal of Psychosomatic Obstetrics and Gynecology, 18*, 45–52.

Epting, L. K., & Overman, W. H. (1988). Sex-sensitive tasks in men and women: A search for performance fluctuations across the menstrual cycle. *Behavioral Neuroscience, 112,* 1304–1317.

Faludi, S. (1991). *Backlash: The undeclared war against American women.* New York: Crown.

Figert, A. E. (1996). *Women and the ownership of PMS: The structuring of a psychiatric disorder.* New York: Aldine DeGruyter.

Frank, R. T. (1931). The hormonal causes of premenstrual tension. *Archives of Neurology and Psychiatry, 26,* 1053–1057.

Fredrickson, B. L., & Roberts, T-A. (1997). Objectification theory: Toward understanding women's lived experiences and mental health risks. *Psychology of Women Quarterly, 21,* 173–206.

Freeman, E. W. (2003). Premenstrual syndrome and premenstrual dysphoric disorder: Definitions and diagnosis. *Psychoneuroendocrinology, 28,* 25–37.

Freeman, E. W., Sondheimer, S. J., & Rickels, K. (1987). Effects of medical history factors on symptom severity in women meeting criteria for premenstrual syndrome. *Obstetrics and Gynecology, 72,* 236–239.

Genther, A. B., Chrisler, J. C., & Johnston-Robledo, I. (1999, August). *Coping, locus of control, and the experience of premenstrual symptoms.* Poster presented at the meeting of the American Psychological Association, Boston, MA.

Giannini, A. J., Price, W. A., Loiselle, R. H., & Giannini, M. D. (1985). Pseudo cholinesterase and trait anxiety in premenstrual tension syndrome. *Journal of Clinical Psychiatry, 46,* 139–140.

Gordon, H. W., & Lee, P. A. (1993). No difference in cognitive performance between phases of the menstrual cycle. *Psychoneuroendocrinology, 18,* 521–531.

Heffernan, V. (2009, July 5). Street smart: *Urban dictionary. New York Times.* Retrieved from http://www.nytimes.com/2009/07/05/magazine/05FOB-medium-t.html.

Houppert, K. (1999). *The curse: Confronting the last unmentionable taboo—menstruation.* New York: Farrar, Straus, & Giroux.

Johnson, S. R., McChesney, C., & Bean, J. A. (1988). Epidemiology of premenstrual symptoms in a nonclinical sample I: Prevalence, natural history, and help-seeking behavior. *Journal of Reproductive Medicine, 33,* 340–346.

Johnson, T. (1987). Premenstrual syndrome as a western culture-specific disorder. *Culture, Medicine, and Psychiatry, 11,* 337–356.

Johnston-Robledo, I., & Chrisler, J. C. (2013). The menstrual mark: Menstruation as social stigma. *Sex Roles, 68,* 9–18.

Johnston-Robledo, I., Sheffield, K., Voigt, J., & Wilcox-Constantine, J. (2007). Reproductive shame: Self-objectification and young women's attitudes toward their bodies. *Women & Health, 46*(1), 25–39.

King, M., Ussher, J. M., & Perz, J. (2014). Representations of PMS and premenstrual women in men's accounts: An analysis of online posts from PMSBuddy.com. *Women's Reproductive Health, 1,* 3–20.

Kissling, E. A. (1996). Bleeding out loud: Communication about menstruation. *Feminism & Psychology, 6*, 481–504.

Kissling, E. A. (2002). On the rag on screen: Menarche in film and television. *Sex Roles, 46*, 5–12.

Kissling, E. A. (2006). *Capitalizing on the curse: The business of menstruation*. Boulder, CO: Lynne Rienner.

Koeske, R. K. (1983). Lifting the curse of menstruation: Toward a feminist perspective on the menstrual cycle. *Women & Health, 8*(2–3), 1–16.

Kuczmierczyk, A. R., Labrum, A. H., & Johnson, C. C. (1992). Perception of family and work environments in women with premenstrual syndrome. *Journal of Psychosomatic Research, 36*, 787–795.

Laws, S. (1990). *Issues of blood: The politics of menstruation*. London: Macmillan.

Lee, S. (2002). Health and sickness: The meaning of menstruation and premenstrual syndrome in women's lives. *Sex Roles, 46*, 25–35.

Markens, S. (1996). The problematic of "experience": A political and cultural critique of PMS. *Gender & Society, 10*, 42–58.

Martin, E. (1988). Premenstrual syndrome: Discipline, work, and anger in late industrial societies. In T. Buckley & A. Gottlieb (Eds.), *Blood magic: The anthropology of menstruation* (pp. 161–181). Berkeley, CA: University of California Press.

Marván, M. L., & Cortés-Iniestra, S. (2001). Women's beliefs about the prevalence of premenstrual syndrome and biases in recall of premenstrual changes. *Health Psychology, 20*, 276–280.

Marván, M. L., & Escobedo, C. (1999). Premenstrual symptomatology: Role of prior knowledge about premenstrual syndrome. *Psychosomatic Medicine, 61*, 163–167.

Nichols, S. (1995). Positive premenstrual experiences: Do they exist? *Feminism & Psychology, 5*, 162–169.

Ornitz, A. W., & Brown, M. A. (1993). Family coping and premenstrual symptomatology. *Journal of Obstetric, Gynecologic, and Neonatal Nursing, 22*, 49–55.

Parlee, M. B. (1973). The premenstrual syndrome. *Psychological Bulletin, 80*, 454–465.

Parlee, M. B. (1987). Media treatment of premenstrual syndrome. In B. E. Ginsburg & B. F. Carter (Eds.), *Premenstrual syndrome: Ethical and legal implications in a biomedical perspective* (pp. 189–205). New York: Plenum.

Pearlstein, T., & Steiner, M. (2008). Premenstrual dysphoric disorder: Burden of illness and treatment update. *Journal of Psychiatry and Neuroscience, 33*, 291–301.

Picone, L., & Kirby, R. J. (1990). Relationship between anxiety and premenstrual syndrome. *Psychological Reports, 67*, 43–48.

Ritenbaugh, C. (1982). Obesity as a culture-bound syndrome. *Culture, Medicine, and Psychiatry, 6*, 347–361.

Rome, E. (1986). Premenstrual syndrome through a feminist lens. In V. E. Olesen & N. F. Woods (Eds.), *Culture, society, and menstruation* (pp. 145–151). Washington, DC: Hemisphere.

Rosewarne, L. (2013). *Periods in pop culture: Menstruation in film and television*. New York: Lexington Books.

Ruble, D. (1977). Premenstrual symptoms: A reinterpretation. *Science, 197,* 291–292.

Sobczak, C. (2014). *Embody: Learning to love your unique body (an quiet that critical voice!)*. Carlsbad, CA: Gurze Books.

Stout, A. L., & Steege, J. F. (1985). Psychological assessment of women seeking treatment for premenstrual syndrome. *Journal of Psychosomatic Research, 29,* 621–629.

Sveinsdottir, H., Lundman, B., & Norberg, A. (2002). Whose voice? Whose experience? Women's qualitative accounts of general and private discussion of premenstrual syndrome. *Scandinavian Journal of Caring Sciences, 16,* 414–423.

Swann, C. J., & Ussher, J. M. (1995). A discourse analytic approach to women's experience of premenstrual syndrome. *Journal of Mental Health, 4,* 359–367.

Taylor, D., & Colino, S. (2002). *Taking back the month: A personalized solution for managing PMS and enhancing your health*. New York: Penguin.

Taylor, D., Golding, J., Menard, L., & King, M. (2001, June). *Sexual assault and severe PMS: Prevalence and predictors*. Paper presented at the meeting of the Society for Menstrual Cycle Research, Avon, CT.

Thornton, L-J. (2013). "Time of the month" on Twitter: Taboo, stereotype, and bonding in a no-holds-barred public arena. *Sex Roles, 68,* 41–54.

Ussher, J. M. (2004). Premenstrual syndrome and self-policing: Ruptures in self-silencing lead to increased self-surveillance and blaming of the body. *Social Theory & Health, 2,* 254–272.

Ussher, J. M. (2013). Diagnosing difficult women and pathologizing femininity: Gender bias in psychiatric nosology. *Feminism & Psychology, 21,* 63–69.

Ussher, J. M., & Perz, J. (2010). Disruption of the silenced self: The case of premenstrual syndrome. In D. C. Jack & A. Ali (Eds.), *The depression epidemic: International perspectives on women's self-silencing and psychological distress* (pp. 435–458). Oxford: Oxford University Press.

Ussher, J. M., & Perz, J. (2013). PMS as a gendered illness linked to the construction and relational experience of hetero-femininity. *Sex Roles, 68,* 132–150.

Warner, P., & Bancroft, J. (1990). Factors related to self-reporting of the premenstrual syndrome. *British Journal of Psychiatry, 157,* 249–260.

Warner, P., Bancroft, J., Dixson, A., & Hampson, M. (1991). The relationship between perimenstrual mood and depressive symptoms. *Journal of Affective Disorders, 23,* 9–23.

Watters, E. (2010). *Crazy like us: The globalization of the American psyche*. New York: Free Press.

Wilson, C. (2004). Court upholds patent for Prozac-related PMS drug. Women's Sports Net. Retrieved from http://womenssportsnet.com/EditModule.aspx?tabid=32&mid=2050&def=News%20Article%20View&ItemId=4905.

Wister, J. A., Stubbs, M. L., & Shipman, C. (2013). Mentioning menstruation: A stereotype threat that diminishes cognition? *Sex Roles, 68*, 19–31.

Woods, N. F., Mitchell, E. S., & Lentz, M. J. (1999). Premenstrual symptoms: Delineating symptom clusters. *Journal of Women's Health & Gender-Based Medicine, 8*, 1053–1062.

Yu, M., Zhu, X., Li, J., Oakley, D., & Reame, N. E. (1996). Perimenstrual symptoms among Chinese women in an urban area of China. *Health Care for Women International, 17*, 161–172.

Chapter 5

Menopause: Deficiency Disease or Normal Reproductive Transition?

Heather Dillaway

Menopause is part of the general aging process (Gannon, 1999; Utz, 2011); it is also a reproductive process experienced *specifically* by women. The term *menopause* refers to the permanent cessation of menstruation and is typically defined by the final menstrual period (FMP; Utz, 2011). Clinical studies suggest that the average age of cessation is between 48 and 52 years old, although women in Western countries can cease menstruation any time between their early forties and late fifties (Mansfield, Carey, Anderson, Barsom, & Koch, 2004; Utz, 2011). Menopause is caused by the fluctuation of hormone levels within the ovaries (Utz, 2011). Despite popular belief, however, the decrease of estrogen is not the sole cause of menstrual cessation; rather, many hormones fluctuate to cause this reproductive transition or "climacteric" (Fausto-Sterling, 1992). These normal hormone fluctuations can occur anywhere from 8 to 10 years prior to menstrual cessation to several years afterward (Fausto-Sterling, 1992). What women experience is not just "menopause" then, but a complex reproductive aging transition that can span multiple decades.

ATTEMPTS TO DEFINE MENOPAUSE AND ITS SYMPTOMS

Physicians and researchers commonly use a three-part clinical definition to make sense of women's experience of reproductive aging (Mansfield et al., 2004). According to clinical guidelines, *menopause* is defined by the *lack* of menstruation for 12 consecutive months and thus can only be defined in retrospect (Dillaway, 2006; Mansfield et al., 2004). *Perimenopause* refers to the period that leads up to menopause, which is the time when signs or symptoms, such as irregular bleeding, hot flashes, and insomnia, may begin (Dillaway, 2006; Mansfield et al., 2004). This stage is sometimes referred to as a menopausal stage simply because it precedes the time when a woman becomes menopausal (McElmurry & Huddleston, 1991). However, women at this stage are not actually going through menopause. *Postmenopause* is the point after which a woman has not had a period for 12 months; often this stage is not diagnosed until one or two years after the cessation of menstruation (Dillaway, 2006; Mansfield et al., 2004; McElmurry & Huddleston, 1991).

The Stages of Reproductive Aging Workshop (STRAW) recently tried to articulate more uniform menopause-related definitions (Harlow et al., 2008; Soules et al., 2001). STRAW definitions suggest, for instance, that perimenopause begins when there are at least seven days in variability between the length of one menstrual cycle and the next, then progresses to a separate stage characterized by skipped periods (at least a 60-day gap between menses), and finally ends at 12 months past the FMP. However, Prior (2005) proposed that perimenopause begins with symptomatic experiences such as hot flashes and increased breast tenderness. She argued that subjective changes precede menstrual irregularity, and that women often find hot flashes and breast tenderness (as well as other signs and symptoms) more problematic than changes in menstrual flow. Individual women also do not always see clear transitions from one menopausal stage to another (Dillaway & Burton, 2011; Mansfield et al., 2004), and some of the STRAW stage definitions have been documented in women in their twenties and thirties, who are not yet perimenopausal (Derry & Derry, 2014). In a longitudinal study of 100 women, some reported remaining in one stage for numerous years and then moving quickly into the next, some flip-flopped between stages over many years, and some progressed quickly through all three stages (Mansfield et al., 2004). Flip-flopping between stages can be quite confusing, especially as women are wondering when perimenopause will end (Dillaway & Burton, 2011). Clinical definitions do not capture the variability in how women define menopause for themselves or how they experience menopausal signs and symptoms. Because of the sole focus on physiology, existing clinical definitions of menopause and its stages are still partial at best. Social science researchers suggested that psychosocial definitions are just as important, such as how a woman herself defines her own stage (Dare, 2011; Lock, 1993; Reynolds, 1997; Utz, 2011).

Defining the signs and symptoms of menopausal transitions has also proven difficult for clinicians and researchers. Medical websites and other authoritative sources, as well as women themselves, often assume a set of symptoms that represent perimenopause, including but not limited to mood changes, memory problems, fatigue, hot flashes, insomnia, vaginal dryness, changes in libido, weight gain, unwanted hair growth, heart palpitations, headaches, and joint pain (Avis et al., 2001; Derry & Dillaway, 2013). Cobb (1993) and Fausto-Sterling (1992) suggested that as many as 100 or more symptoms have been attributed to menopause. Epidemiological studies have not shown evidence of universal perimenopausal symptoms despite cultural lore and biomedical assumptions (Avis et al., 2001). Only bleeding changes, hot flashes, vaginal dryness, and perhaps insomnia are more frequently reported by perimenopausal or menopausal women than by premenopausal women (Derry & Dillaway, 2013; NIH, 2005). In Europe and the United States, approximately 70% of women experience hot flashes during perimenopause (Ayers, Forshaw, & Hunter, 2010); thus, the hot flash is the symptom most frequently attributed to reproductive aging, even though it can be attributed to other conditions as well. Perhaps we blame more on perimenopause and menopause than we should (Ayers et al., 2010; Fausto-Sterling, 1992; Lonborg & Travis, 2007); perhaps there are very few bodily symptoms that can be tied specifically to menopause (and not, instead, to other life situations at midlife or to continual conditions across women's life course). For instance, in a study of insomnia during perimenopause, Vigeta, Hachul, Tufik, and de Oliveira (2012) found that many women who reported an increase in sleep disturbance also reported insomnia during earlier life stages. It was only after the effects of insomnia were more noticeable in their daily lives (at midlife) that they sought medical treatment for this symptom. McHugh (2007) suggested that vaginal dryness may just indicate that women's bodies are not ready for sexual intercourse and that women take longer to become moist as they grow older; thus, vaginal dryness is neither a permanent condition for most middle-aged women, nor is it always directly attributable to menopause. The uncertainty about attribution of symptoms to menopause can be difficult for women as they attempt to evaluate and make sense of their own midlife experiences.

Despite debates over how to define each stage of reproductive aging and whether bodily signs and symptoms can be attributed to this transition, biomedical and feminist researchers agree that menopause is a time of transition and border crossing (Avis & McKinlay, 1991; Daly, 1997; Dare, 2011; Lyons & Griffin, 2003; Meyer, 2003). However, the biomedical literature suggests that menopause primarily represents deficiency, whereas feminist literature proposes that menopause represents a normal health experience that women may experience as positive, neutral, or negative, depending on their individual life circumstances. These conflicting characterizations result partially from different empirical emphases; biomedical research focuses on biological or bodily change and presents a medicalized view of menopause, whereas feminist research highlights the social, cultural, and developmental contexts for menopause. This chapter presents each of these perspectives and discusses their value in helping us to understand individual women's experiences.

THE MEDICALIZATION OF MENOPAUSE: BIOMEDICAL PERSPECTIVES ON REPRODUCTIVE AGING

The dominant perspective on menopause is biomedical and based on the idea that menopause is a cluster of symptoms caused by a "deficiency" in reproductive hormones (Dickson, 1990; Lyons & Griffin, 2003; Meyer, 2003; Niland & Lyons, 2011; Utz, 2011). Medical texts suggest that the ovaries become "unresponsive" and therefore "regress" as a result of the "withdrawal" of estrogen at menopause (Martin, 1992, p. 26; Niland & Lyons, 2011). Ovarian failure and a deficiency of reproductive hormones are seen as the biological causes of any physical, physiological, or psychological changes during this time of life, and these changes are defined as negative (Dickson, 1990; Lyons & Griffin, 2003; MacPherson, 1981; Martin, 1992; Meyer, 2003; Niland & Lyons, 2011; Utz, 2011). Within this perspective, women are reduced to "the internal secretions of their reproductive organs" (Dickson, 1990, p. 17). This focus on biology (narrowly defined) eventually leads medical professionals to feel responsible for fixing women's "deteriorating" bodies and simultaneously encourages women to seek medical treatment to "replace" or "restore" their hormones (Martin, 1992; Meyer, 2003; Niland & Lyons, 2011; Utz, 2011).

Medicalization bolsters and facilitates the biomedical perspective of women's deficiency (Meyer, 2003; Utz, 2011). Riessman (1983, p. 4) defined "medicalization" as the process by which behaviors or conditions take on medical meanings—"that is, defined in terms of health and illness" (see also Meyer, 2003; Niland & Lyons, 2011; Utz, 2011). It is a process in which "medical practice becomes a vehicle for eliminating or controlling problematic experiences that are defined as deviant, for the purpose of securing adherence to social norms" (Riessman, 1983, p. 4). Medicalization can be (a) conceptual, in that medical vocabulary is used to define a problem; (b) institutional, when medical providers legitimate a program or problem, or (c) interactional, at the level of doctor–patient encounters, when actual diagnosis and treatment of a problem occurs (Niland & Lyons, 2011; Riessman, 1983; Utz, 2011). A consequence of medicalization is the "de-skilling of the populace," as experts begin to "manage" and "mystify" human experiences (Riessman, 1983, p. 4). Thus, menopausal women must consult experts to understand experiences that historically they may have understood better themselves.

We can view the process of medicalization through the development and normalization of medical treatment for menopause (Ferguson & Parry, 1998; Niland & Lyons, 2011; Utz, 2011). An analogy was made in the mid-1960s by Robert Wilson (1966, p. 17), one of the leading promoters of estrogen replacement therapy, between diabetes and menopause:

> In the course of my work, spanning four decades and involving hundreds of carefully documented clinical cases, it became evident that menopause . . . is in fact a deficiency disease. . . . To cure diabetes, we supply the lacking substance in the form of insulin. A similar logic can be applied to menopause—the missing hormone can be replaced.

Wilson (1966) concluded that estrogen replacement could eliminate menopause and keep women "feminine forever." He saw menopause as the death of womanhood and linked this death to estrogen deficiency. Wilson clearly defined menopause as a pathological state—a state of illness rather than health—and also defined a treatment plan for restoring women to health; both helped in the medicalization of reproductive aging.

Even as Wilson's work has been discredited by later work and menopause is no longer defined as the end of womanhood, biomedical researchers still uphold estrogen as crucial for the physical health of women (Meyer, 2003; Murtaugh & Hepworth, 2003). In this view, when estrogen levels decline below those of the reproductive years, a woman becomes vulnerable to a range of chronic illnesses, including heart disease, osteoporosis, and Alzheimer's disease (Meyer, 2003; Murtaugh & Hepworth, 2003; Niland & Lyons, 2011). Menopause then becomes a precursor for a range of other diseases and, if women do not take hormones, they will be at greater risk for these diseases (Meyer, 2003; Niland & Lyons, 2011). This means that the exact reasons for the medicalization of menopause might change over time, but the equation of menopause with deficiency and bodily decay continues within biomedicine today.

Some feminist scholars have argued that, before Wilson's work and the introduction of artificial estrogens, menopause was defined more "naturally" and was seen in the context of a larger reproductive process that "healthy" women experience (Utz, 2011). However, another argument could be that, before the development of hormone therapies, menopause was simply a more hidden or ignored reproductive process that most women ("healthy" or not) dealt with in private. Regardless of whether that is true, the advent, widespread prescription, and normalization of hormone therapies cemented the medicalization of menopause (Meyer, 2003; Niland & Lyons, 2011; Utz, 2011). Medicalization originated primarily in the United States, but now there is evidence that women in Europe, Australia, New Zealand, as well as other parts of the world have started to accept medicalized views of menopause (Meyer, 2003). Some scholars infer that medicalization spreads through the marketing and prescription of hormone therapies (Meyer, 2003; Niland & Lyons, 2011; Utz, 2011; Wilbush, 1993). Although the percentage of women taking hormones is still highest in the United States, hormone use has also been on the rise in these other countries (Meyer, 2003).

EVIDENCE OF RECENT DEMEDICALIZATION?

With the exception of a drop in hormone therapy use in the 1970s (due to early fears about its side effects) and in the early 2000s (after the Women's Health Initiative findings about side effects, which are discussed below), hormone therapy use has risen steadily since the 1960s and has only recently leveled off in the face of alternative remedies and highly publicized risks of traditional therapies. Beginning in the 1990s, professional guidelines increasingly recommended offering hormone replacement therapy (HRT) to all perimenopausal women for disease prevention. For example, even the National Committee for Quality Assurance (2001), the U.S. federal agency that provides standards for medical practice, recommended that women be encouraged to use HRT. Although there was no conclusive research evidence to support such extensive prescription, and despite the growing discussion of the risks of HRT (Derry & Dillaway, 2013), medical professionals routinely treated perimenopausal signs and symptoms with prescription hormone supplements. In the United States, HRT prescriptions increased from 58 million in 1995 to 90 million in 1999 (Hersh, Stefanick, & Stafford, 2004). Growing critiques of the (over)medicalization of menopause, however, led to suspicions about the benefits and risks of hormone use. HRT was portrayed as the answer to bodily discomforts during menopause and postmenopause, but findings from the national Women's Health Initiative (WHI) study and an early end to the WHI study called this into question (Spake, 2004).

The WHI clinical trials were designed to examine whether hormone therapies are safe and effective for postmenopausal women in the face of increasing critiques and growing evidence of risks (Derry & Dillaway, 2013). The U.S. National Institutes of Health established the WHI in 1991 and began a WHI study of HRT in the fall of 1997. In that study, 16,608 postmenopausal women between the ages of 60 and 79 were randomly assigned to take a combination of estrogen and progestin (Spake, 2004). The WHI study specifically investigated the effects of HRT on women's rates of heart disease and various cancers, including breast cancer (thought to be the major potential adverse outcome from HRT). A global index also measured whether the overall effect of HRT was helpful or harmful when a number of diseases were considered simultaneously (Derry & Dillaway, 2013). The research was scheduled to be completed in 2005, however all trials finished early.

In July 2002, WHI researchers reported the first major findings of the study, which indicated that there were serious health risks associated with the long-term combined use of progestin and estrogen that greatly outweighed any health benefits to women (Derry & Dillaway, 2013). A slightly increased and statistically significant risk of breast cancer among women taking estrogen and progestin was the major reason for stopping part of the WHI study in 2002 (Minkin & Giblin, 2004). Many WHI trials ended after the release of the 2002 data; participants on estrogen only, however, were instructed to continue. WHI results from March 2004 suggested increased risk of coronary artery disease among continuing participants, and reports at that time suggested more overall harm than benefit from hormone use (Chlebowski et al., 2003; Derry & Dillaway, 2013; MacLennan, 2008; Manson et al., 2003).

Considerable numbers of women stopped taking HRT when they heard about the findings (Bestul, McCollum, Hansen, & Saseen, 2004; Dentzer, 2003; Pace, 2006; Spake, 2004). MacLennan (2008, p. 13) suggested that as many as two-thirds of women stopped taking their prescriptions right after the release of the WHI results, often without consulting their providers first. Prescription rates also fell because of decisions by individual women as well as by their doctors; thus a slight demedicalization of menopause occurred at that point, as both women and doctors quickly steered away from hormone use (Bestul et al., 2004) in response to considerable media coverage of the WHI results (Colombo et al., 2010; MacLennan, 2008; Pace, 2006).

A cover article in *U.S. News and World Report* characterized menopausal women as in a "hormone conundrum," confused in the face of problematic symptoms and inconclusive data on the risks and benefits associated with HRT (Spake, 2004, p. 60). Colombo et al. (2010) suggested that widespread (yet unbalanced) media coverage led women to receive incomplete information about the WHI study and prevented them from making fully informed decisions about whether to keep using or discontinue HRT. Health care providers were faced with the same incomplete information. Upon review of the released WHI findings, the U.S. Food and Drug Administration (FDA) concluded that HRT should be used only for treatment of hot flashes, vaginal dryness, and osteoporosis, at the lowest dose and for the shortest period of time (Derry & Dillaway, 2013; U.S. FDA, 2003). Further, an FDA advisory stated that hormone medications should not be referred to as "hormone replacement therapy" because no evidence existed that a replacement of hormones is necessary (Derry & Dillaway, 2013). "Hormone therapy" (HT) is now the phrase and acronym used to refer to traditional hormone supplements prescribed for alleviation of women's symptoms. This change in terminology is reflective of a change in perspective (however slight) on how necessary hormone supplementation is during menopause and postmenopause (Brett & Keenan, 2006; Burke et al., 2003).

The original WHI research reports and the FDA guidelines both concluded that the risk of harm is small enough to warrant use for symptomatic postmenopausal women who will gain a clear benefit. The results are still inconclusive about perimenopausal use, but clinicians and biomedical researchers still generally hail HT as a way to alleviate menopausal symptoms (particularly hot flashes) and improve quality of life (Derry & Dillaway, 2013; MacLennan, 2008; Taylor & Manson, 2011; Williams et al., 2007). However, the WHI results, especially as portrayed in some professional articles and in the popular media, have led many women to stop using HT more quickly, make more complex decisions about whether their symptoms warrant HT, or look for alternative remedies. Directly after the WHI results were released, studies estimated that the use of diet, exercise, multivitamins, herbal supplements, and other complementary and alternative medicine (CAM) approaches were preferred over HT by 45% to 80% of women (Brett & Keenan, 2006; Burke et al., 2003). Yet, alternative treatments are not seen as providing the relief that traditional hormone supplements do (Taylor & Manson, 2011; Williams et al., 2007); consequently physicians do still frequently prescribe HT. Nonetheless, one of the important effects of the WHI and other follow-up studies is that clinical recommendations are now that HT should be used only for a "limited duration" (Taylor & Manson, 2011, p. 262); that is, women should not remain on HT prescriptions indefinitely. This represents a concrete change in treatment regimens and encourages women and their doctors to think about other ways to alleviate menopausal symptoms. For example, in a recent survey of over 3,000 perimenopausal women, Williams and colleagues (2007) found that, of those women who sought and accepted treatment for symptoms, about one-third used traditional hormone therapies only; other women used CAM, and some women used both forms of treatment.

Whether the fallout from the WHI studies led to a permanent demedicalization of menopause is debatable. Berger (2004, p. 1) suggested that perhaps "the rush away from the drugs" ended fairly quickly and that large numbers of women are still given prescriptions for HT. The biomedical perspective continues to represent the dominant model of menopause, which means that the equation of menopause with deficiency and disease still exists (Meyer, 2003; Niland & Lyons, 2011; Utz, 2011). Medicalization is still a strong influence on contemporary women and health care providers. Yet, even though these shifts may not represent demedicalization of menopause, women and their doctors may be recognizing the limits of biomedical knowledge of, and traditional medical solutions for, menopause. It is now more common for health professionals to tell women that menopause is natural and normal, even if they also suggest that it is related to negative health effects (Derry & Dillaway, 2013; Meyer, 2003). At the very least, there is some sentiment that the strictly biomedical or medicalized view of menopause is faulty.

FEMINIST CRITIQUES OF MEDICALIZATION

For at least four decades, feminist scholars have written about the effects of the medicalization of menopause on individual women (Hyde, Nee, Howlett, Drennan, & Butler, 2010; Lyons & Griffin, 2003; MacPherson, 1981; Utz, 2011; Voda, 1992). Some have argued that feminist researchers have concentrated their energy on refuting the biomedical perspective to the detriment of building their own complete, alternative perspective (Koeske, 1983; Lyons & Griffin, 2003; Oakley, 1998). Some authors (Gullette, 1997; Lyons & Griffin, 2003) have suggested that the biomedical discourse is a "master narrative" because it represents the only "fully constituted" perspective on reproductive aging. Because this perspective is masked as "information" and women have little access to resistant discourses, they believe they have "no choice but to take [the information] to heart, repeat [it] as truth" (Gullette, 1997, p. 190). The more exposure individual women have to medical providers and medical institutions, the more likely they may be to adhere to negative views of menopause (Brumberg, 1997; Conrad, 2007; Dillaway, 2005a). Although family and reproductive contexts may make menopause seem positive or neutral at times, exposure to biomedical ideas may cause negativity. Women find it difficult to resist the power of these pervasive negative definitions (Barbre, 1998; Hyde, Nee, Howlett, Drennan, & Butler, 2010; Lyons & Griffin, 2003; Utz, 2011; Winterich & Umberson, 1999). Hyde et al. (2010, p. 805) concluded that "the cultural authority of biomedicine shaped participants' experiences of the body and how they constituted their health identity," even among those women in their study who "strongly contested biomedical definitions of their situation." Biomedical practitioners' definitions have a strong normalizing power in how the body is perceived and experienced, because of the authority that biomedical perspectives have in the face of a lack of comprehensive, resistant perspectives (Gullette, 1997; Hyde et al., 2010; Lyons & Griffin, 2003; Niland & Lyons, 2011).

Feminist critics have suggested that the biomedical perspective and medicalization reflect stereotypes about gender and aging rather than science (Derry & Dillaway, 2013; Kaufert & Gilbert, 1986; MacPherson, 1981; Utz, 2011; Voda, 1992). Many authors have pointed out that scientific descriptions of menopause have not been objective and are related to gendered and ageist views about women's worth (Derry & Dillaway, 2013; Martin, 1992; Niland & Lyons, 2011). Feminists and other social science and humanities scholars have questioned the idea that the FMP or "ovarian failure" signifies the most important experience of menopause (Ferguson & Parry, 1998; Rostosky & Travis, 1996; Utz, 2011), and they have noted that women begin experiencing changes in hormonal production in their thirties and may continue to do so throughout their fifties and sixties (Greer, 1993; McElmurry & Huddleston, 1991). According to feminists and other social scientists, to concentrate on a single event (the FMP) and call it "menopause" is to exclude from analysis as many as 30 (or more) years of "reproductive aging" (Fausto-Sterling, 1992; Greer, 1993; McElmurry & Huddleston, 1991). In addition, increased menstrual cycle variability and missed cycles are defined as abnormal during perimenopause (Santoro, 2005) but not during adolescence, when they also occur frequently. A medicalized view of menopause does not recognize the true continuity and change across women's life course (Lyons & Griffin, 2003) and instead defines women by their reproductive capacity and fertility, despite the fact that, on average, women live considerably more years of their lives in a nonreproductive capacity than in a reproductive one. Other feminist scholars (Fausto-Sterling, 1992) have appropriately noted that biomedical and other essentialist approaches also ignore a wide variation in menopausal experiences among different groups of women (Avis et al., 2001; Mansfield et al., 2004).

Furthermore, woman-centered, cross-cultural researchers have often proposed that menopausal symptoms are more the result of sociocultural attitudes and ideologies than of biology (Beyenne, 1986; Lock, 1993; Rostosky & Travis, 1996; Wasti, Robinson, Akhtar, & Badaruddin, 1993). Lock (1993) made this clear in her comparative study of menopausal women in North America and Japan. She found that "menopause is neither fact nor universal event but an experience that we must interpret in context" (p. 370). For example, whereas North American ideology dictates youth as the norm, this is not the case in Japan, where "middle-aged" individuals actually form the "backbone" of society, "support[ing] both old and young, keep[ing] the economy growing and build[ing] the new Japan—men and women alike" (p. 370). Constricting gender ideology does exist in Japan, of course, but Japanese women conceptualize the lifecycle as "part of a larger cyclical continuum rather than as a path of no return that fragments youth from old age" (Lock, 1993, p. 378). Lock also found fewer reports of symptoms, such as hot flashes, among Japanese women. Similarly, Buck and Gottlieb (1991, p. 43) discovered discrepancies in symptom reporting and attitudes about menopause between Mohawk women in Canada and other Canadian women, and concluded that the "expression of symptoms at menopause varies with the social context within which it takes place." Beyenne (1986, pp. 58–59) explored how menopause "presents neither a life crisis nor psychological or physiological problems" for Mayan and Greek women. Both the Mayan and

Greek groups viewed menopause as a natural transition "that all women go through," "unrecognizable" except for signifying "the end of menstruation and childbearing" (p. 63).

Other anthropological studies suggest that increased medicalization of menopause in North America leads to more negative views among individual women in that setting as well (Lock, 1993). Lock (1993) and Utz (2011) mentioned the importance of "local biologies," in that women think about and experience physical or physiological changes at midlife differently, depending on their expectations for reproductive aging, their knowledge about the menopausal transition, and other psychosocial life contexts.

The view that women's reproductive aging might also involve a "normal" transition to a stage of life that has the potential for expanded opportunities, new identities, and a chance to reevaluate oneself in a different, *more positive* way is rarely addressed within mainstream discourse (Chrisler, 2007; Gray, 1996; Weed, 1999). The dominant (biomedical) perspective pays little attention to women's own views of their menopause experiences, which is why we hear less about menopause as a "normal," "natural" reproductive transition. In response, there are recent feminist efforts to move *beyond* the refutation of the biomedical model of menopause to understand other psychosocial contexts for this reproductive transition.

FEMINIST RESEARCH ON OTHER PSYCHOSOCIAL CONTEXTS: MENOPAUSE IS MORE THAN JUST NEGATIVE CHANGE

A burgeoning feminist literature proposes a different perspective on "normal" menopausal change and further demonstrates the need to look for broader, more complex knowledge of menopause as a reproductive transition. That is, feminist scholars have recognized that menopause is more than just a collection of uncomfortable signs and symptoms. For instance, feminist scholars have suggested that increasing numbers of women see menopause as a positive or neutral transition because of certain life contexts (Barbre, 1993; Gannon, 1999; Lock, 1993; Lyons & Griffin, 2003; Winterich & Umberson, 1999). For instance, women may welcome menopause as relief from the threat of pregnancy and the burdens of menstruation and contraception (Dillaway, 2005b; Gannon & Ekstrom, 1993; Lyons & Griffin, 2003; Voda, 1992). The baby boomers are the first generation to have had widespread access to the birth control pill and other advances in contraceptive technologies that enable women to avoid biological motherhood (Dillaway, 2005b; Utz, 2011). Contemporary women, then, may elect to end their reproductive years long before menopause. Within this context, menopause may be positive or insignificant for many individuals. Regardless of the bodily changes they may face during menopause, then, individuals may view menopause as ushering in a "good" life stage, one that is better and more carefree than the one before it.

Family Contexts for Menopause

Other research indicates that some family contexts can make the menopausal transition seem neutral, positive, or negative. For instance, women at midlife are often caring for their parents, partners, and children (often simultaneously); menopause can pale in importance to these care-giving responsibilities (Dare, 2011; Dillaway, 2005b; Winterich & Umberson, 1999). Women told Winterich and Umberson (1999, p. 61) that menopause was "last on [their] list" of things to worry about and "no big deal" in the context of other family problems (e.g., divorce, children "acting out," or family death) (see also Dillaway, 2005b, 2012). Dare (2011) also found that experiencing divorce and the aging and death of parents weighed much more heavily on women than menopause. Thus, family contexts can make women feel neutral or even positive about menopause. Bodily change may be noticed but might not be something for which women take time to seek medical help, given their busy and complicated family lives.

There also are instances in which menopause seems more negative, given certain family contexts. Winterich and Umberson (1999) and Mansfield, Koch, and Gierach (2003) reported that husbands sometimes have negative views of menopause or know little about the experience overall. Even husbands who want to be supportive lack the information to do so or feel unsure about how to help (Mansfield et al., 2003). Further, women sometimes want to share perimenopausal experiences with their partners, but they avoid doing so because it is "a private thing" (Walter, 2000, p. 117). Due to their lack of information and to women's reticence about sharing experiences, husbands' interactions with their wives can cement negative meanings about menopause and encourage women to think about menopause as a collection of treatable symptoms.

We do know from previous research on social support that the older women are, the less likely they are to receive support from their spouses (Schwarzer & Gutierrez-Dona, 2005). Partners can be supportive during other reproductive events (e.g., pregnancy, birth, breastfeeding) but, because more secrecy surrounds menopause, Mansfield et al. (2003) suggested that male partners may be less supportive at midlife than at previous stages (if only because they lack information about how to help). Negative images of menopause (or a lack of support for women at menopause) within families may affect women in adverse ways, lead women to their own negative views, and incline them toward a medicalized view of menopause (Mansfield et al., 2003). In this case, individual women may turn to medical relief for symptoms in order to appease intimate partners. On the other hand, we know that sharing health experiences with intimate partners leads to better physical and emotional well-being (Mansfield et al., 2003; Reid, 2004; Walter, 2000). "Women who are moving through the menopausal transition, even those who experience few adverse physical or emotional changes, still need to negotiate a change in status or a 'redefinition of self,' and married women may benefit from social support provided by their husbands during this transition" (Mansfield et al., 2003, p. 103). Sharing health experiences in a positive way can increase individuals' reports of marital satisfaction as well (Reid, 2004), because family relationships are molded alongside health experiences.

Reproductive Histories

Women's feelings about menopause also cannot be separated from decisions that women and their partners make about whether to become parents. In some social contexts, menopause may take on more negative meanings, as seen in trends toward delayed childbearing and rising concerns about infertility (Dillaway, 2012). Loss of fertility may be an important issue for a woman who has delayed childbearing until her thirties or forties and then discovers that she is having trouble conceiving. These women do not want to be finished with childbearing, both emotionally and in terms of life goals. Other women may never have actively made the decision to stop having children (even if, in some cases, it has been more than 10 or 15 years since their youngest child was born). For these women, the onset of menopause may make it feel like they never had the choice to finalize their decision themselves—the onset of menopause took that final decision out of their hands (Dillaway, 2012).

Women with fertility difficulties may feel that menopause has robbed them of their final chance to become biological parents. In cases of divorce and remarriage or delayed first marriage (especially if a new intimate partner desires children), menopause may also take on a negative light. Conversely, some women who assume they are no longer fertile become pregnant accidentally during perimenopause, especially if they have stopped using birth control. Thus, menopause can be neutral, positive, or negative for women as a result of earlier reproductive difficulties and reproductive histories. Coping with menopause may not seem as difficult as coping with infertility or miscarriage, and menopause may be a relief for a woman with a long history of difficulty becoming pregnant, who now has closure and can put decisions about infertility treatment and hopes for a family to rest (Dillaway, 2012).

Connections between Menopause and Aging

Whether or not women equate menopause with aging is also important for how they view and experience menopause as a transition. Hall (1999, pp. 17–18) discussed an interview she conducted with one menopausal woman who explained:

> Those night sweats—and other symptoms I began to notice—suddenly made me feel old. One day I'm a young woman in her prime, and the next day I'm worrying about whether or not I'm prepared for retirement and thinking about getting my affairs in order.

Because of its conflation with chronological aging, the onset of menopause may have resembled a "death sentence" for many women in the past (Hall, 1999; Weed, 1999). Furthermore, some people have a misconception that all women used to die before menopause, and thus postmenopausal women are currently living beyond what nature prescribes (Weed, 1999). Even if menopause is no longer a death sentence in our imaginations, we are still confronted with a reiteration of the idea that "old guys can be gorgeous, but old women pollute the landscape, so mask them, keep their 'decay' out of sight" (Gray, 1996, p. 186; see also Greer, 1993; Jarrell, 1999; Zones, 2000). The message is that women lose their "feminine," "healthy," and "sexy" attributes in midlife and begin a continual decline after that. "After 50," women supposedly take on "the grandma look [becoming] women in buns, girdles, and orthopedic shoes" (Jarrell, 1999, p. 2; Utz, 2011). This situation arises directly from the fusion of a sexist and ageist culture, one that insists on viewing older people as "ill" or "sick" (Carmody, 1993; Gray, 1996; Zones, 2000) and women primarily as "mothers" (and, if not mothers, then sex objects) (Dillaway, 2005a).

The image of femininity *is* primarily associated with youth, physical beauty, fertility, and reproductive capabilities in Western industrialized countries (Brumberg, 1997; Dickson, 1990; Greer, 1993; Wilson, 1966; Worcester & Whatley, 1992). Women may believe that bodily changes must be slowed down or halted; gray hair, wrinkles, dentures, age spots, drowsiness, thickening of the waistline, sagging abdomens and breasts, sagging muscles, or crinkling skin and bifocal glasses seriously challenge one's self-identity (Berkun, 1986; Brumberg, 1997; Grambs, 1989; Zones, 2000). Women have been taught since girlhood to control their bodies (Brumberg, 1997; Dinnerstein & Weitz, 1998; Zones, 2000), which could make menopause and midlife bodily changes anxiety producing. The fear of "being let down by their bodies if they must maneuver in a world that favors youth" may be strong (Berkun 1986, p. 383).

On the other hand, age-based norms are changing as the baby boomers age. For example, baby boomers may identify and behave in the same ways they did when they were chronologically younger. For example, they participate in similar leisure activities, wear similar clothing, and are physically and socially active (Featherstone & Hepworth, 1991; Muhlbauer

& Chrisler, 2007; Utz, 2011). As a result, some scholars now suggest that there is no current cultural consensus about what it means to be a midlife, mature, or menopausal woman, and women no longer routinely report feeling old at midlife (Dillaway, 2005a; Muhlbauer & Chrisler, 2007; Utz, 2011).

In addition, women are increasingly in the paid labor force and have other meaningful social roles during midlife, so menopause has less potency as a cultural marker of entry into a negative life stage. In fact, menopause may parallel women's greatest accomplishments in paid work. "Aging" stars (e.g., Meryl Streep, Helen Mirren, Diane Keaton) or "older" women in politics (e.g., Hillary Clinton) call into question the idea that older women are merely stereotypical grandmothers who are past their prime (Dinnerstein & Weitz, 1998; Featherstone & Hepworth, 1991; Muhlbauer & Chrisler, 2007). Thus, they may experience chronological aging or reproductive aging (or both) as less stressful and more representative of new possibilities than previous generations did. Self-esteem for contemporary middle-aged and older women may depend not only on physical appearance and biology, but also on nonreproductive, nonfamilial accomplishments—as is the case for men. These developments could make the current cohort of menopausal women more positive about experiences of reproductive aging than previous generations of women who had fewer opportunities outside the home (Grambs, 1989; Muhlbauer & Chrisler, 2007). The disruption of the equation of midlife and aging, then, may lessen women's negative attitudes toward menopause and decrease some of women's attention to negative bodily experiences. All of these psychosocial contexts will mediate how women view and experience menopausal signs and symptoms and whether they will adhere to a purely medicalized view of menopause. When we consider other psychosocial contexts for menopause, we realize that menopause is more than just a collection of treatable symptoms (and that symptoms may be seen through particular life contexts as well). Thus, contemporary women may think more carefully before wholeheartedly adopting a biomedical perspective as their own.

COPING STRATEGIES AND SELF-CARE AT MENOPAUSE, IN THE FACE OF DUELING PERSPECTIVES

Regardless of how women feel about reproductive aging as a transition, there is no doubt that perimenopause and menopause involve biopsychosocial changes that women must navigate. Most women report experiencing some signs and symptoms, even if they vary in frequency, severity, and cause. Depending on how women feel about other parts of their lives (e.g., family situations, work status, relationships, aging) and how exposed they are to (negative) biomedical perspectives on menopause and aging (Brumberg, 1997; Hyde et al., 2010; Kafanelis, Kostanski, Komesaroff, & Stojanovska, 2009; Lyons & Griffin, 2003), they also may feel more or less positive about reproductive aging. Coping with bodily changes and possible identity transitions at menopause is easier if one feels more comfortable with one's body and has a positive concept of one's life stage, as well as accurate and comprehensive information about health-promoting practices. If a woman believes that she is experiencing a change that is already defined as negative, or if it has negative implications for her self-image, then she may feel troubled by menopause. In this case she may feel more anxiety and distress and may engage in more reactive strategies for dealing with bodily signs and symptoms (Ayers at el., 2010; Bosworth, Bastian, Rimer, & Siegler, 2003; Hunter & Mann, 2010; Kafanelis et al., 2009; Reynolds, 1997). Women may react to menopause using a narrow, medicalized view—even if they want to resist that view—because they have little knowledge of comprehensive alternative perspectives (Hyde et al., 2010; Kafanelis et al., 2009; Lyons & Griffin, 2003). Cultural or biomedical attitudes that overestimate the likelihood of troubling symptoms and underestimate the possibility of good coping strategies may make the situation more difficult (Ayers et al., 2010; Derry & Dillaway, 2013; Gullette, 1997; Hyde et al., 2010; Lyons & Griffin, 2003).

Despite the negative biomedical perspectives on reproductive aging, however, there are an increasing variety of coping strategies and alternative remedies for promoting and improving health during menopause, and these strategies and remedies may increase in popularity as individual women find out that menopause and its bodily changes can be taken in stride. As individual women increasingly take a neutral or positive stance toward reproductive aging (and aging in general), it is important to cover the range of possible coping strategies that women may use during this transition. Women always engage in a variety of self-help techniques to cope with distress. Self-help techniques for hot flashes might include, but are not limited to, dressing in layers, carrying a fan, identifying and avoiding individual triggers of hot flashes (e.g., caffeine, spicy food, alcohol, sugar, physical exertion, stress), use of CAM, and talking with supportive female friends (Derry & Dillaway, 2013; Kafanelis et al., 2009). In this way women can reduce the frequency and severity of hot flashes and deal with them more positively and actively if these symptoms are physically bothersome or embarrassing on a day-to-day basis. Women often complain as much about the public nature of hot flashes as the bodily sensation of them (Dillaway, 2011); thus, reducing the chances that they will experience hot flashes in public is often one of the primary goals women have.

Proactive, health-promoting behaviors of women between the ages of 40 and 70 have increased dramatically in the past 5 to 10 years, perhaps in part because of the flurry of attention to the WHI findings, but probably

also because midlife is becoming a time of new possibilities and new successes for women (Derry & Dillaway, 2013; Muhlbauer & Chrisler, 2007).
Multivitamins and minerals, herbal and dietary supplements, home remedies, and various CAM strategies are increasingly used by women for the
relief of signs and symptoms attributed to perimenopause or menopause
(Brett & Keenan, 2006; Kafanelis et al., 2009; Williams et al., 2007). Research
does indicate that some relief might be gained from dietary modification
and lifestyle changes, such as reduction in smoking, caffeine, and alcohol
use; stress management; and increased exercise (Fiona & Davis, 2010;
Kafanelis et al., 2009). Although studies are still inconclusive about the effects of CAM, women sometimes report benefits of supplements, mind-
body therapies, and Eastern medicine, and these practices have not been
found to do any harm (Innes, Selfe, & Vishnu, 2010; Low Dog, 2005; Scheid,
Ward, Cha, Watanabe, & Liao, 2010; Testerman, Morton, Mason, & Ronan,
2004).

Individual women may need to sort through whether their troubling
symptoms are really due to hormonal changes related to perimenopause
or menopause, or if they are attributing their symptoms to menopause
because of stereotypes about reproductive aging as a transition (Derry &
Dillaway, 2013). The belief that menopausal symptoms are negative and
representative of decline may amplify the psychosocial experience of
menopause and make proactive or inventive coping strategies less likely
(Ayers et al., 2010; Hyde et al., 2010; Kafanelis et al., 2009; Lyons & Griffin,
2003). Women should not expect to experience bodily problems at perimenopause or menopause that cannot be overcome (Derry & Dillaway,
2013). If individual women think of menopause as part of a predictable,
biopsychosocial continuum and a normal, reproductive life course, then
coping with a bothersome sign or symptom may seem easier and make
the transition seem less jarring and more normal (Kafanelis et al., 2009).
Kafanelis suggested that self-awareness and gathering comprehensive information about one's life stage is critical; then women can actively cope
with any bodily signs and symptoms they may face and better resist
purely negative (biomedical) definitions of their experiences.

CONCLUSIONS

Menopause is a "complex transition involving biological, psychological,
sociological, and cultural variables" (Lock, 1986, p. 1; see also Fausto-
Sterling, 1992). Individual women regard menopause, as they do most
life changes, in a variety of ways. Research on menopause has often been
"discipline-oriented" and "hence designed to answer specific, narrowly-
defined problems" or support specific perspectives (Lock, 1986, p. 1).
Biomedical perspectives that ignore psychosocial experiences of menopause are flawed, and feminist perspectives that simply refute

medicalization and ignore the bodily experience of menopause are also flawed. Therefore, researchers need to analyze menopause as a complicated biopsychosocial experience that has been partially defined by these perspectives but that also is much broader than either of those perspectives (Derry, 2002).

Considering the pervasiveness of the biomedical model, we might ask more about what implications it has for women who are going through the menopausal transition (Hyde et al., 2010; Kafanelis et al., 2009; Utz, 2011). "Locating women's 'problems' in their bodies" and biological capacities "detracts from the recognition" that there are other "potent context(s)" for menopause (Rostosky & Travis, 1996, p. 302). Holding steadfast to a biomedical perspective discourages in-depth explorations of how women's existing life situations impact their menopause experiences. Systematic feminist analyses of other psychosocial life contexts (such as the ones outlined above) can produce a more complete understanding of what menopause and midlife really represent for individual women. Yet psychosocial research cannot give us the complete picture of menopause.

Some scholars have argued that most feminist researchers have avoided in-depth empirical explorations of the physical or bodily experience of menopause for fear of reifying the very biomedical equations they have worked to dismantle (Koeske, 1983; Oakley, 1998). Likewise, some have noted that most feminists have not sufficiently studied women's apprehensions about menopause (Dillaway, 2005b). Almost 20 years ago, Oakley (1998, p. 140) argued that there is "little attempt to explore topics that women themselves think are important," which suggests that bodily changes during menopause may be more important to some menopausal women than feminists have generally acknowledged. Yet, those bodily changes may be perceived differently by individual women than clinicians and biomedical researchers think is the case, and therefore we need to spend more time thinking about both what women have gained from medicalization as well as what they have lost.

Women are not gaining adequate information from their health care providers about the variety of treatment options, and providers do not ask patients about their expectations for symptom relief (Ma, Dreiling, & Stafford, 2006). Ma et al. (2006) suggested that, perhaps due to medicalization, providers have limited preparedness to guide patients' decision making about symptom management. In addition, if the trend is toward the demedicalization of menopause after the WHI, feminist researchers need to pay much more attention to what this means for individual women. An additional issue that warrants more in-depth investigation is women's increased use of CAM to manage menopausal symptoms and maintain their health (Low Dog, 2005; Ma et al., 2006; Testerman et al., 2004; Williams et al., 2007).

Finally, we still have only partial definitions of what menopause really means for women today. Until we gain answers to more of these questions and truly weigh the impact of medicalization against women's desires for alternative perspectives (and know what those alternatives are), we lack a full understanding of the meanings and experiences of menopause or the impact of the corresponding discourses or perspectives on women's self-concept and quality of life.

REFERENCES

Avis, N., & McKinlay, S. (1991). A longitudinal analysis of women's attitudes toward the menopause: Results from the Massachusetts Women's Health Study. *Maturitas, 13,* 65–79.

Avis, N., Stellato, R., Crawford, S., Bromberger, J., Ganz, P., Cain, V., & Kagawa-Singer, M. (2001). Is there a menopausal syndrome? Menopausal status and symptoms across racial/ethnic groups. *Social Science and Medicine, 52,* 345–356.

Ayers, B., Forshaw, M., & Hunter, M. (2010). The impact of attitudes toward the menopause on women's symptom experience: A systematic review. *Maturitas, 65,* 28–36.

Barbre, J. W. (1993). Meno-boomers and moral guardians: An exploration of the cultural construction of menopause. In J. Callahan (Ed.), *Menopause: A midlife passage* (pp. 23–35). Bloomington: Indiana University Press.

Berger, L. (2004, June 6). Hormone therapy: The dust is still settling. *New York Times.* Retrieved from http://www.nytimes.com/2004/06/06/health/two-years-after-on-hormone-therapy-the-dust-is-still-settling.html.

Berkun, C. (1986). In behalf of women over 40: Understanding the importance of the menopause. *Social Work, 31,* 378–384.

Bestul, M. B., McCollum, M., Hansen, L. B., & Saseen, J. J. (2004). Impact of the Women's Health Initiative trial results on hormone replacement therapy. *Pharmacotherapy, 24,* 495-499.

Beyenne, Y. (1986). Cultural significance and physiological manifestations of menopause: A biocultural analysis. *Culture, Medicine, and Psychiatry, 10,* 47–71.

Bosworth, H. B., Bastian, L. A., Rimer, B. K., & Siegler, I. C. (2003). Coping styles and personality domains related to menopausal stress. *Women's Health Issues, 13,* 32–38.

Brett, K. M., & Keenan, N. L. (2006). Complementary and alternative medicine use among midlife women for reasons including menopause in the United States: 2002. *Menopause, 14,* 300–307.

Brumberg, J. J. (1997). *The body project: An intimate history of American girls.* New York: Random House.

Buck, M., & Gottleib, L. (1991). The meaning of time: Mohawk women at midlife. *Health Care for Women International, 12,* 41–50.

Burke, G. L., Legault, C., Anthony, M., Bland, D. R., Morgan, T. M., Naughton, M. J., . . . Vitolins, M. Z. (2003). Soy protein and isoflavone effects on vasomotor symptoms in peri- and postmenopausal women: The Soy Estrogen Alternative Study. *Menopause, 10*, 147–153.

Carmody, D. (1993, September 15). At lunch with Betty Friedan: Trying to dispel 'the mystique of age' at 72. *New York Times.* Retrieved from http://www.nytimes.com/1993/09/15/garden/at-lunch-with-betty-friedan-trying-to-dispel-the-mystique-of-age-at-72.html.

Chlebowski, R., Hendrix, S., Langer, R., Stefanick, M., Gass, M., Lane, D., . . . McTiernan, A.; WHI Investigators. (2003). Influence of estrogen plus progestin on breast cancer and mammography in healthy postmenopausal women. *Journal of the American Medical Association, 289*, 3243–3253.

Chrisler, J. C. (2007). Body image issues of women over 50. In V. Muhlbauer & J. C. Chrisler (Eds.), *Women over 50: Psychological perspectives* (pp. 6–25). New York: Springer.

Cobb, J. (1993). *Understanding menopause.* New York: Penguin.

Colombo, C., Mosconi, P., Buratti, M. G., Liberati, A., Donati, S., Mele, A., & Satolli, R. (2010). Press coverage of hormone replacement therapy and menopause. *European Journal of Obstetrics & Gynecology and Reproductive Biology, 153*, 56–61.

Conrad, P. (2007). *The medicalization of society: On the transformation of human conditions into treatable disorders.* Baltimore, MD: Johns Hopkins University Press.

Daly, J. (1997). Facing change: Women speaking about midlife. In P. Komesaroff, P. Rothfield, & J. Daly (Eds.), *Reinterpreting menopause: Cultural and philosophical issues* (pp. 159–175). New York: Routledge.

Dare, J. S. (2011). Transitions in midlife women's lives: Contemporary experiences. *Healthcare for Women International, 32*, 111–133.

Dentzer, S. (2003). Science, public health, and public awareness: Lessons learned from the Women's Health Initiative. *Annals of Internal Medicine, 138*, 352–353.

Derry, P. (2002). What do we mean by the "biology of menopause"? *Sex Roles, 46*, 13–23.

Derry, P., & Derry, G. (2014). Analysis of the STRAW operational definition of the early menopausal transition. *Women's Reproductive Health, 1*, 21–30.

Derry, P., & Dillaway, H. (2013). Rethinking menopause. In M. Spiers, P. Geller, & J. Kloss (Eds.), *Women's health psychology* (pp. 440–466). Hoboken, NJ: Wiley.

Dickson, G. (1990). A feminist poststructuralist analysis of the knowledge of menopause. *Advanced Nursing Science, 12*, 15–31.

Dillaway, H. (2005a). (Un)Changing menopausal bodies: How women think and act in the face of a reproductive transition and gendered beauty ideals. *Sex Roles, 53*, 1–17.

Dillaway, H. (2005b). Menopause is the "good old": Women's thoughts about reproductive aging. *Gender & Society, 19*, 398–417.

Dillaway, H. (2006). When does menopause occur, and how long does it last? Wrestling with age- and time-based conceptualizations of reproductive aging. *Feminist Formations, 18*, 31–60.

Dillaway, H. (2011). Menopausal and misbehaving: When women "flash" in front of others. In C. Bobel & S. Kwan (Eds.), *Embodied resistance: Breaking the rules in public spaces* (pp. 197–208). Nashville, TN: Vanderbilt University Press.

Dillaway, H. (2012). Reproductive history as social context: Exploring how women converse about menopause and sexuality at midlife. In J. DeLamater & L. Carpenter (Eds.), *Sex for life: From virginity to Viagra, how sexuality changes throughout our lives* (pp. 217–235). New York: New York University Press.

Dillaway, H., & Burton, J. (2011). "Not done yet?! How women discuss the "end" of menopause. *Women's Studies, 40*, 149–176.

Dinnerstein, M., & Weitz, R. (1998). Jane Fonda, Barbara Bush, and other aging bodies: Femininity and the limits of resistance. In R. Weitz (Ed.), *The politics of women's bodies* (pp. 189–204). New York: Oxford University Press.

Fausto-Sterling, A. (1992). *Myths of gender* (rev. ed.). New York: Basic Books.

Featherstone, M., & Hepworth, M. (1991). The mask of ageing and the postmodern life course. In M. Featherstone, M. Hepworth, & B. Turner (Eds.), *The body: Social process and cultural theory* (pp. 371–389). London: Sage.

Ferguson, S., & Parry, C. (1998). Rewriting menopause: Challenging the medical paradigm to reflect menopausal women's experiences. *Frontiers, 19*, 20–41.

Fiona, J., & Davis, S. (2010). Menopause. In L. Borgelt, M. B. O'Connell, J. Smith, & K. Calis (Eds.)., *Women's health across the life span* (pp. 249–265). Bethesda, MD: American Society of Health-System Pharmacists.

Gannon, L. (1999). *Women and aging: Transcending the myths*. New York: Routledge.

Gannon, L., & Ekstrom, B. (1993). Attitudes toward menopause: The influence of sociocultural paradigms. *Psychology of Women Quarterly, 17*, 275–288.

Grambs, J. D. (1989). *Women over forty: Visions and realities* (rev. ed.). New York: Springer.

Gray, F. (1996, March 26). The third age. *New Yorker*, 186–192.

Greer, G. (1993). *The change: Women, aging, and the menopause*. New York: Knopf.

Gullette, M. M. (1997). Menopause as magic marker: Discursive consolidation in the United States and strategies for cultural combat. In P. Komesaroff, P. Rothfield, & J. Daly (Eds.), *Reinterpreting menopause: Cultural and philosophical issues* (pp. 176–199). New York: Routledge.

Hall, L. (1999, November–December). Taking charge of menopause. *FDA Consumer*, 17–21.

Harlow, S., Mitchell, E., Crawford, S., Nan, B., Little, R., & Taffe, J. (2008). The ReSTAGE collaboration: Defining optimal bleeding criteria for onset of early menopausal transition. *Fertility and Sterility, 89*, 129–140.

Hersh, A., Stefanick, M., & Stafford, R. (2004). National use of postmenopausal hormone therapy: Annual trends and response to recent evidence. *Journal of the American Medical Association, 291*, 47–53.

Hunter, M. & Mann, E. (2010). A cognitive model of menopausal hot flushes and night sweats. *Journal of Psychosomatic Research, 69*, 491–501.

Hyde, A., Nee, J., Howlett, E., Drennan, J., & Butler, M. (2010). Menopause narratives: The interplay of women's embodied experiences with biomedical discourses. *Qualitative Health Research, 20*, 805–815.

Innes, K., Selfe, T., & Vishnu, A. (2010). Mind-body therapies for menopausal symptoms: A systematic review. *Maturitas, 66*, 135–149.

Jarrell, A. (1999, November 28). Noticed; Models give aging a sexy new look. *New York Times.* Retrieved from http://www.nytimes.com/1999/11/28/style/noticed-models-defiantly-gray-give-aging-a-sexy-new-look.html.

Kafanelis, B. V., Kostanski, M., Komesaroff, P. A., & Stojanovska, L. (2009). Being in the script of menopause: Mapping the complexities of coping strategies. *Qualitative Health Research, 19*, 30–41.

Kaufert, P., & Gilbert, P. (1986). Women, menopause, and medicalization. *Culture, Medicine, and Psychiatry, 10*, 7–21.

Koeske, R. D. (1983). Lifting the curse of menstruation: Toward a feminist perspectives on the menstrual cycle. *Women & Health, 8*, 1–15.

Lock, M. (1986). Ambiguities of aging: Japanese experience and perceptions of menopause. *Culture, Medicine, and Psychiatry, 10*, 23–46.

Lock, M. (1993). *Encounters with aging: Mythologies of menopause in Japan and North America.* Berkeley: University of California Press.

Lonborg, S. D., & Travis, C. B. (2007). Living longer, healthier lives. In V. Muhlabuer & J. C. Chrisler (Eds.), *Women over 50: Psychological perspectives* (pp. 53–78). New York: Springer.

Low Dog, T. (2005). Menopause: A review of botanical dietary supplements. *American Journal of Medicine, 118*, 98S–108S.

Lyons, A. C., & Griffin, C. (2003). Managing menopause: A qualitative analysis of self-help literature for women at midlife. *Social Science & Medicine, 56*, 1629–1642.

Ma, J., Dreiling, R., & Stafford, R. S. (2006). US women desire greater professional guidance on hormone and alternative therapies for menopause symptom management. *Menopause, 13*, 506–516.

MacLennan, A. H. (2008). Hormone replacement therapy: A 2008 perspective. *Obstetrics, Gynaecology and Reproductive Medicine, 19*, 13–18.

MacPherson, K. (1981). Menopause as disease: The social construction of a metaphor. *Advanced in Nursing Research, 3*, 95–113.

Mansfield, P. K., Carey, M., Anderson, A., Barsom, S. H., & Koch, P. B. (2004). Staging the menopausal transition: Data from the Tremin research program on women's health. *Women's Health Issues, 14*, 220–226.

Mansfield, P. K., Koch, P. B., & Gierach, G. (2003). Husbands' support of their perimenopausal wives. *Journal of Women and Health, 38*, 97–112.

Manson, J., Hsia, J., Johnson, K., Rossouw, J., Assaf, A., Lasser, N., . . . Cushman, M.; Women's Health Initiative Investigators. (2003). Estrogen plus progestin and the risk of coronary heart disease. *New England Journal of Medicine, 349,* 523–534.

Martin, E. (1992). *The woman in the body: A cultural analysis of reproduction* (2nd ed.). Boston: Beacon Press.

McElmurry, B., & Huddleston, D. (1991). Self-care and menopause: Critical review of research. *Health Care for Women International, 12,* 15–26.

McHugh, M. C. (2007). Women and sex at midlife: Desire, dysfunction, and diversity. In V. Muhlbauer & J. C. Chrisler (Eds.), *Women over 50: Psychological perspectives* (pp. 26–52). New York: Springer.

Meyer, V. F. (2003). Medicalized menopause, U.S. style. *Health Care for Women International, 24,* 822–830.

Minkin, M. J., & Giblin, K. L. (2004). *Manual of management counseling for the perimenopausal and menopausal patient: A clinician's guide.* New York: Parthenon.

Muhlbauer, V., & Chrisler, J. C. (2007). Introduction. In V. Muhlbauer & J. C. Chrisler (Eds.), *Women over 50: Psychological perspectives* (pp. 1–5). New York: Springer.

Murtaugh, M. J., & Hepworth, J. (2003). Menopause as a long-term risk to health: Implications of general practitioner accounts of prevention for women's choice and decision-making. *Sociology of Health & Illness, 25,* 185–207.

National Committee for Quality Assurance. (2001). *HEDIS 2001: Specifications for survey measures* (vol. 3). Washington, DC: Author.

National Institutes of Health (NIH). (2005, March 21–23). NIH state-of-the-science conference statement on management of menopause-related symptoms. *NIH Consensus Statements Scientific Statements, 22,* 1–38.

Niland, P., & Lyons, A. C. (2011). Uncertainty in medicine: Meanings of menopause and hormone replacement therapy in medical textbooks. *Social Science & Medicine, 73,* 1238–1245.

Oakley, A. (1998). Science, gender, and women's liberation: An argument against postmodernism. *Women's Studies International Forum, 21,* 133–146.

Pace, D. T. (2006). Menopause: Studying the research. *Nurse Practitioner, 31,* 17–23.

Prior, J. (2005). Ovarian aging and the perimenopausal transition. *Endocrine, 26,* 297–300.

Reid, A. (2004). Gender and sources of subjective well-being. *Sex Roles, 51,* 617–629.

Reynolds, F. (1997). Psychological responses to menopausal hot flushes: Implications of a qualitative study for counseling interventions. *Counseling Psychology Quarterly, 10,* 309–321.

Riessman, C. K. (1983). Women and medicalization: A new perspective. *Social Policy, 14,* 3–18.

Rostosky, S., & Travis, C. (1996). Menopause research and the dominance of the biomedical model 1984–1994. *Psychology of Women Quarterly, 20,* 285–312.

Santoro, N. (2005). The menopausal transition. *American Journal of Medicine, 118,* 8S–13S.

Scheid, V., Ward, T., Cha, W., Watanabe, K., & Liao, X. (2010). The treatment of menopausal symptoms by traditional East Asian medicines: Review and perspectives. *Maturitas, 66,* 111–130.

Schwarzer, R., & Gutierrez-Dona, B. (2005). More spousal support for men than for women: A comparison of sources and types of support. *Sex Roles, 52,* 523–532.

Soules, M., Sherman, S., Parrott, E., Rebar, R., Santoro, N., Utian, W., & Woods, N. (2001). Stages of reproductive aging workshop (STRAW). *Journal of Women's Health and Gender-Based Medicine, 10,* 843–848.

Spake, A. (2004, March 15). The hormone conundrum. *U.S. News & World Report,* 60–63.

Taylor, H. S., & Manson, J. E. (2011). Update in hormone therapy use in menopause. *Journal of Clinical Endocrinology and Metabolism, 96,* 255–264.

Testerman, J. K., Morton, K. R., Mason, R. A., & Ronan, A. M. (2004). Patient motivations for using complementary and alternative medicine. *Complementary Health Practice Review, 9,* 81–92.

U.S. Food and Drug Administration. (2003). *Menopause and hormones.* Retrieved from http://www.fda.gov/womens/menopause/mht-FS.html.

Utz, R. L. (2011). Like mother, (not) like daughter: The social construction of menopause and aging. *Journal of Aging Studies, 25,* 143–154.

Vigeta, S. M. G., Hachul, H., Tufik, S., & de Oliveira, E. M. (2012). Sleep in postmenopausal women. *Qualitative Health Research, 22,* 466–475.

Voda, A. (1992). Menopause: A normal view. *Clinical Obstetrics and Gynecology, 35,* 923–933.

Walter, C. A. (2000). The psychosocial meaning of menopause: Women's experiences. *Journal of Women & Aging, 12,* 117–131.

Wasti, S., Robinson, S. C., Akhtar, Y., Khan, S., & Badaruddin, N. (1993). Characteristics of menopause in three socioeconomic groups in Karachi, Pakistan. *Maturitas, 16,* 61–69.

Weed, S. (1999). Menopause and beyond: The wise woman way. *Journal of Nurse-Midwifery, 44,* 267–279.

Wilbush, J. (1993). The climacteric kaleidoscope: Questions and speculations. *Maturitas, 16,* 157–162.

Williams, R. E., Kalilani, L., DiBenedetti, D. B., Zhou, X., Fehnel, S. E., & Clark, R. V. (2007). Healthcare seeking and treatment for menopausal symptoms in the United States. *Maturitas, 58,* 348–358.

Wilson, R. (1966). *Feminine forever.* New York: M. Evans/Lippincott.

Winterich, J., & Umberson, D. (1999). How women experience menopause: The importance of social context. *Journal of Women & Aging, 11,* 57–73.

Worcester, N., & Whatley, M. (1992). The selling of HRT: Playing on the fear factor. *Feminist Review, 41,* 1–27.

Zones, J. S. (2000). Beauty myths and realities and their impacts on women's health. In M. B. Zinn, P. Hondagneu-Sotelo, & M. Messner (Eds.), *Gender through the prism of difference* (2nd ed., pp. 87–103). Boston: Allyn and Bacon.

Chapter 6

Menopause and Sexuality: Resisting Representations of the Abject Asexual Woman

Jane M. Ussher, Janette Perz, and Chloe Parton

In Western cultures, the aging reproductive body is the epitome of the abject. Older women are all but invisible within cultural representations of idealized femininity, and silence surrounds women's embodied experiences of aging (Hillyer, 1998). When the menopausal or postmenopausal woman is represented, she is routinely shown as the crone, the hag, or the dried-up grandmother figure, her body covered, and her sexuality long left behind. If she *is* depicted as sexual, this in itself makes her an object of fascination because of the contradiction of age and sexuality; women who present a sexually desirable visage postmenopause apparently defy the ravages of time (Rostosky & Travis, 2000) or are caricatured as "cougars," their sexuality ridiculed and derided (McHugh & Interligi, 2015).

The master narrative of decline propagated by biomedicine reinforces this representation of the abject menopausal woman by positioning her as "suffering," "hormonal," "diseased," "abnormal," "asexual," and in need of treatment (Trethewey, 2001). It was the gynecologist Robert Wilson, in his highly influential book *Feminine Forever*, first published in 1966, who enshrined the myth of menopausal asexuality and deficiency as medical truth and normalized the practice of a medically managed midlife. Wilson described menopause thus: "No woman can escape the horror of this living decay . . . even the most valiant woman can no longer hide the fact that she is, in effect, no longer a woman . . . dowager's hump, ugly body contours, flaccidity of the breast, and atrophy of the genitals" manifest her sexual decline (p. 43). Reductions in estrogen at menopause were described by Wilson as stripping out the very essence of womanhood, and the replacement of the "lost" hormones was deemed the solution, because "women have a right to remain women. They should not have to live as sexual neuters for half their lives" (p. 25). Hormone replacement therapy (HRT; now known simply as hormone therapy [HT]) was thus recommended for all women as "menopause prevention" and to ensure that a woman was "capable of being physically and emotionally fulfilled by her husband or lover" (p. 65); HRT was said to produce a "sexually restored woman" (p. 65) and maintain her "total femininity" (p. 19).

Following Wilson's pronouncements, which were echoed in the mass media, women took to HT in droves. Prescriptions for HT in the United States tripled between 1967 and 1975 (Seaman & Seaman, 1975), and the myth of menopausal asexuality was born. However, Wilson's principal research, on which he based his book, was an uncontrolled study of 304 women, ages 40 to 70, who were taking HT (Ussher, 2006). When large-scale, randomized, controlled trials of HT were finally conducted in the United Kingdom (Beral, Banks, Bull, & Reeves, 2003) and the United States (Writing Group for the Women's Health Initiative Investigators, 2002) decades later, there was no evidence of HT having a significant positive effect on sexuality, but there was a significant increased risk of breast cancer (by 26%), heart disease (by 29%), and strokes (by 41%), and later research identified an increased risk of ovarian cancer (Beral & Million Women Study Collaborators, 2007). This led to a dramatic reduction in the numbers of women taking HT for "menopause prevention"; rates in the United Kingdom dropped from 2 million in 2002 to 1 million in 2005 (BBCNews, 2007), and in the United States from 28% to 12% to 17% (Kelly et al., 2005; Kim, Alley, Hu, Karlamangla, Seemsn, & Crimmins, 2007). Women were clearly making their own assessments of the risks and benefits of HT and determining their embodied experience for themselves without medical management (Lewin, Sinclair, & Bond, 2003), accepting menopause as a normal developmental phase that does not need to be "prevented."

What about Wilson's notion that menopause turns women into neuters, their sexuality stripped away by falling estrogen? The evidence is negligible. It is widely accepted that physical changes associated with sexual *functioning* do occur for many women postmenopause, including vaginal dryness, changes in sexual arousal, and reduced elasticity of the vagina, particularly after periods of sexual abstinence (Leiblum, 1990; Nappi & Lachowsky, 2009). These physical changes have been linked to alterations in sex steroids, autonomic nerves, and arterial flow to the genitals (Bachmann & Leiblum, 2004; Dennerstein, Lehert, Burger, & Guthrie, 2005). However, the evidence for a direct association between hormonal changes and sexual *desire, response,* or *activity* is unpersuasive, as no direct relation has ever been reported between hormonal changes and vaginal lubrication, sexual interest, or sexual activity (Avis, Stellato, Crawford, Johannes, & Longcope, 2000; Bancroft & Graham, 2011). Large-scale population studies suggest that women's sexual *activity* and *desire* do not inevitably decline with age; indeed, some women report improved sexual desire and functioning at midlife and beyond (Dennerstein, 1996; Dillaway, 2005; Hinchliff & Gott, 2008; Koch & Mansfield, 2002; Koch, Mansfield, Thurau, & Carey, 2005; Mansfield, Koch, & Voda, 1998). However, for some women, physical, psychological, and relational changes that happen during naturally occurring menopause (Cawood & Bancroft, 1996; Dennerstein et al., 2005; Koster & Garde, 1993; Osborn, Hawton, & Oath, 1988) or during early menopause induced by illnesses such as cancer (Gilbert, Ussher, & Perz, 2011) can have a dramatic effect on sexual desire and experience. But this is not because of hormonally induced "atrophy and decay."

This chapter presents a critical examination of the body of research on changes to sexuality during and after the menopausal transition. We challenge the biomedical model of sexual decline and deficiency, wherein women's sexuality is tied to an abject aging body, and normalize the physical changes that some women experience following menopause—whether menopause occurs early or at midlife. We argue that sexuality can continue to be a positive experience for women throughout adult life and into older age; however, the continuation of sexual desire and pleasure is a product of an interaction of embodied, cultural, and psychological factors. This includes the experience of embodied changes within the context of a woman's personal life circumstances; the influence of cultural representations of sex, aging, and menopause; and women's psychological negotiation of sex and bodily changes, which occur within a relational context.

We draw on a range of sources to substantiate our argument, including previously published research and theory on women's experiences of sexuality during menopause and beyond, interviews we have conducted with women at midlife, and two studies we have conducted on sexual changes after cancer, which draw upon accounts where early menopause was a consequence of cancer treatment (for details of the methodology of each study, see Parton, 2014; Perz & Ussher, 2008; Ussher, Perz, & Gilbert, 2012; Ussher, Perz, Gilbert, Wong, & Hobbs, 2013). Where our interview data have been published previously, we provide a direct reference for the quotes; in instances where no reference is provided, we are drawing on previously unpublished interview extracts that were collected as part of our research.

We begin with an examination of the psychological factors associated with sexuality during menopause, including the role of well-being and the negotiation of cultural representations of sex and menopause.

PSYCHOLOGICAL FACTORS: WELL-BEING AND CONSTRUCTIONS OF SEX AND MENOPAUSE

Sex is not simply a physical experience: A woman's feelings about herself and her psychological well-being can have a significant influence on her continued interest and engagement in sex at midlife (Cawood & Bancroft, 1996; Osborn et al., 1988). Indeed, psychological well-being is a more important predictor than hormonal status of sexual activity at midlife, with women who are experiencing psychological distress less likely to be interested in sex (Bancroft & Graham, 2011; Schnatz, Whitehurst, & O'Sullivan, 2010). It has previously been reported that mood is a more important predictor of women's sexual interest and arousal in midlife women than it is at a younger age (Graham, Sanders, Milhausen, & McBride, 2004), which suggests that depression experienced during menopause may have a greater effect on women's sexuality than it does at other times in life. However, menopause is not inevitably associated with reductions in psychological well-being, as a prior depressive episode is the strongest predictor of midlife depression (Avis, Brambilla, McKinlay, & Vass, 1994). Although women are more likely than men to experience depression at any time in the lifecycle (Ussher, 2011), the rates of depression actually *fall* with age: thus the notion of the menopausal woman being in a state of "psychological turmoil" that requires medical intervention (Wilson, 1966) is a myth. For example, in a study of 2,000 Australian women aged 45 to 55, participants reported that most of the time they felt clear-headed (72%), good natured (71%), useful (68%), satisfied (61%), confident (58%), loving (55%), and optimistic (51%) (Dennerstein, 1996). This is confirmed by a study of 103 women aged 40 to 59 living in New York, where the majority felt very happy (72%) and said that this time in their lives was not confusing (64%) (McQuaide, 1998). So mood may affect sexual desire, but most menopausal women feel good and many feel better than they did in their younger years (Perz & Ussher, 2008).

Constructions of Sex and Sexuality

Well-being is not the only psychological factor associated with sexuality during menopause. It has been reported that older women's attitudes toward sex are more important than "biomedical influences" in maintaining desire (DeLamater & Sill, 2005, p. 138). For example, in a longitudinal study of 602 midlife women, Thomas, Chang, Dillon, and Hess (2014) found that, although *believing* that sex is important was a significant predictor of continued sexual activity, sexual functioning was not, which suggests that "the quality of sex does not affect whether a woman will continue to have sex over time" (p. 633). There is consistent evidence that older women consider sex to be an important part of their lives and that a significant proportion continue to be sexually active as they age (Hinchliff & Gott, 2008; Nicolosi et al., 2006; Winn & Newton, 1982). Accounts of sex as important were common in our interviews with women, across both heterosexual and lesbian relationships: "Sex has always been important to me. I'm lucky my partner is still loving, patient, and supporting."

> While my partner has always been my love, she is very much the center of my life. We make more time in our life to have kisses, cuddles, and hold hands. I never leave the house without telling her "I love you." . . . Sexuality is important in my relationship to express my love and support for my beautiful woman.

There is another side to this issue, however. Women who consider sex to be important may experience distress following the embodied changes that can occur at menopause and the impact those changes had on their sexual response. In this vein, some of the women we interviewed variously described embodied sexual changes as "depressing," "confusing," "frustrating," and "demoralizing" (Ussher et al., 2013, p. 459). Some heterosexual women may continue to engage in sexual intercourse when they have little desire or pleasure because they view coital sex as important to their relationship (Jensen et al., 2004; Stephens, 2001). For example, a woman we interviewed said:

> I've had less than five orgasms in 12 months. . . . I worry about how my partner must feel as I struggle to appear interested when we have sex. We are close but I know he would like more from me.

This comment confirms previous accounts of heterosexual women who experience sex as a "nuisance" and "not pleasurable" after menopause, but feel that they "have to have it for your husband's sake" (Stephens, 2001, p. 661). Winterich (2003, p. 633) found that many midlife heterosexual women had internalized the notion of sex as intercourse, and, as a result, continued with sexual practices that were now painful because of their vaginal dryness. Those women were adhering to the coital imperative (McPhillips, Braun, & Gavey, 2001), which emphasizes penile–vaginal contact and positions women who cannot, or will not, engage in this practice as sexually dysfunctional (Tiefer, 2001) or as negating the needs of their men (Ayling & Ussher, 2008). The consequence of the coital imperative is that discussion of sexual discomfort or lack of interest is difficult, as coital sex is seen as central to heterosexual relationships and often defined as "real sex" (McPhillips et al., 2001), as well as something that men want and need (Hollway, 1989; Zilbergeld, 1992). In this vein, one of our participants told us that "it was harder for me to tell [him] about how painful it was when it was happening as I couldn't have sort of made him stop and say, 'This hurts me too much,' because I think he would have felt *really* bad about that." Conversely, the coital imperative can result in the cessation of sex if coital sex is avoided in the context of sexual discomfort following menopause. For example, one woman told us: "Because I don't want to have sexual intercourse, then it has stopped me doing all the other loving things, such as hugging, touching, teasing, in case they encourage him to want to go further. I do things like pretend to be asleep rather than have sex." If this couple had been able to explore noncoital sexual practices, they might have continued a sexual relationship in the absence of intercourse.

Sex is not always constructed as important. Some menopausal women have little interest in sex, and so they are not troubled by reductions in sexual desire or activity. As one of our interviewees, aged 55, described it, "I almost feel like sexless in a sense. I'd rather have a cup of tea and a book and be by myself." Other women in their mid-forties told us: "Being sexuality active or not does not define me or my relationship. It's just not that important to me anymore"; "I know my husband still loves me and cares for me. We are getting older and realize sex is not the most important thing in a relationship. We know we love each other no matter what happens." It has previously been reported that midlife and older women are less likely than younger women to be upset by changes in sexual desire (Bancroft, Loftus, & Long, 2003). Indeed, some women have reported that changes in sexual desire at midlife are positive things; in the case of one woman interviewed by Winterich and Umberson (1999), this was because she felt free of the sex drive that had previously dominated her life:

> It was absolutely wonderful because you finally get to a point of life where . . . your sex drive that drives you to distraction and it's just sort of like, you finally get to a point where you're really satisfied . . . you don't have to be distracted with other people (laughs)! (p. 70)

Similarly, one of the women we interviewed commented that she had made too many major life decisions in the past on the basis of romantic or sexual attraction; she now made decisions that suited herself: "When you're younger . . . there's that real primal looking for a partner thing. It's such a huge, about 50%, of your life, isn't it? All of that's gone now, and I can do what I really want to do, and that's one of the best things about middle age" (Ussher, 2006, p. 145). This puts Wilson's proclamations about sex and HT in perspective: Some midlife women do not want to be sexually "restored" and would avoid HT for this very reason: "And the thing they all talk about is how it (HT) really increases your sexual interest. It brings it back . . . and I just laughed, I said, 'Well, that's not a plus!'" (laughs) (Winterich & Umberson, 1999, p. 70).

Meaning of Menopause

The meaning of menopause to women can also influence their beliefs about and experience of embodied and sexual changes. For example, in a study of 474 Danish women, menopausal hormonal status did not predict a reduction in sexual desire; however, the *expectation* that menopause caused decreased sexuality did produce a reduction (Koster & Garde, 1993). As reported in previous research (Dillaway, 2005; Stephens, 2001; Winterich, 2003), some women we interviewed mentioned a sense of freedom at the end of menstruation and fertility, which was positive for their sexuality: "On the one hand it's relief [laughs] that stage is past and um, huge relief at not having to go through the monthly ritual of having a period anymore."

> In certain ways I think there's a lot of sexual freedom still comes with that next stage of your life. . . . You don't have to worry that if you happen to forget taking the pill or do something which you could end up pregnant at 48 years of age. I see a lot of freedom moving through this stage. (Ussher, 2006, p. 154)

In a similar vein, a woman interviewed by Dillaway (2005, p. 416) said: "Menopause [is] wonderful. It's like years ago, taking off your bra! No more Tampax." Midlife and menopause were thus conceptualized as positive experiences and associated with freedom, as many women we interviewed described themselves as "more confident sexually," having a "happy window," or feeling more "in tune with my body."

> Yes, you do feel much more free. You're so flat out fulfilling roles or playing parts I think when you're younger, sort of acting out a role, which is a bit crazy isn't it, and by the time you've lasted this long you don't find you've got to do any of those things.

Other women we talked to thought of menopause as a normal part of life and accepted the changes that accompanied it: "Midlife hasn't been a struggle because you just take what you've got and keep going." Expectations of menopause are frequently more negative than the reality (Hunter & O'Dea, 1997; Stephens, 2001), and many women are surprised to find that they do not conform to negative cultural constructions of menopausal women as "big, oldish grandmas" (Stephens, 2001, p. 658) or as having "wrinkly, short hair, everybody has their hair short and permed," as one of our participants commented.

However, for some women, the subjective experience of menopause, and the embodied changes that accompany it, can become the site for the body's "dys-appearance" (Leder, 1990, p. 106), as aspects of the body come into awareness because of changes or dysfunction (Gilbert, Ussher, & Perz, 2013). Thus, taken-for-granted sexual desire or response may come into consciousness for the first time because of its absence. This is illustrated in the following account from one of our participants, who described increased "awareness" of her body following menopause:

> It just goes back to the menopause thing the part of your body that was kind of active and informed you on a daily basis what it was up to and on a monthly basis what it was up to has gone silent. It's gone silent because it's not there. [Pause] a lot of people talk about the sense of reduced femaleness or something like that but I'm, not sure how I feel about that. I can understand that people might feel that way but, and there's a, sometimes a slight sense of it, but not a distressing sense of it. An *awareness* rather than an upset [our emphasis].

Although that awareness was not associated with distress in the account above, the dys-appearing body may be experienced negatively if menopause is premature, or medically induced (Nappi & Lachowsky, 2009), and therefore defies the boundaries of normality. For example, in a study of women who experienced menopause following hysterectomy, one woman described feeling as if she had a "black hole inside" that stopped her from wanting to "make love" (Pearce, Thøgersen-Ntoumani, Duda, & McKenna, 2014, p. 742). In our interviews with women who experienced early menopause following cancer treatment, we heard similar accounts: "Terrible! I am young and had not expected the side effects sexually that come from menopause and treatments . . . very sad"; "It was totally unexpected . . . made me feel that I had lost something very precious. I just wanted to be normal again" (Ussher et al., 2013, p. 460). This loss was described by one woman we interviewed as loss of "all the things that keep you going and feeling like you're a sexual *animal*." Other women reflected negatively on their fertility status, in line with previous reports that absence of fertility can impact self-identity and sexual relationships (Greil, Slauson-Blevins, & McQuillan, 2010; Perz, Ussher, & Gilbert, 2014). One woman told us, "Shit. I'm barren"; another said, "I don't like the sterility of it." For other women, menopause signifies being "old," which is experienced negatively: "I think I got quite caught up in the menopause, and the ovariectomy and that really impacted me a lot, sexually. . . . It's more just feeling old."

> Devastating. Devastating. I'm not ready to feel 80. I'm getting used to it now, it took me a little while, it just, yeah the whole [breathes],

the whole menopause thing I wasn't ready for menopause. It was devastating.

In combination, these accounts draw attention to the importance of self-perception of changes that occur during menopause and at midlife. For some women, menopause is embraced, and embodied changes are experienced as positive; for others who adopt a medicalized viewpoint or experience menopausal changes prematurely, menopause can signify loss and aging, and changes are experienced negatively. It is women's thoughts and feelings in the context of cultural representations of menopause that are at play here, not a woman's "faulty" body or her "raging hormones."

FEELING SEXY OR FRUMPY? BODY IMAGE AND THE MALE GAZE

Changes in skin tone and texture, changes in hair color and weight, and the development of wrinkles are another set of bodily changes that mark women's experience of aging, and these often become apparent around the time of menopause. These changes can have a significant influence on women's sexual desire and activity in a cultural context where the appearance of youth is associated with sexual attractiveness (McHugh & Interligi, 2015). Accepting the signs of an aging body and the development of a positive body image at midlife and beyond have been associated with continued sexual activity (Fooken, 1994) as well as greater sexual desire, response, and activity (Mansfield, Koch, & Voda, 2000). As two of our research participants told us: "I'm more comfortable with my body and self since the onset of menopause—I think because I'm on a big health kick and am in better shape than before—also less willing to let little things upset me, so if anything, our sexual relationship is better"; "my sexuality has changed for the better, I feel better about myself, more accepting of my body and sexuality." These comments confirm previous reports that between one-quarter and one-third of women feel more positive and comfortable in their bodies *after* menopause (Bellerose & Binik, 1993; Dillaway, 2005; Koch et al., 2005), which is associated with improved sexual enjoyment. As a woman interviewed by Dillway (2005, p. 407) commented, "I look in the mirror and I say, 'My, you've gotten sexier since you've gotten here [i.e., to this stage of life] (laugh). More sexy and more good looking." Another woman Dillaway interviewed said, "I am much more open than I used to be sexually (because) I don't give a shit anymore" (p. 408). This echoes the comments of a woman interviewed by Price (2006, p 46), who said that she felt "more free, adventurous, and open about what I want" sexually postmenopause.

There is evidence that many women experience less appearance anxiety and self-objectification as they age (Tiggemann & Lynch, 2001), as they construct alternative definitions of female beauty and attractiveness (Clarke,

2002) and as they experience incongruence between self-perceptions of the body and cultural norms (Banister, 1999). The relationship between self-perception of the body and sexual activity is circular, as sexually active women have also been reported to feel more sexually attractive (Bancroft et al., 2003). So maintaining a sexual relationship and feeling desired by a partner (Koch et al., 2005) can contribute positively to a woman's perception of her body and to her sexual desire at midlife. At the same time, sexual desire does not have to be present for women to feel attractive, as some women who report loss of sexual desire still feel positive about their bodies at midlife (Hinchliff, Gott, & Wylie, 2009).

At the same time, some women have been reported to attribute negative changes in sexual response at menopause to changed appearance (Mansfield et al., 2000), as reflected in comments by some of our research participants: "I've felt quite unattractive, I feel like I have no interest from my partner"; "I feel a lot less desirable and that affects my confidence hugely. It makes me avoid sex at times." Women's concerns about the aging body are not surprising; in a culture that values youth and beauty, changes to appearance over time signify mortality, disintegration, and decay, which lead to feelings of loss for the youthful body—even if a woman is comfortable with her midlife self. As one of our interviewees commented, "I look in the mirror and I can't believe that that same face is me. That wrinkled old lady type look. I don't feel that." In a study of postmenopausal women, aged 61 to 92, living in Canada, Clarke (2002) found that many women accepted wrinkles, describing them as "badges of merit" and an intrinsic part of their identities. However, this was not a universal view. For example, a Canadian woman interviewed by Banister (1999) commented, "Other women I know say, 'I've earned all the grey hair I have and I've earned every wrinkle.' I don't want to earn those things. Thank you very much!'" (p. 754).

Other women describe facial hair as a threat to femininity and sexuality, signifying a body that is out of control, or sexually undesirable, as is evidenced by the following accounts of our interviewees: "There's obviously issues around bone density, growing moley things with hair sprouting out of them on my face [laughs . . . laughs softly]"; "I would go with the menopause if it didn't make the hair grow on my face so much [laughing]" (Parton, 2014, p. 181). Many women are also unhappy about increased weight in later life. As one woman interviewed by Clarke (2002, p. 435) commented: "I especially don't like the fact that I'm fat . . . I don't even mind so much getting wrinkles, it's the fat that bothers me. It really does." This was also borne out by a number of our interviews: "I have to work harder to stay slim. I can't stand my spreading waistline."

But what has worried me for many, many years is the weight thing. I just can't seem to lose it and when I do I can't keep it off. I think it just must be in my genes to gain weight easily. That's really the only thing. Looking matronly, I don't want to. (Ussher, 2006, p. 151)

In their longitudinal study of midlife women, Thomas and colleagues (2014) reported that lower body mass index was one of two predictors of continued sexual activity; the other was viewing sex as important, as discussed above. This suggests that increased body weight, as well as perceptions of weight gain, can influence women's sexuality.

One of the consequences of the physical changes that begin in midlife and continue as women age is that women can no longer meet gendered beauty ideals (Dillaway, 2005), and, as a result, they can experience a movement toward the margins of sexual desirability. The shift from visible to invisible at midlife was illustrated in the comment by one American woman: "I remember when I was younger having a flat tire on the highway. I can't tell you how many cars stopped to help me. . . . Five years ago I had a flat, and they just whizzed by" (Kagawa-Singer et al., 2002, p. 79). Concerns about the aging body can be experienced by both heterosexual and lesbian women (McHugh & Interligi, 2015), but there is some evidence that lesbians are less dissatisfied with their bodies than heterosexual women and less concerned about being rejected by a female partner due to aging (Sharp, 1997; Winterich, 2007). This suggests that it is invisibility in relation to the "male gaze" (Berger, 1979) that can result in anxiety for women who want to maintain their position as an object of the sexual interest of men. For example:

I worry that as I become more obviously older—if my skin changes and I if I don't continue to die my hair—will men see me as a sexual object? Will P. (her partner) stop finding me attractive? If I am really in the final stages of menopause and no longer menstruating, would he find me unattractive? Would that turn him off? I do think about that. But I don't feel that change. I worry about—is it going to be projected onto me—but it's not that I feel it. (Jones, 1994, p. 55)

This woman was not saying that she feels less attractive, but that she worries she will be *seen* as less attractive by her partner, as no longer a "sex object." This may be at odds with what her partner actually thinks. In a study of the relational context of body image, Markey, Markey, and Birch (2004) found that women *thought* their husbands were much more dissatisfied with their bodies than the husbands actually were. In our own research, many women reported that they were concerned about weight gain or other bodily changes after menopause, but that their partners had reassured them that they were still attractive: "My partner tells me I am beautiful, and so I have to believe it"; "I was worried my partner would not find me attractive after menopause, but it has strengthened our relationship and made me feel more confident sexually and physically that he obviously does find me attractive." Others felt invisible in relation to the male gaze but were untroubled by it: "Men might not look at me anymore, but I feel great in myself, more sexy in fact, which is such an irony, isn't it?" (Ussher, 2006, p. 157).

However, the fact that this invisibility *can* be experienced as an annihilation of the self is evidenced by the comments of two of our interviewees:

> Yes, after the age of 40 I noticed that I became invisible to men and I'd heard about that and I thought, well I don't really care because I'm married anyway, I shouldn't care, but I do care. I still want to be attractive to men, I still want men to notice me, I want men to try and get onto me. . . . And for some reason they just don't, especially men my age or older. You see them looking through you to the young babe behind you, the young 20 year olds and probably even up to 30 year olds, and it's the most horrible feeling. (Ussher, 2006, p. 148)
>
> And I'd love to think that I could pull the guys still because I had no trouble when I was younger. I think if I went out to a night-club now I'd just be sitting there like a shag on a rock and no one would come up to me. Maybe a 70-year-old guy would. (Ussher, 2006, p. 149)

These accounts confirm previous reports that many women are still affected by cultural notions of beauty and desirability as they age, despite the silence that surrounds older women's sexuality in cultural discourse (Dillaway, 2005; Hillyer, 1998). However, these changes in appearance that women report are not due to the biological event of menopause, rather, they are due to the aging process—as premenopausal women at midlife have been found to report similar concerns about the aging body (Giesen, 1989). This has led to the conclusion that sociocultural factors, in particular ageism and sexism, play a more important role in determining body image at midlife than do the physiological changes of menopause (Koch et al., 2005). The importance of the interpretation of midlife invisibility in specific cultural contexts was highlighted in the comparative study of Japanese and American women conducted by Kagawa-Singer et al. (2002). Although both groups of women reported feeling invisible, only the American women experienced this as negative and felt that their identity was being invalidated. In contrast, the Japanese women saw invisibility as a desirable objective, a valued state of being, which allowed them to be freed of their obligations as wives and mothers and able to express their creative desires in ways that were more "transparent," "invisible," or "pure" (Kagawa-Singer et al., 2002, p. 84). In a study of Rajput women in northern India, a context where women emerge from Purdah and move freely about their village at midlife, no longer being seen as a sex object, menopause was found to be experienced as a positive, symptom-free experience (Flint & Samil, 1990).

DESIRE OR DIFFICULTY? THE RELATIONAL CONTEXT OF SEXUALITY AT MIDLIFE

Biomedical models implicitly conceptualize women's sexuality at midlife as an individual experience, located in the workings of the (dys)functional body, but feminist critics argue that women's experience of menopausal embodiment and sexuality is located in the social and relational context of their lives (Dillaway, 2008; Koch et al., 2005; Stephens, 2001). This is a viewpoint shared by many midlife women who conceptualize desire in the context of their intimate relationship (Goldhammer & McCabe, 2011) and attribute sexual changes that occur at menopause to their relationship (Dillaway, 2005; Hyde, Nee, Drennan, Butler, & Howlett, 2011). It is also supported by empirical research, which shows that the presence of a sexual partner is a significant predictor of women's desire in later life (DeLamater & Sill, 2005) and that the quality of a sexual relationship is a more important predictor than hormonal status of continued engagement and enjoyment of sex (Cawood & Bancroft, 1996; Dennerstein et al., 2005; Osborn et al., 1988).

Relationship factors can influence women's sexuality at menopause in a number of ways—both positively and negatively. Relationship change, such as entering into a new relationship (Dennerstein, 1996; Hinchliff, Gott, & Ingleton, 2010; Winterich, 2003), children leaving home, or improvement in positive feelings toward a partner (Dennerstein et al., 2005; Koch & Mansfield, 2002), have been associated with renewed sexual activity for women. As one 54-year-old woman told us, "My new partner has commented that we have the best sex he has had." Another 53-year-old said that her "husband was generally not interested in sex," but her "new partner was much more interested in sex" and it was "very good." A 60-year-old woman interviewed by Winterich (2003) described having had a low libido with her ex-husband "because he was a bad lover . . . with no skill at all," but in her new sexual relationship with a woman "the drive came back to active levels again" (p. 636). This confirms the notion that many women have responsive sexual desire, which is triggered by sexual interaction with a partner, rather than a stable trait within the woman herself (Bancroft & Graham, 2011). Feeling desired by a partner is thus central to many women's sexual desire (Graham et al., 2004), and the desire to be desired is often difficult to distinguish from the desire to have sex (Meana, 2010). In our research, we found evidence that partner desire is the reason why many women were continuing to enjoy sexual activity following menopause; as one woman said, "Your partner's response affects yours."

Others told us: "He shows he loves me more often, both in and out of the bedroom"; "My husband still loves me and desires me so that has made me feel appreciated by him and I love him even more." These accounts illustrate the way that a partner's response can influence how a woman feels about herself, with positive consequences for sexual desire and response.

At the same time, being in a long-term relationship is a predictor of decreased sexual activity, regardless of age (Dennerstein et al., 2005; McCabe & Goldhammer, 2012). As a high percentage of menopausal women are in long-term relationships, overfamiliarity, institutionalization of the relationship, and couples adopting desexualized roles all may contribute to any sexual changes that occur (Meana, 2010). One 49-year-old woman we interviewed adopted such an explanation to describe her acceptance of sexual changes after menopause:

> Well, that's right, you just accept the [sexual] changes and that and how things are. If you were in a new relationship, you'd be bonking every day but you know, when you've been together 35 years, you don't need to do it every day. I wouldn't want to [laughter].

However, this is not to suggest that long-term relationships are inevitably asexual. A number of large-scale population studies of midlife women have reported *no* reduction in sexual interest or activity for the majority of participants, regardless of relationship length (Dennerstein, 1996; Koch & Mansfield, 2002; Thomas et al., 2014). This is illustrated by the comment of one of our 66-year-old interviewees who told us that she still experienced sexual interest and desire after 30 years of marriage and described herself and her husband as "rutting rabbits." Other women described having experienced "greater understanding," "more love and comfort," and "greater intimacy" over time in their relationships, which had a positive impact on their sexual desire.

A partner's negative response to embodied changes experienced during or after menopause can impact a woman's response to these changes, as well as her level of sexual desire and activity. For example, some women we interviewed told us that their relationship had experienced difficulty, or broken down, following embodied sexual changes that resulted from early menopause. Comments included: "It was all very difficult, and placed a big strain on my relationship"; "My husband did not react well and subsequently left" (Ussher et al., 2012, p. 462). Having previously had sexual difficulties made continued sexual activity in the face of embodied change less likely, as one of our participants commented:

> Our sex life was not great before—now it is nonexistent. Despite trying to still see myself as [a] normal sexual being, the "closed door"

attitude of my partner has hurt me and I now struggle with my self-esteem—I am now 68, but still, I am told, an attractive woman. I find it very hard to retain this belief at times.

Sexual problems experienced by male partners (Deeks & McCabe, 2001; Hinchliff et al., 2010) have also been associated with women's decreased sexual interest or activity at midlife. Rates of men's erectile difficulties increase with age (DeLamater & Sill, 2005) and can result in the cessation of sex in heterosexual couples, as a number of our participants commented: "My husband's had a lot of problems with it, with getting an erection, so our sex life is over"; "His testosterone levels have dropped to pretty well much nothing and he just can't get an erection, so there's no, we haven't had sex for about two, two and a half years." These women *were* experiencing reductions in sexual activity at midlife—but it had nothing to do with the loss of their own "raging hormones," rather it had to do with their male partner's embodied changes.

Renegotiation of Sexuality: A Relational Experience

A couple's communication and the ability to explore a range of sexual practices in the face of embodied changes that may occur during or after menopause are key to maintaining sexual activity (Winterich, 2003). Many women we interviewed reported renegotiation of sexual activities to minimize pain or discomfort caused by vaginal dryness or in response to their partner's erectile dysfunction (Gilbert et al., 2013; Ussher et al., 2013). Their accounts confirm previous reports of some women who prefer to engage in noncoital sexual activities after menopause because of sexual discomfort (Mansfield et al., 1998; Winterich, 2003) and suggest that the "coital imperative" can be resisted and the meaning of "sex" redefined to encompass noncoital sex, intimacy, and other activities normally positioned outside of the sexual domain (Ussher et al., 2013). For example, many women described engaging in noncoital genital contact after menopause, such as mutual masturbation and oral sex, sometimes describing it as like "being teenagers again" (Ussher et al., 2013, p. 457); "Learning different techniques on how to do hand jobs and, and just things like that is interesting and fun, and our sex life is very good."

> We were like, oh, two puppies playing together, even though I'm 59 and he's 74. And even sort of simulated sex we'd get on top of each other and not actually have sex but, you know, sort of loving each other in a sex position. (Ussher, Perz, & Gilbert, 2014, p. 213)

One 49-year-old woman told us that she had initially bought a vibrator to "keep all the (vaginal) muscles working" (Ussher et al., 2013, p. 458), but that she and her husband also "had a bit of fun with it and now and again I'd think through the day, 'Oh, I should go and do that.'" Other women described developing a focus on nongenital intimacy, including accounts of more cuddling, kissing, massage, and touching following menopause: "Well, I guess we sleep together, so that's a good thing [chuckles], and cuddle up, and touch, and that sort of thing is always good."

> If he passes me in the kitchen or in the house somewhere he'll just put his hand out, or sometimes in the car he just puts his hand out and touches my leg or something like that. There's, there's a great sense of, it's a tactile relationship, even though the, that strong physical urges aren't there.

Partner response was key to this renegotiation, and a number of our participants told us that they discussed noncoital sexual practices with their partner: "[he said] I'm just there when, you know, I'm ready to just go along with what you, your needs are, as well as my own."

> We were looking at a different version of a sex life than what we would have had in the past or would have wanted in the past. And maybe the fact that I went through menopause and had started to accept the fact that, that physical sex, penetration, all those things were just not there as much as they had been or nor did I want them as much as I had.

Women in lesbian relationships have been reported to be more able to discuss the impact of bodily changes at midlife on their sexuality (Winterich, 2003) and to negotiate different ways of pleasuring each other, largely because they shared a broader definition of "sex," which is not tied to penetration. In our research, we found that lesbian participants were more likely to report renegotiating sexual activities following vaginal dryness that accompanied menopause. As one woman told us:

> We tend to be very open communicators in the bedroom. We're also probably on the fringe of on the top echelon of wanting to explore and to try different things. So we'll see, we tend to see if a) does it work, b) does it feel good, c) if both a and b work well that's great. If A and B don't work well then we don't do that one again. We stop. (Ussher et al., 2014, p. 214)

Similarly, a woman interviewed by Winterich (2003), whose partner experienced vaginal dryness that made her sensitive to touch, said "There are moments when we can be really loving . . . but we're just not at the point of orgasm all the time" (p. 638).

In combination, these accounts suggest that biomedical research that focuses on coital sexual functioning and uses engagement in coital sex as a primary indicator of sexual activity is producing only a partial and distorted picture of women's sexuality after menopause. It also demonstrates that women are able to adopt nonmedical strategies to address any embodied changes experienced by themselves, or their partner, including challenging the very definition of "sex" and exploring a range of sexual activities. Nevertheless, coital sex is important to many women, and a number of women have described overcoming changes in vaginal lubrication through the use of topical hormonal cream or lubricants (Dillaway, 2005; Hyde et al., 2011). For example, two women we interviewed said: "I use this local hormonal cream, which is not a lubricant but it just helps to reduce the dryness"; "I had suppositories as well, to make me more wet." These accounts do not imply that women are internalizing a biomedical view of the menopausal body, however, because these interviewees are not attempting to "prevent" menopause or describing their bodies as dysfunctional. Rather, they are living proof that women can continue to desire and enjoy sex at menopause and beyond, and that they can utilize topical aids to assist with their sexual pleasure and functioning.

CONCLUSION

It is important to acknowledge the embodied changes that many women experience during and after menopause. However, such changes need not be problematic or have any effect on women's sexual desire or activity. It is the cultural context within which such changes are experienced, and the meaning given to them by the woman and her partner (based on gendered discourses of sex and aging), that will determine whether the changes are seen as "symptoms" and whether they have a negative impact on sexual desire or activity. Women's interpretation of this cultural context also determines whether or not they adopt a biomedical model in understanding their experiences, and thus turn to HT as a "cure," or whether they embrace any changes as part of this period of life and either renegotiate sex or accept a changed sexual life. Some women experience increased sexual desire and pleasure during menopause and feel more positive and confident in their bodies. Other women experience acute loss about embodied changes and changes to their sexual life. However, it is not menopause that is the source of their distress, rather, it is representations of the abject, aging woman and the narrow constructions of heterosex that lead to invisibility and dysfunction. These are ideas that women can resist in order to enjoy a positive sexual life at menopause and beyond—if sex is something that they want.

Recognizing embodied change during menopause, as well as the impact of such change on sexuality, does not inevitably lead to a medicalized solution for those who wish to ameliorate women's distress. There is a growing body of self-help literature (e.g., Boston Women's Health Book Collective, 2006; Brayne, 2012) that normalizes and provides holistic advice about menopausal changes, including nonmedical solutions that women can adopt. In our own research, we have found that providing women with information about sexual changes that occur after cancer-induced menopause, as well as strategies for exploring noncoital sex (e.g., oral sex, massage, mutual masturbation, sex toys), was effective in increasing sexual satisfaction, facilitating couples' communication about sex, and normalizing sexual changes (Perz, Ussher, & the Australian Cancer and Sexuality Study Team, forthcoming). This information was effective when it was provided in either a self-help written form (Centre for Health Research, 2010) or through a one-off session of counseling that accompanied the written information. Cognitive behavior therapy, with a focus on challenging negative thoughts about menopausal changes and developing positive self-care strategies, is also effective in reducing women's distress (Hunter, 2012). This suggests that psychoeducational or counseling interventions can be beneficial in addressing embodied changes that may impact sexuality at menopause, if they operate within a sex-positive approach that emphasizes older women's agency (McHugh & Interligi, 2015) rather than a medicalized model of deficit and decay. There is also consistent evidence that exercise is a positive strategy for maintaining women's physical and psychological well-being (Reed et al., 2014; Woods, 2014) and alleviating embodied sexual changes during menopause (Dbrowska, Droszdzol, Skrzypulec, & Plinta, 2010; Duijts et al., 2012; Lara et al., 2012). These strategies do not conceptualize menopause as a pathological state that needs to be prevented or treated; rather, they help women to live with, and accept, the menopausal body and even embrace the changes that midlife brings. This can lead to a positive experience of sexual embodiment:

> I feel as if I've finally come alive after fifty years of living in a daze. I am so *in* my body these days—not looking at it from the outside with a critical eye, but really in it, inhabiting myself for the first time. I feel so strong and free as a result, as if I could do anything. (Ussher, 2006, p. 160)

This is as far from Wilson's notion of menopausal "atrophy and decay" as could be imagined.

REFERENCES

Avis, N., Brambilla, D., McKinlay, S. M., & Vass, K. (1994). A longitudinal analysis of the association between menopause and depression. Results from the Massachusetts Women's Health Study. *Annals of Epidemiology, 4*(3), 214–220.

Avis, N. E., Stellato, R., Crawford, S., Johannes, C., & Longcope, C. (2000). Is there an association between menopause status and sexual functioning? *Menopause, 7*(5), 297–309.

Ayling, K., & Ussher, J. M. (2008). "If sex hurts, am I still a woman?" The subjective experience of vulvodynia in hetero-sexual women. *Archives of Sexual Behavior, 37*(2), 294–304.

Bachmann, G. A., & Leiblum, S. R. (2004). The impact of hormones on menopausal sexuality: A literature review. *Menopause, 11*(1), 120–130.

Bancroft, J., & Graham, C. A. (2011). The varied nature of women's sexuality: Unresolved issues and a theoretical approach. *Hormones and Behavior, 59*(5), 717–729.

Bancroft, J., Loftus, J., & Long, J. S. (2003). Distress about sex: A national survey of women in heterosexual relationships. *Archives of Sexual Behavior, 32*(3), 193–208.

Banister, E. M. (1999). Women's midlife experience of their changing bodies. *Qualitative Health Research, 9*(4), 520–537.

BBCNews. (2007). HRT linked to ovarian cancer. Retrieved from http://news.bbc .co.uk/1/hi/health/6182445.stm.

Bellerose, S., & Binik, Y. (1993). Body image and sexuality in oophorectomized women. *Archives of Sexual Behavior, 22*(5), 435–459.

Beral, V., Banks, E., Bull, D., & Reeves, G. (2003). Breast cancer and hormone replacement therapy in the million women study. *Lancet, 362*(9382), 419–447.

Beral, V., & Million Women Study Collaborators. (2007). Ovarian cancer and hormone replacement therapy in the million women study. *Lancet, 369*(9547), 1703–1710.

Berger, J. (1979). *Ways of seeing*. London: Penguin.

Boston Women's Health Book Collective. (2006). *Our bodies, ourselves: Menopause*. New York: Simon and Schuster.

Brayne, S. (2012). *Sex, meaning and the menopause*. London: Continuum.

Cawood, E. H. H., & Bancroft, J. (1996). Steroid hormones, the menopause, sexuality and well-being of women. *Psychological Medicine, 26*(05), 925–936.

Centre for Health Research. Univeristy of Western Sydney. (2010). *Sexuality, intimacy and cancer: A self-help guide for people with cancer and their partner*. Retrieved from http://www.uws.edu.au/chr/centre_for_health_research /research/cancer_and_sexuality

Clarke, L. H. (2002). Beauty in later life: Older women's perceptions of physical attractiveness. *Canadian Journal on Aging, 21*(3), 429–442.

Dbrowska, J., Drosdzol, A., Skrzypulec, V., & Plinta, R. (2010). Physical activity and sexuality in perimenopausal women. *European Journal of Contraception and Reproductive Health Care, 15*(6), 423–432.

Deeks, A. A., & McCabe, M. (2001). Sexual function and the menopausal woman: The importance of age and partner's sexual function. *Journal of Sex Research, 38*(3), 219–225.

DeLamater, J. D., & Sill, M. (2005). Sexual desire in later life. *Journal of Sex Research*, 42(2), 138–149.

Dennerstein, L. (1996). Well-being, symptoms and the menopausal transition. *Maturitas*, 23, 147–157.

Dennerstein, L., Lehert, P., Burger, H., & Guthrie, J. (2005). Sexuality. *American Journal of Medicine*, 118(12, Suppl 2), 59–63.

Dillaway, H. E. (2005). Menopause is the "good old": Women's thoughts about reproductive aging. *Gender & Society*, 19(3), 398–417.

Dillaway, H. E. (2008). "Why can't you control this?" How women's interactions with intimate partners define menopause and family. *Journal of Women & Aging*, 20(1–2), 47–64.

Duijts, S. F. A., Van Beurden, M., Oldenburg, H. S. A., Hunter, M. S., Kieffer, J. M., Stuiver, M. M., . . . Aaronson, N. K. (2012). Efficacy of cognitive behavioral therapy and physical exercise in alleviating treatment-induced menopausal symptoms in patients with breast cancer: Results of a randomized, controlled, multicenter trial. *Journal of Clinical Oncology*, 30(33), 4124–4133.

Flint, M., & Samil, R. S. (1990). Cultural and subcultural meanings of the menopause. In M. Flint, F. Kronenberg & W. Utian (Eds.), *Multi-disciplinary perspectives on menopause* (pp. 134–197). New York: Annals of New York Academy of Sciences.

Fooken, I. (1994). Sexuality in the later years—the impact of health and body-image in a sample of older women. *Patient Education and Counseling*, 23(3), 227–233.

Giesen, C. B. (1989). Aging and attractiveness: Marriage makes a difference. *International Journal of Aging & Human Development*, 29(2), 83–94.

Gilbert, E., Ussher, J. M., & Perz, J. (2011). Sexuality after gynaecological cancer: A review of the material, intrapsychic, and discursive aspects of treatment on women's sexual-wellbeing. *Maturitas*, 70(1), 42–57.

Gilbert, E., Ussher, J. M., & Perz, J. (2013). Embodying sexual subjectivity after cancer: A qualitative study of people with cancer and intimate partners. *Psychology & Health*, 28(6), 603–619.

Goldhammer, D. L., & McCabe, M. P. (2011). A qualitative exploration of the meaning and experience of sexual desire among partnered women. *Canadian Journal of Human Sexuality*, 20(1–2), 19.

Graham, C. A., Sanders, S. A., Milhausen, R. R., & McBride, K. R. (2004). Turning on and turning off: A focus group study of the factors that affect women's sexual arousal. *Archives of Sexual Behavior*, 33(6), 527–538.

Greil, A. L., Slauson-Blevins, K., & McQuillan, J. (2010). The experience of infertility: A review of recent literature. *Sociology of Health & Illness*, 32(1), 140–162.

Hillyer, B. (1998). The embodiment of old women: Silences. *Frontiers*, 19(1), 48.

Hinchliff, S., & Gott, M. (2008). Challenging social myths and stereotypes of women and aging: Heterosexual women talk about sex. *Journal of Women & Aging*, 20(1–2), 65–81.

Hinchliff, S., Gott, M., & Ingleton, C. (2010). Sex, menopause and social context: A qualitative study with heterosexual women. *Journal of Health Psychology, 15*(5), 724–733.

Hinchliff, S., Gott, M., & Wylie, K. (2009). Holding onto womanhood: A qualitative study of heterosexual women with sexual desire loss. *Health, 13*(4), 449–465.

Hollway, W. (1989). *Subjectivity and method in psychology: gender, meaning and science.* London: Sage.

Hunter, M., & O'Dea, I. (1997). Menopause: Body changes and multiple meanings. In J. M. Ussher (Ed.), *Body talk: The material and discursive construction of sexuality, madness and reproduction* (pp. 199–222). London: Routledge.

Hunter, M. S. (2012). Cognitive behavioral interventions for the treatment of menopausal symptoms. *Expert Review of Obstetrics & Gynecology, 7*(4), 321.

Hyde, A., Nee, J., Drennan, J., Butler, M., & Howlett, E. (2011). Women's accounts of heterosexual experiences in the context of menopause. *International Journal of Sexual Health, 23*(3), 210–223.

Jensen, P. T., Groenvold, M., Klee, M. C., Thranov, I., Petersen, M. A., & Machin, D. (2004). Early-stage cervical carcinoma, radical hysterectomy, and sexual function. *Cancer, 100*(1), 97–106.

Jones, J. (1994). Embodied meaning: Menopause and the change of life. *Social Work in Health Care, 19*(3–4), 43–65.

Kagawa-Singer, M., Wu, K., Kawanishi, Y., Greendale, G. A., Kim, S., Adler, S. R., & Wongvipat, N. (2002). Comparison of the menopause and midlife transition between Japanese American and European American women. *Medical Anthropology Quarterly, 16*(1), 64–91.

Kelly, J. P., Kaufman, D. W., Rosenberg, L., Kelley, K., Cooper, S. G., & Mitchell, A. A. (2005). Use of postmenopausal hormone therapy since the Women's Health Initiative findings. *Pharmacoepidemiology and Drug Safety, 14,* 837–842.

Kim, K. J., Alley, D., Hu, P., Karlamangla, A., Seeman, T., & Crimmins, E. M. (2007). Changes in postmenopausal hormone therapy use since 1988. *Women's Health Issues, 17,* 338–341.

Koch, P. B., & Mansfield, P. K. (2002). Women's sexuality as they age: The more things change, they more they stay the same. *SIECUS Report, 30*(2), 5–9.

Koch, P. B., Mansfield, P. K., Thurau, D., & Carey, M. (2005). "Feeling frumpy": The relationships between body image and sexual response changes in midlife women. *Journal of Sex Research, 42*(3), 215–223.

Koster, A., & Garde, K. (1993). Sexual desire and menopausal development. A prospective study of Danish women born in 1936. *Maturitas, 16,* 49–60.

Lara, L. A. D. S., Montenegro, M. L., Franco, M. M., Abreu, D. C. C., Rosa e Silva, A. C. J. D. S., & Ferreira, C. H. J. (2012). Is the sexual satisfaction of postmenopausal women enhanced by physical exercise and pelvic floor muscle training? *Journal of Sexual Medicine, 9*(1), 218–223.

Leder, D. (1990). *The absent body.* Chicago: University of Chicago Press.

Leiblum, S. R. (1990). Sexuality and the midlife woman. *Psychology of Women Quarterly, 14,* 495–508.

Lewin, K. J., Sinclair, H. K., & Bond, C. M. (2003). Women's knowledge and attitudes towards hormone replacement therapy. *Family Practice, 20,* 112–119.

Mansfield, P. K., Koch, P. B., & Voda, A. M. (1998). Qualities midlife women desire in their sexual relationships and their changing sexual response. *Psychology of Women Quarterly, 22*(2), 285–303.

Mansfield, P. K., Koch, P. B., & Voda, A. M. (2000). Midlife women's attributions for their sexual response changes. *Health Care for Women International, 21*(6), 543–559.

Markey, C., Markey, P., & Birch, L. (2004). Understanding women's body satisfaction: The role of husbands. *Sex Roles, 51*(3), 209–216.

McCabe, M. P., & Goldhammer, D. L. (2012). Demographic and psychological factors related to sexual desire among heterosexual women in a relationship. *Journal of Sex Research, 49*(1), 78–87.

McHugh, M., & Interligi, C. (2015). Sexuality and older women: Desirability and desire. In V. Muhlbauer, J. C. Chrisler, & F. L. Denmark (Eds.), *Women and aging: An international, intersectional power perspective* (pp. 89–116). New York: Springer.

McPhillips, K., Braun, V., & Gavey, N. (2001). Defining (hetero)sex: How imperative is the coital imperative? *Women's Studies International Forum, 24,* 229–240.

McQuaide, S. (1998). Women at midlife. *Social Work, 43*(1), 21–31.

Meana, M. (2010). Elucidating women's (hetero)sexual desire: Definitional challenges and content expansion. *Journal of Sex Research, 47*(2–3), 104–122.

Nappi, R. E., & Lachowsky, M. (2009). Menopause and sexuality: Prevalence of symptoms and impact on quality of life. *Maturitas, 63*(2), 138–141.

Nicolosi, A., Laumann, E., Glasser, D., Brock, G., King, R., & Gingell, C. (2006). Sexual activity, sexual disorders and associated help-seeking behavior among mature adults in five Anglophone countries from the Global Servey of Sexual Attitudes and Behaviors (GSSAB). *Journal of Sex & Marital Therapy, 32*(4), 331–342.

Osborn, M., Hawton, K., & Oath, D. (1988). Sexual dysfunction among middle aged women in the community. *British Medical Journal, 296,* 959–962.

Parton, C. (2014). *Women's experiences of sexual embodiment in the context of cancer.* Unpublished Ph.D. thesis, University of Western Sydney.

Pearce, G., Thøgersen-Ntoumani, C., Duda, J. L., & McKenna, J. (2014). Changing bodies: Experiences of women who have undergone a surgically induced menopause. *Qualitative Health Research, 24*(6), 738–748.

Perz, J., & Ussher, J. M. (2008). The horror of this living decay: Women's negotiation and resistance of medical discourses around menopause and midlife. *Women's Studies International Forum, 31,* 293–299.

Perz, J., Ussher, J. M., & the Australian Cancer and Sexuality Study Team. (forthcoming). A randomised trial of a minimal intervention for sexual concerns after cancer: A comparison of self-help and professionally delivered modalities [under review].

Perz, J., Ussher, J., & Gilbert, E. (2014). Loss, uncertainty, or acceptance: Subjective experience of changes to fertility after breast cancer. *European Journal of Cancer Care, 23*(4), 514–522.

Price, J. (2006). *Better than I ever expected: Straight talk about sex after sixty.* Emeryville, CA: Seal Press.

Reed, S. D., Guthrie, K. A., Newton, K. M., Anderson, G. L., Booth-Laforce, C., Caan, B., . . . Lacroix, A. Z. (2014). Menopausal quality of life: RCT of yoga, exercise, and omega-3 supplements. *American Journal of Obstetrics and Gynecology, 210*(3), 244.e241–244.e211.

Rostosky, S. S., & Travis, C. B. (2000). Menopause and sexuality: Ageism and sexism unite. In C. B. Travis & J. W. White (Eds.), *Sexuality, society, and feminism* (pp. 181–209). New York: American Psychological Association.

Schnatz, P. F., Whitehurst, S. K., & O'Sullivan, D. M. (2010). Sexual dysfunction, depression, and anxiety among patients of an inner-city menopause clinic. *Journal of Women's Health, 19*(10), 1843–1849.

Seaman, B., & Seaman, G. (1975). *Women and the crisis in sex hormones.* New York: Bantam.

Sharp, C. E. (1997). Lesbianism and later life in an Australian sample: How does development of one affect anticipation of the other? *Journal of Gay, Lesbian and Bisexual Identity, 2*(3–4), 247–263.

Stephens, C. (2001). Women's experience at the time of menopause: Accounting for biological, cultural and psychological embodiment. *Journal of Health Psychology, 6*(6), 651–663.

Thomas, H. N., Chang, C. H., Dillon, S., & Hess, R. (2014). Sexual activity in midlife women: Importance of sex matters. *JAMA Internal Medicine, 174*(4), 631–633.

Tiefer, L. (2001). The selling of "female sexual dysfunction." *Journal of Sex and Marital Therapy, 27*(5), 625–628.

Tiggemann, M., & Lynch, J. E. (2001). Body image across the life span in adult women: The role of self-objectification. *Developmental Psychology, 37*(2), 243–253.

Trethewey, A. (2001). Reproducing and resisting the master narrative of decline: Midlife professional women's experiences of aging. *Management Communication Quarterly, 15*(2), 183–226.

Ussher, J. M. (2006). *Managing the monstrous feminine: Regulating the reproductive body.* London: Routledge.

Ussher, J. M. (2011). *The madness of women: Myth and experience.* London: Routledge.

Ussher, J. M., Perz, J., & Gilbert, E. (2012). Changes to sexual well-being and intimacy after breast cancer. *Cancer Nursing, 35*(6), 456–464.

Ussher, J. M., Perz, J., & Gilbert, E. (2014). Women's sexuality after cancer: A qualitative analysis of sexual changes and renegotiation. *Women and Therapy, 37,* 205–221.

Ussher, J. M., Perz, J., Gilbert, E., Wong, W. K. T., & Hobbs, K. (2013). Renegotiating sex after cancer: Resisting the coital imperative. *Cancer Nursing, 36*(6), 454–462.

Wilson, R. (1966). *Feminine forever*. New York: M. Evans.

Winn, R., & Newton, N. (1982). Sexuality in aging: A study of 106 cultures. *Official Publication of the International Academy of Sex Research, 11*(4), 283–298.

Winterich, J. A. (2003). Sex, menopause, and culture: Sexual orientation and the meaning of menopause for women's sex lives. *Gender & Society, 17*(4), 627–642.

Winterich, J. A. (2007). Aging, femininity, and the body: What appearance changes mean to women with age. *Gender Issues, 24*(3), 51–69.

Winterich, J. A., & Umberson, D. (1999). How women experience menopause: The importance of social context. *Journal of Women & Aging, 11*(4), 57–73.

Woods, N. F. (2014). Trial suggests yoga and exercise lead to modest improvements in menopause-related quality of life: Longer term studies are needed. *Evidence Based Medicine, 19*(5), 173.

Writing Group for the Women's Health Initiative Investigators. (2002). Risks and benefits of estrogen plus progesterone in healthy menopausal women: Principal results from the Women's Health Initiative randomized controlled trial. *Journal of the American Medical Association, 288*(3), 321–333.

Zilbergeld, B. (1992). *The new male sexuality*. New York: Bantam Books.

Chapter 7

Women's Sexual Problems: Is There a Pill for That?

Leonore Tiefer

The second half of the 20th century witnessed many social events that radically transformed both public and private sexual life (e.g., the contraceptive pill, the rise of sexualized media, changes in dating patterns, the growth of tourism, the HIV-AIDS epidemic, cable television, the home videocassette industry, the Internet, and above all, the women's; lesbian, gay, bisexual, and transgender; and civil rights social movements).

One of the most influential, however, is often overlooked—the rise since 1980 of an aggressive, medicalized, sexuopharmaceutical industry with its penetration into academic sexology through underwriting professional activities (e.g., journals, conferences, research) and its penetration into everyday sexual life via medicalized media and direct-to-consumer advertising campaigns. This topic is absent from recent handbooks on sexuality (Aggleton & Parker, 2012) and body studies (Turner, 2012), where, despite works on seemingly everything under the sun, there is nothing about the sexuopharmaceutical industry or the rise of pharmaceuticalization (Abraham, 2010; Williams, Martin, & Gabe, 2011).

This chapter begins with some background on the rise of the medicalization of sexuality and describes the new sexuopharmaceutical industry and its discourses. Then, in keeping with the theme of this book, I examine how this new industry does women's sexual lives a grave disservice in a variety of significant ways.

MEDICALIZATION AND PUBLIC HEALTH SEXOLOGY (19TH TO EARLY 20TH CENTURIES)

Although sex advice texts have existed throughout history (e.g., the *Kama Sutra*), the identification of physicians and biomedical researchers as sex experts dates to the late 19th century when doctor/authors such as Richard Krafft-Ebing in Germany and Havelock Ellis in England inaugurated a new era of medical sexual authority. An outpouring of authors and lecturers followed (including some women physicians and researchers), along with technical journals, international congresses, and the whole apparatus of professionalization (McLaren, 1999; Robinson, 1976; Weeks, 1981). Focused on deviant behaviors and identities, the new "sexologists" challenged old taboos and created new norms for sexual identities, marital and premarital sexual practices, sexual partner choice, frequency and intensity of desire, use of stimulants, modesty, masturbation, and more. The sexual landscape changed, and they were in part responsible.

Deviations from the new norms came to be viewed not as bad because they were immoral, polluted, and debauched (i.e., sinful), but as bad because they were abnormal, unnatural, and perverted (i.e., sick). Social scientists call this discourse of health and biomedical expertise "medicalization" (Conrad, 1980), and it has been a major trend over the past century (Nye, 2003). Scholars have tracked medicalization in the 20th century as it transformed people's understanding and approach to many aspects of everyday life, such as mood, sleep, appetite, emotions, alcohol use, activity level, weight, aging, pregnancy, menstruation, child development, drug use, mental state, and sociability (Conrad, 2007). By now it is difficult to think of any part of everyday life that does not have a "health" angle. Deviations from "health" norms are usually identified as either symptoms of illness or as risk factors for illness. Some would say that a sense of being at risk has replaced our personal sense of well-being, and articles in medical journals are awash in a "risk epidemic" (Skolbekken, 1995). The public monitors its own (and its family's) psychology and behavior obsessively, a situation labeled by Robert Crawford (1980) as "healthism."

MEDICALIZATION AND THE FIRST WAVE OF THE WOMEN'S MOVEMENT (EARLY 20TH CENTURY)

In the early 20th century, the first wave of the women's movement and sexual reformers in England and Germany used the discourses of human rights (including homosexual rights) and medicalization to *support* female emancipation. Although this material is well known to feminist historians, sexuality textbooks usually ignore the widespread sexual experimentation in the first decades of the 20th century and suggest that the first and only sexual revolution occurred in the 1960s. Yet, many first wave feminists were tireless activists on behalf of sex reform, including women's rights (to have pleasure or to say "no") in the bedroom, divorce and marriage reform, birth control and abortion rights, eugenic issues, and "bastardy reform" (Hall, 2011). Even issues of bisexuality and masturbation were written and spoken about by feminists at early 20th-century congresses and in publications of socialist and sexologist groups at that time.

Justification for sexual emancipation was argued on the bases of both rights and health. Although the scientific arguments fall short of what serves as evidence in our era, those early works sold like hotcakes and were liberating to women, such as my mother, born in 1913, who kept a copy of Marie Stopes's 1918 "sex manual," *Married Love*, in our New York apartment long after her marriage in 1937.

WHY DOES THE MEDICALIZATION OF SEX CARRY SO MUCH WEIGHT?

Most aspects of sexual conduct and experience are now medicalized, and social norms for sexual behavior and desire are considered health norms. Every healthy adult is supposed to want, have, and enjoy diverse sexual activities; have a sexual identity; and express "modern" attitudes toward bodies, stimulation techniques, and pleasure. In the 21st century, this biomedical lens on sex seems totally "natural" (Tiefer, 1994, 2004). I believe that the adoption of medicalization has occurred for two primary reasons: the lasting influence of religious history and the invisibility of social construction.

First, the centuries-old relation of sex with religion, taboo, and shame has created a sexually ignorant and anxious public, despite the appearance of a sexually permissive culture. Mainstream religions have construed sexual conduct as hugely important, yet, at the same time, they condemn too much or the wrong kind of sexual knowledge and activity as sinful. School-based education about sex is limited because of religious politics. Ordinary people who want and need to know about sex are often anxious and tongue-tied, and they come to depend on "experts" for information and advice. Clerical experts were supplanted by medical and scientific experts, and the vocabulary of sin and shame has been replaced by the vocabulary of health and science, though much of the normative structure (what is considered good sex and what is considered bad) remains the same (Rubin, 1984).

Second, sex easily lent itself to medicalization because the process of the social construction of sexual norms and meanings is hidden behind myths about naturalness and biology (Weeks, 1985). Only cross-cultural and transhistorical research can show how desires and satisfactions are continuously (re)shaped and modified by changing social expectations. As Simone de Beauvoir[1] memorably said about becoming a woman, we are not "born sexual" but rather we "become sexual" as we learn one set of meanings for our physical and emotional experiences, and then "become sexual" again and again as we age (or emigrate or educate ourselves) and as social values change. What we are born with are human capacities for sensation and action that are available to be shaped and labeled as sexual. What we do with those capacities depends on where we are socially located and who we are. Sexuality is, if anything, a way to describe the results of human potentials rather than the product of a DNA-driven "instruction manual."

The medicalization framework, however, defines sex not as a hobby, an expression of emotion, a set of learned behaviors, an aspect of spiritual transcendence, a complex psychophysical activity, a political minefield, a way to express or experience love, or a collection of widely diverse cultural displays, all of which would highlight its cultural embeddedness, but rather as a genitally focused, biological, universal, evolutionary script driven by an instinctive need akin to respiration, digestion, or sleep. From this reductionistic viewpoint, a life or marriage without sex is not healthy, sexual choreography must include genital activities, orgasm is the apogee of sex, too little (or too much or the wrong kind of) sex is not normal, sex contributes to well-being and longevity, and so forth. In our current gene-crazy, brain-crazy culture (Shorter, 2013), anything sexual that can be pegged to biology (e.g., identity, partner choice, drive) has a credibility that the discourse of learning and choice utterly lacks. Science does not and cannot back up this bias, but that is beside the point. The rhetoric is so prevalent that the model seems self-evident.

MEDICALIZATION OF SEX IN THE ERA OF THE *DIAGNOSTIC AND STATISTICAL MANUAL OF MENTAL DISORDERS*

People want advice and information. Sexual health experts proliferated throughout the 20th century, offering therapeutic advice based in "common sense," or in social work, medicine, psychology, psychiatry, gynecology, or marriage counseling (Bailey, 1989). The popularity of "sexual science" was shown by the avalanche of media attention paid to the large interview-based Kinsey Reports in 1947 and 1953. People were riveted by these new statistics on what people do, how many times, and at what ages and doubtlessly hoped to find some personal guidance or reassurance. Although Kinsey went to great lengths to characterize his research as descriptive and not prescriptive, many health experts used his data as a basis for their advice writings.

Slowly, through the 1950s and 1960s, media censorship of sexual topics diminished as a result of judicial freedom-of-speech decisions, which greatly affected professionals as well as the public. Social science and psychotherapy organizations focused on sex were founded in the 1960s and 1970s to capitalize on the publication of Masters and Johnson's best sellers, *Human Sexual Response* (1966) and *Human Sexual Inadequacy* (1970). The first described psychophysiological changes in the body during intercourse and masturbation, and the second offered an innovative behavioral treatment program.

Human Sexual Response, in particular, by creating a genital and physiological roadmap for normal sexual response (the iconic "human sexual response cycle"), went a long way toward medicalizing sexual discourse. Masters and Johnson claimed that their research had proven that women and men had identical (not just equivalent) physiological sexual function, and they defined an arousal/orgasm pattern that was presumably fixed, lifelong, universal, and applicable to all people whether gay or straight, young or old, urban or rural, religious or atheist, sensual or cerebral. They reported not just *a* sexual response, but *the* sexual response. The use of universalizing language and the absence of subjective or cultural considerations are landmark features of medicalization.

Psychiatrists publicized Masters and Johnson's human sexual response cycle through their official psychopathology classification manual, the *Diagnostic and Statistical Manual of Mental Disorders* (*DSM*), also used by psychologists, social workers, and other health and mental health professionals. The third edition of the *DSM*, published in 1980, expanded the list of mental disorders from 134 pages to 494 pages. It adopted the human sexual response cycle as the framework for sexual function nomenclature, and it specified deviations from that pattern (e.g., inhibited arousal, inhibited orgasm, premature ejaculation, erectile dysfunction) as abnormal and problematic (i.e., sexually dysfunctional). This was a huge leap forward for the medicalization of sex. As the *DSM* gained popularity because of global trends in the insurance and research industries, the human sexual response cycle began essentially to define normal and abnormal sex; it was used not only in clinical settings but also was quoted in every textbook and training program for health and mental health professionals. Even if people did not know the phrase *human sexual response cycle*, the idea that "correct sex" consisted of genital arousal, orgasm, erection, and lubrication on every occasion was ubiquitous. The performance focus of the *DSM* and the absence of anything about pleasure or meaning, subjective experience or priorities, communication or diverse preferences, lifecycle stage, or lifestyle created lingering problems and biases.

The fifth edition of the *DSM*, published in 2013 and now up to 947 pages, seemed to eliminate the human sexual response cycle (HSRC) model. Sexual dysfunctions were listed alphabetically instead of in their HSRC sequence, and there is no mention of a "normal" sexual response cycle. However, the omissions remain, and the volume and categories are all so complicated that I wonder if anyone is going to be able to find the advertised changes and distinctions from previous editions.

From the 1980s on, more and more constituencies have used the *DSM* sexuality nomenclature to teach, diagnose, research, and treat. A new helping profession called *sex therapy* emerged, with journals, organizations, annual conferences, and treatment sessions that were reimbursed by private insurers if the therapist had professional qualifications and used official (i.e., *DSM*) diagnoses. Sex therapists wrote and edited casebooks and research papers using the medical model framework and nomenclature. Pleasure-centered, cultural, or spiritual sexuality discourses were marginalized in sex therapy, even as feminist researchers showcased the ubiquity of variables such as body self-consciousness, changing dating standards, and sexual violence.

Medical researchers and clinicians (especially urologists) became interested in "sexual medicine" in the 1990s due to new medical and business environments. Health care delivery and physician compensation models changed in ways that encouraged new specialty areas. Perhaps most influential of all, the pharmaceutical industry responded to a regulatory environment that changed with new congressional emphases. As of 1997, legal direct-to-consumer advertising opportunities stimulated the industry to focus on promoting products to the largest possible markets for "lifestyle" conditions such as baldness, acne, and sexual function. An entire global multibillion-dollar business pivoted in a very short period of time.

Sex therapists were recruited throughout the 1990s to help develop clinical trial questionnaires for measuring sexual distress and satisfaction and to partner with physicians in new sexual dysfunction clinics. The focus of academic sexology shifted heavily into performance measurement and drug trial issues. When a huge publicity wave accompanied the approval of Viagra by the U.S. Food and Drug Administration (FDA) in 1998, a new "sexuopharmaceutical" era was officially ushered in. Some people have equated sexuality medicalization with the sexuopharmaceutical era, but as I hope I have shown, drugs have joined a medical model approach to sex that has been the core of medicalization for decades.

THE HUNT FOR THE FEMALE VIAGRA

Soon after Viagra was approved in 1998 for the treatment of erectile dysfunction, the news media began asking, "Where is the Viagra for women?" Although in 2004 and 2010 pharmaceutical companies brought their clinical trial results for "female sexual dysfunction" drugs to the FDA, there is no "female Viagra" as of this writing (late 2014). Both proposed drugs were rejected on safety and efficacy grounds, and the second drug has even been rejected a second time.

In 2004, the FDA rejected a testosterone patch called Intrinsa, which was manufactured by Procter & Gamble, the world's largest consumer goods company. Testosterone had never been approved for men's sexual problems (a fact that I imagine would surprise most people), but it was nonetheless widely promoted as "the hormone of desire," and Procter & Gamble eagerly capitalized on this mythical status. The 20th century had been full of hormone stories, some positive but many negative and even scary. At the time Intrinsa was being considered, steroid hormones for women were feared because the 2002 Women's Health Initiative (WHI) had shown risks of cancer related to postmenopausal hormone use. At the 2004 FDA hearing for Intrinsa, consulting experts said they did not want to risk "another WHI." Intrinsa was later approved in the United Kingdom, but without the promotional energy of direct-to-consumer drug advertising (which is illegal everywhere other than the United States and New Zealand, another fact not generally known by the public), it was not widely prescribed. The drug was ultimately removed from use in Europe and the United Kingdom in 2012, and journalists speculated that the reason was limited sales. The 2004 FDA hearing was featured in a 2011 American documentary film titled *Orgasm, Inc.*, which shows the years' long, behind-the-scenes efforts of pharmaceutical companies in the early 2000s to find a diagnosis and fund clinical trials on women's sexuality that would successfully capitalize on the popularity of Viagra with men.

In 2010, Boehringer-Ingelheim (B-I), a German pharmaceutical company, brought its drug application to the FDA, this time not for a hormonal treatment, but for a central nervous system pill called flibanserin, which would affect the serotonin and dopamine receptors in brain cells and perhaps cause an increase in sexual interest. This model piggybacked on the popular "chemical imbalance" theory, which claimed, without scientific evidence, that low levels of serotonin or dopamine were responsible for mood disorders.

Prior to the FDA hearing, B-I hired the Ogilvy Public Relations Company to create an extensive media campaign (i.e., "Sex Brain Body: Make the Connection") to frame low sexual desire as a prevalent and underrecognized neurotransmitter disorder (hypoactive sexual desire disorder). B-I and Ogilvy hired Lisa Rinna, a television soap opera star, to make media

appearances to describe her tragic loss of desire and its gratifying restora-
tion (though she never mentioned how it was restored as no drug had yet
been approved). B-I also funded documentary-like cable television info-
mercials that endorsed a brain deficiency theory of low sexual desire.
Nevertheless, the FDA again rejected the flibanserin application on the
grounds of a poor risk-to-benefit ratio (i.e., safety concerns that were not
outweighed by the slight increases in sexual desire measured by self-
report questionnaires).

In 2011, B-I sold the rights to flibanserin to Sprout Pharmaceuticals,
which conducted additional studies and resubmitted the application.
Nonetheless, in 2013 the application was again rejected by the FDA. Not
content to rest their case on the scientific evidence, in 2014 Sprout hired
Edelman Public Relations, the world's largest PR firm, to create a new
campaign (i.e., "Even the Score") to bring political pressure on the FDA.[2]
A new website and publicity campaign (i.e., "26:0") urged the public to
complain about alleged gender bias by the FDA, Sprout's explanation for
why drugs have been approved to treat men's but not women's sexual
dysfunction. This campaign, which grossly misrepresents the facts as well
as the gender politics, gained traction throughout the summer of 2014,
capitalizing on the plans for an FDA meeting on female sexual dysfunction called for October 2014 to discuss the status of the diagnosis and clinical trials. This shows the lengths to which the industry will go in pursuit
of sales.

Feminist health groups, including the "New View Campaign," which
challenged Intrinsa in 2004 and flibanserin in 2010, mobilized resistance.
This entire story can be read on the FDA 2014 page of the New View
website.[3]

Intrinsa and flibanserin are only the tip of the iceberg in terms of sexuality drugs for women. There have been many drugs tested but then
dropped, and several are still in the development pipeline. Readers can
follow the stories of the new products in the business and medical press
(e.g., Scudellari, 2014).

MEDICALIZATION UNDERMINES UNDERSTANDING SEX

Many aspects of the medicalization of sex need to be challenged because
of their negative impact on sexual life. Some problems are conceptual,
some political, and some practical, but they all detrimentally affect wom-
en's sexual lives.

Perhaps the most important, albeit the most abstract, is the conceptual
aspect. The medicalization perspective profoundly shapes how we con-
strue sexuality (e.g., what kind of a thing it is, what we should expect,
how much variation there is, who should be the experts, what kind of
public and professional education there should be). Medicalization

directs sexuality education, research, professional training, and clinical intervention toward aspects of sexuality thought to be primary (i.e., biological, physiological, universal, evolutionary, health-related) and sidelines other aspects (e.g., cultural, political, relational, learned, diverse, subjective). A quick overview of sexuality education websites and books shows this bias, which enforces the discourse of normalcy. A person would be hard pressed to find material that describes the reality and consequences of diverse genital anatomies, different kinds of orgasms, lifetime changes in arousal patterns, or varied feelings about genital smells and fluids, for example. There is simply no research from this angle.

But medicalization does not just shape education and policy, it also deeply affects personal expectations and priorities. By defining sexual experience and satisfaction as a narrow physiological norm of functioning (i.e., routine genital arousal and orgasm), medicalization profoundly influences what people think sex is for and how we assess our own private and personal emotional and physical experiences. By creating a mindset that focuses on universal performance standards, medicalization creates anxiety over potential sexual inadequacies and deviations from "normal" functioning. As with all forms of self-consciousness, this creates a judgmental attitude incompatible with relaxation and pleasure that is doomed to find fault and disappointment. Dysfunction is practically inevitable in such an atmosphere.

In its emphasis on built-in universal physiology, medicalization ignores sexual mind–body diversity and thus harms people whose bodies or experiences differ from the "norm." We know that bodies function diversely from a lifetime of witnessing others' reactions to cold or hunger or fear or sleep deprivation. We know people's appetites vary from their different reactions to intoxicants, sweets, or spices. We know people have different abilities to concentrate on music or ignore noise. We know some people are touchy-feely, whereas others need their personal space. We know people differ widely in modesty and in their comfort with or enjoyment of nudity. We know people differ in their tolerance of strong bodily odors. All of these factors affect the sensory experience of sexual intimacy and the consequent intensities of arousal. By insisting that sex is "built-in" rather than an acquired accumulation of meanings and experiences, medicalization obscures the true social construction of sexual life.

The human sexual response cycle model is based on a penetrative model of penis-in-vagina reproductive sexuality. If reproduction is not the purpose of sexual activity, however, there is no necessary choreography or physiological sequencing for enjoyment, expression, or experience. Women's sexual emancipation requires awareness of the subtle pressures of arousal-orgasm norms. Feminists are concerned about inequality and have long complained that most intercourse choreography, derived from the reproductive model, is organized around men's erection, orgasm, and pleasure. This has become especially clear since the approval of Viagra. It is taken for granted that men will want to use Viagra to continue having erections and intercourse as part, or the central part, of sexual activity. The consequences of this assumption have led to a landscape of prescription and nonprescription vaginal lubricants so that women will be able to perform penetrative sexuality at any age. The reality of this as a cultural norm, rather than an evolutionary one, is often hidden.

UNINTENDED CONSEQUENCES OF MEDICALIZATION

The medical model introduces coercive genital performance norms into sexual experience in a way I describe as the "McDonaldization of Sex," which refers to a standardized script and quantified goals. These days a sexual experience is rated as "successful" if it culminates in both parties experiencing orgasm, a script seen as "fair." This (mis)appropriation of feminist political rhetoric has become a self-fulfilling prophecy in an era when a sexual encounter has become something of a competitive performance rather than an exploration of individuality and mutuality. Much qualitative research on sexuality, largely ignored by mainstream sexology conferences and journals, shows that all women do not have the same sexual goals, they do not all rate orgasm at the top of the pleasure list, and they express much diversity in both cognitive and sensual elements. However, the use of biology as the bedrock aspect of sex in the medicalization model mistakenly results in identifying satisfaction with physical goals that can be measured and quantified—of which, of course, there are very few. As a result, satisfaction becomes about genital arousal and orgasm rather than about a plethora of subjective indicators.

The individual and social harms created by medicalization are extensive. They include the escalation of costly and unproductive workups for "female sexual dysfunction" in the growing industry of sexual health clinics. Medical workups, not usually covered by health insurance, can include physical and pelvic examination, extensive blood work, vaginal pH measures, vaginal and clitoral ultrasound blood flow measures, vulvar sensitivity tests, and testing of the circumvaginal musculature with intravaginal silicone balloons. It is extremely rare, however, that any of these tests uncovers a medical cause for lost desire, failed orgasm, sexual aversion, extreme self-consciousness or ticklishness, disgust at being touched, or any of the other scores of complaints women have about their sexual lives. The workups are a form of medical hocus-pocus that provides a smokescreen of scientificism (i.e., the illusion that all this equipment is measuring the sexual "reality" of the body).

The resources directed into medical research and services are, of course, not matched by comparable resources for sex and relationship education, media literacy, or consumer literacy, all subjects that women require in order to understand themselves and their sexual options. The public is poorly educated, for example, not only about sexual development and the diversity of sexual response and experience, but the public also lacks awareness of the widespread prevalence of conflicts of interest and pseudoscience in contemporary sexology, which has allowed these to become major drivers of the "hunt for the pink Viagra" in the past decade. As a sex therapist for over 40 years, I can honestly say that most people know very little about sex: The more important the topic is, the less common sense they seem to bring to it.

Medicalization, then, which was supposed to replace stigma with science and speculation with evidence, seems, in the case of sexuality, to have introduced a new set of norms and even oppressions. Once there is a consensus that sexuality is a matter of health, rather than hobby, expression of emotion or culture, or optional interpersonal priority, then biological research, authority of medical experts, and more and more medical institutionalization occurs. It is difficult to get all those messages out of one's head, and the advice to "relax" and "get into the moment" and "let your body go" and "just enjoy what happens" is superficial and inadequate. Adding "correct sexual response" to all the other "shoulds" operating in the bedroom for women (e.g., looking and smelling good in every nook and cranny of the body, proper balance of behavioral assertion and diffidence, modesty, technical smoothness, awareness of danger, precautions against pregnancy and sexually transmitted disease risk, focus on satisfying her partner) makes sexual encounters more fraught than ever.

CONCLUSION

The story of medicalization, though it was seen as a beacon of "scientific hope" by feminists in the early 20th century, has not produced the kind of emancipatory results we would like in the 21st century. The role of science in the exposure of myths has been replaced, it seems, by the role of medicalization in the creation of new myths. Science itself may be neutral, but what and who are studied (or ignored), and how they are studied (or dismissed), serve the interests of institutions with agendas other than women's liberation. Show me the pharmaceutical company truly interested in women's sexual well-being, and I will show you a company that has a narrow portfolio focused on medical conditions such as multiple sclerosis and spinal cord injuries, rather than on blockbuster drugs for the masses. And even in those narrow instances, the attention would be on reducing pain or physical blocks rather than "stimulating" desire or arousal or anything else. I do not know of such a pharmaceutical company.

Looking for pills for most women's sexual problems is so short-sighted as to be absurd. What women need for good sex lives are accurate information, good sex partners, sexual safety, freedom from media pressure, health and energy, appropriate health care, and an atmosphere of common sense about their bodies and their capacities. Uncommon common sense, it would seem, is what women really need.

NOTES

1. From https://philosophynow.org/issues/69/Becoming_A_Woman_Simone _de_Beauvoir_on_Female_Embodiment.
2. From www.eventhescore.org.
3. From www.newviewcampaign.org.

REFERENCES

Abraham, J. (2010). Pharmaceuticalization of society in context: Theoretical, empirical, and health dimensions. *Sociology, 44*, 603–622.

Aggleton, P., & Parker, R. (Eds.) (2010). *Routledge handbook of sexuality, health, and rights*. London: Routledge.

American Psychiatric Association. (1980). *Diagnostic and statistical manual of mental disorders* (3rd ed.). Washington, DC: Author.

American Psychiatric Association. (2013). *Diagnostic and statistical manual of mental disorders* (5th ed.). Washington, DC: Author.

Bailey, B. L. (1989). *From front porch to back seat: Courtship in twentieth-century America*. Baltimore, MD: Johns Hopkins University Press.

Conrad, P. (1980). *Deviance and medicalization: From badness to sickness*. Philadelphia, PA: Temple University Press.

Conrad, P. (2007). *The medicalization of society*. Baltimore, MD: Johns Hopkins University Press.

Crawford, R. (1980). Healthism and the medicalization of everyday life. *International Journal of Health Services, 10*, 365–388.

Hall, L. A. (2011). *The life and times of Stella Browne, feminist and free spirit*. New York: I. B. Tauris.

Masters, W. M., & Johnson, V. E. (1966). *Human sexual response*. Boston: Little Brown.

Masters, W. M., & Johnson, V. E. (1970). *Human sexual inadequacy*. Boston: Little Brown.

McLaren, A. (1999). *Twentieth century sexuality: A history*. Oxford: Blackwell.

Nye, R. (2003). The evolution of the concept of medicalization in the late 20th century. *Journal of the History of the Behavioral Sciences, 39*, 115–129.

Robinson, P. (1976). *The modernization of sex*. New York: Harper.

Rubin, G. S. (1984). Thinking sex: Notes for a radical theory of the politics of sexuality. In C. Vance (Ed.), *Pleasure and danger: Exploring female sexuality* (pp. 267–319). London: Routledge.

Scudellari, M. (2014, July). That loving feeling. *Scientist*. Retrieved from http:// www.thescientist.com/?articles.view/articleNo/40272/title/That-Loving -Feeling/.

Shorter, E. S. (2013). *How everyone became depressed*. New York: Oxford University Press.

Skolbekken, J. A. (1995). The risk epidemic in medical journals. *Social Science and Medicine, 40*, 291–305.

Stopes, M. (1918). *Married love*. New York: Critic and Guide.

Tiefer, L. (1994). *Sex is not a natural act, and other essays*. Boulder, CO: Westview.

Tiefer, L. (2004). *Sex is not a natural act, and other essays* (2nd ed.). Boulder, CO: Westview.

Turner, B. S. (Ed.) (2012). *Routledge handbook on body studies*. London: Routledge.

Weeks, J. (1981). *Sex, politics, and society: The regulation of sexuality since 1800*. London: Longman.

Weeks, J. (1985). *Sexuality and its discontents: Meanings, myths, and modern sexualities*. London: Routledge & Kegan Paul.

Williams, S. J., Martin, P., & Gabe, J. (2011). The pharmaceuticalization of society? A framework for analysis. *Sociology of Health and Illness, 33*, 710–725.

Chapter 8

The Thin Ideal: A "Wrong Prescription" Sold to Many and Achievable by Few

Mindy J. Erchull

It has been argued that body dissatisfaction among women, particularly Western women, is so widespread that it has become a "normative discontent" (Rodin, Silberstein, & Streigel-Moore, 1984). A few minutes in a checkout line at a grocery store can reinforce this idea as one is confronted with headlines on magazine covers such as "Diets that Work: Celebrity Weight-loss Secrets to Help You Slim Down Fast—Without Starving!" (*OK! USA*, April 21, 2014), "Flat Belly, Sleek Legs, Tight Butt in Just 3 Steps" (*Shape*, October 2014), and "Thinspiration! Three New Celeb Diets for You to Try" (*Reveal*, July 5–11, 2014). These headlines imply that (a) women should be thin, (b) women need to diet and lose weight to be thin, and (c) women need to reshape particular body parts. And these are just three headlines—one could fill a book with countless eye-catching blurbs and the underlying messages they send to women about their bodies and the cultural expectations about them.

This chapter discusses the "thin ideal," a key element of this normative discontent experienced by women, how it is related to a culture of objectification and sexualization, methods girls and women use to try to conform to the thin ideal, and the complex relation between thinness and health. In reality, the message that thinness and weight loss are good things can really be quite problematic. A cultural focus on thinness is associated with poor quality of life, body dissatisfaction, malnutrition, and eating disorders.

THE THIN IDEAL

In order to understand the thin ideal, it is important first to realize that people are constantly being influenced by social norms. Social norms are the rules, whether explicitly stated or implicitly implied, in a given society, culture, or social group that tell people what is acceptable and expected in terms of values, beliefs, and behaviors (Kelley, 1955). Individuals who conform to the norms for their group are accepted and even rewarded. Those who do not conform to these norms are seen as different and, sometimes, deviant. Every culture has beauty norms or standards—relatively narrow representations of how individuals should look (Zones, 2000). As with other social norms, conforming to these standards signals an understanding of cultural values and a desire to be part of a particular social group. Similarly, when people conform to beauty norms, they receive social rewards (Wooley, Wooley, & Dyrenforth, 1979). There are appearance norms for both men and women, but the consequences of not conforming to these norms are typically more severe for women than for men (Wolf, 1991); indeed, attending to how one looks has even been described as a core part of femininity (Mahalik et al., 2005).

Mahalik and colleagues (2005) identified both thinness and investing in one's appearance as core feminine norms, and Calogero and Thompson (2010) identified thinness as the most consistent beauty standard for women over the past 50 years. The thin ideal has become a very specific beauty norm for women, and a large body of research has shown that internalization of this cultural norm is relatively common (Karazsia, van Dulmen, Wong, & Crowther, 2013). In fact, even girls just starting elementary school have reported a desire to be thinner (Lowes & Tiggemann, 2003). This is highly problematic, however, as ideals are aspirational and hard to achieve at the best of times, and the thin ideal is nearly impossible for women to achieve, let alone maintain (Chrisler, 2008, 2012). Norms, however, are meant to be what is actually done by most. Unfortunately, norms can also be made up of what is expected of most, even if it is not achievable, and this is the case with the thin ideal and beauty norms. An unrealistic standard has become the core expectation for women's appearance.

Thinness on its own is hard to achieve, but the modern thin ideal is more complex than just wanting to be slim. Western beauty ideals, particularly for young White women, include a thin body with no obvious body fat and well-defined, but sleek, muscle tone (Calogero, Boroughs, & Thompson, 2007; Thompson & Tantleff, 1992). Trends indicate an ever-increasing pursuit of a muscular ideal among women (Garner, 1997), an ideal that has been more commonly associated with men's body image concerns (Thompson & Cafri, 2007). Thinness and muscularity can each, on its own, be very difficult to achieve, but expecting them to coexist adds additional challenge. The reality is that muscle takes up space and can make the body appear less thin. Given this, conforming to these two appearance standards at the same time can be nearly impossible.

Another near impossible juxtaposition of appearance norms is the juxtaposition of the thin ideal with the ideal of full, voluptuous breasts. Because breasts are composed, in part, of body fat, this is another combination of beauty ideals that nearly none can conform to without surgical intervention (Harrison, 2003). The thin ideal, something already unachievable for many, is now far more complex. Women are now being told to be thin, fit, and sleekly muscled with voluptuous breasts. This means that women are essentially being told to reduce their caloric intake, increase their physical activity, and undergo surgery to achieve an "ideal" body that does not really exist in nature. Is it any wonder that discontent with one's body is experienced as normative?

MEDIA REPRESENTATIONS OF THE THIN IDEAL

Although women are sometimes explicitly told to lose weight, work out, dress differently, or consider cosmetic surgery (all explicit confirmations of beauty norms), more often information about beauty norms, and specifically the norm of thinness, is conveyed in more subtle ways through both interpersonal interactions and media representations of women. In fact, many have studied the role the media can play in the development, perpetuation, and internalization of the thin and the more recent thin/fit ideal. This is key as thinness is a dominant theme in representations of women across forms of media, including movies, television, music videos, and magazines (Levine & Harrison, 2004).

One way in which the media influence women is by serving as an information source for what social norms, including beauty norms, are. People can look to the media to learn how they are expected to behave in certain situations, how they should dress, and what they should look like. This is because, according to social learning theory, humans often learn through observation and imitation (Bandura, 1977). The fact that we do not always need to learn through firsthand experience is a wonderful boon as it can save tremendous time and effort, allowing us to accomplish more and integrate more information into our understanding of the complex world in which we live. At the same time, this method of learning is only useful if we have information sources that provide accurate, high-quality information.

When it comes to representations of women's bodies, the media are providing skewed information (Kilbourne, 1999). Models, for example, are, on average, far thinner than the average woman, and photoshopping is routinely used in print media to "improve" the look of models. Body doubles are often used in movies because even actresses who are praised for their beauty do not meet the body ideals deemed necessary for certain shots. Thus, girls and women are being shown a body ideal as desired, expected, and, perhaps, even typical that is actually largely unattainable. They are learning that they should want and work toward this ideal body—a body most can never achieve. Cultivation theory focuses particularly on the impact of television on people's attitudes, beliefs, and behaviors (Gerbner, Gross, Morgan, & Signorielli, 1994). The idea here is not just that we can learn from what we see; rather, greater exposure to images and themes makes it more likely that they will influence how we see the world, what we judge as typical, and what we desire. Although this theory centers on television as a key media source, the underlying idea can apply to all media sources. Essentially, what we are exposed to on a regular basis becomes more real and more realistic to us; demarcations between fiction and reality blur, and these ideals, which are really the exceptions, become the norms.

These unrealistic ideals can then serve as a source for social comparison, and this is yet another way that the media influence girls and women. Research has shown that one way people gain knowledge about themselves is by engaging in social comparison, both with others they know personally and with more abstract representations of others (e.g., characters in movies, models in advertisements; Festinger, 1954). When a woman compares herself to another and perceives herself as better off, thereby making a downward social comparison, she will typically feel good about herself and may experience a boost to her self-esteem. When she compares herself and judges herself as lacking in comparison to another (an upward social comparison), she is likely to experience decreased self-esteem and a lowered sense of well-being. As most women do not, and cannot, look like the women in the media (we are not photoshopped in our daily lives, we do not have body doubles to stand in for us, and we may just be built differently than others at a biological level), women are certain to feel dissatisfied with their appearance if they have accepted the idea that these images represent a desired and desirable ideal.

There is not just a theoretical link between media filled with idealized, thin women and the actual thoughts and behaviors of women, however; there are also a great deal of data from many studies to support this relation (e.g., Ferguson, 2013; Grabe, Ward, & Hyde, 2008). For example, exposure to images of women who conform to the thin ideal (or at least appear to conform after photo-editing or computer manipulation of the images) has been shown to result in increased body dissatisfaction (Dittmar,

Halliwell, & Stirling, 2009; Harrison, Taylor, & Marske, 2006). Researchers have found that women who watch more television are more likely to perceive themselves as overweight—regardless of their actual weight—than are those who watch less often (McCreary & Sadava, 1999). Behavior has also been shown to be related to consumption of media that depict a thin ideal: Women who were shown thin ideal images subsequently ate less in the presence of others than did those who did not see thin ideal images of women (Harrison et al., 2006).

Perhaps some of the most compelling evidence for the impact of the media comes from a study conducted in Fiji in the 1990s. Fiji, like other island cultures in the South Pacific, has traditionally seen plump bodies as beautiful. Television was introduced to Fiji in 1995, and, in the years following the introduction of Western television shows, the desire for thinness increased among Fijian girls. There has also been a corresponding increase there in both disordered eating attitudes and behaviors since 1995 (Becker, 2004; Becker, Burwell, Herzog, Hamburg, & Gilman, 2002).

It is important to note, however, that not everyone who is exposed to idealized media images of women becomes dissatisfied with their own appearance or desires greater thinness. Some research indicates that dissatisfaction with one's own body is more likely to result if women are already dissatisfied with their appearance in some way (Ferguson, 2013). Other research has indicated that the thin ideal is not endorsed by all. For example, Black women are less likely than White women to endorse the thin ideal (Capodilupo, 2014), and Latinas who immigrated to the United States endorse a larger body ideal than either European American women or Latinas born in the United States (Lopez, Blix, & Blix, 1995). To understand these findings, it is important to realize the role that internalization of media images and the thin ideal can play in women's relationships with their bodies.

Internalization is a process of adopting sociocultural standards as personal standards and ideals as goals (Thompson, Heinberg, Altabe, & Tantleff-Dunn, 1999). In terms of the thin ideal, this means that women learn, through myriad sources, that thinness is deemed desirable and ideal and begin to hold this view themselves. They internalize the ideal of thinness and strive to meet the goal of conforming to the ideal body type. Research has indicated that those who are more exposed to the thin ideal through media are more likely to idealize thinness (Harrison & Cantor, 1997). It is important to note, however, that they do not just idealize thinness; they also assume that their lives will be better if they are thinner and look more like the women they encounter in the media (Engeln-Maddox, 2006). We tend to assume that "what is beautiful is good" (Dion, Berscheid, & Walster, 1972; Langlois et al., 2000), and, if women think thin is beautiful (i.e., if they have internalized the thin ideal), they associate thinness with all manner of positive things. These include greater romantic success, increased interpersonal skills, and employment advancement; and media sources such as magazines and television commercials often make this explicit (Chrisler, 2012). This is highly problematic, however, as internalization of media ideals of female beauty has been associated with many negative consequences.

SELF-OBJECTIFICATION

One of the most frequently researched negative consequences of the internalization of the beauty ideal is the experience of self-objectification (Fredrickson & Roberts, 1997). To understand self-objectification, we first have to realize that our culture is one in which women are routinely sexualized and objectified. Sexual objectification is when women are made into sex objects for consumption by others. Essentially, women are reduced to their appearance and taught that it is, largely, the source of their value. This objectification of women is reflected in the media to which we are all exposed on a routine basis, as when we see a magazine display while standing in line at a grocery store, view advertisements on websites we visit, or watch television or a movie with friends and family. Through repeated exposure to these media, we can internalize these images and messages, as described above. Doing so can result not only in internalizing these messages about women's roles and women's bodies, but it can also result in internalizing an observer's perspective in relationship to our own bodies.

The process of stepping outside of oneself and surveying one's own body as an outsider would is engaging in self-objectification (Fredrickson & Roberts, 1997; McKinley & Hyde, 1996). Although it is normal to survey one's appearance occasionally to make sure one meets whatever standards have been deemed appropriate (e.g., no clothes on inside out, no toilet paper stuck to one's shoe), doing so routinely can be problematic for a number of reasons. This routine behavior, sometimes called the adoption or internalization of the male gaze, is known as self-surveillance; that surveillance is judgmental and results in body shame.

Engaging in self-objectification, or body surveillance, can be detrimental because it reduces one's ability to focus on other things. The human mind is wonderful and can handle multiple tasks and many pieces of information at a given point in time. However, there is a finite amount of attention we have to use at any one moment (Pashler, 1994). If we shift attention to checking out how our bodies look to others, we have to remove attention from something else. If we are making a quick check before we leave the house or a public restroom, this is usually not seriously detrimental, but if we do it while taking a math test or during a job interview, we are reducing our ability to succeed to the best of our potential. In fact, research has indicated that increased levels of self-objectification among college women are associated with decreased performance on math tests (Fredrickson, Roberts, Noll, Quinn, & Twenge, 1998; Hebl, King, & Lin, 2004).

Much of the research on self-objectification has focused on ongoing, or trait, levels of self-objectification (Moradi & Huang, 2008; Tiggemann, 2011). Rather than asking whether self-objectification increases in a given situation (e.g., when wearing a swimsuit), researchers have looked at typical levels of self-objectification that women report across situations on a daily basis. Although levels of self-objectification vary among individuals, it is a fairly common experience for women. This ongoing trait form of self-objectification has been consistently linked to a number of negative psychological outcomes, including decreased self-esteem, depression, sexual dysfunction, and disordered eating (Moradi & Huang, 2008; Tiggemann, 2011). More recent research has even shown a link between self-objectification and both dissociation and self-harm (Erchull, Liss, & Lichiello, 2013). These negative outcomes are not linked to short-term re-allocation of mental energies, however. Rather, they are understood as resulting from how women react to what they find when they engage in body surveillance.

If a woman typically self-objectifies, that means she mentally steps outside of her body to check it out as an observer would. When she does this, given that she has probably internalized cultural beauty norms and the thin ideal and that hardly anyone fits these standards, she does not like what she sees. She will, therefore, likely experience body shame or discomfort with her appearance as a result of not conforming to the beauty ideal she has internalized as her standard. This experience of body shame as a result of a negative self-evaluation after surveying one's body is what is believed to result in the increased levels of psychological disorders, at both clinical (i.e., meets criteria for a psychiatric diagnosis) and subclinical levels.

Perhaps the best-researched negative outcomes of self-objectification include body dissatisfaction, negative eating attitudes, and both clinical and subclinical levels of disordered eating (Moradi & Huang, 2008; Tiggemann, 2011). Body dissatisfaction is the extent to which individuals feel satisfied or dissatisfied with their bodies or specific body parts (Thompson et al., 1999), and it is very common. Research indicates that approximately one-half of women and girls, at least in the United States, are dissatisfied with their body size and want to be thinner (Bearman, Presnell, Martinez, & Stice, 2006; Smolak, 2012; Tantleff-Dunn, Barnes, & Larose, 2011). This is why body dissatisfaction among women has been referred to as a normative discontent (Rodin et al., 1984; Tantleff-Dunn et al., 2011).

For some, negative feelings about their bodies do not end with a sense of being dissatisfied with their bodies; they are also ashamed. As noted above, body shame can result when people evaluate their appearance against standards they hold for how women (and they themselves) should look (Fredrickson & Roberts, 1997; McKinley & Hyde, 1996; Moradi & Huang, 2008), and research indicates that women who highly value thinness and other aspects of physical attractiveness are more likely to report having experienced body shame (Calogero & Thompson, 2009; Noll & Fredrickson, 1998).

EATING DISORDERS AND DISORDERED EATING

Much research has shown that body shame is an important variable in the sequence between internalization of the beauty ideal and subsequently experiencing negative outcomes such as disordered eating (Moradi & Huang, 2008; Tiggemann, 2011). Anorexia nervosa (AN) and bulimia nervosa (BN) are the most commonly discussed eating disorders, and both are related to body dissatisfaction and self-objectification. AN is characterized by unrealistic evaluations of the body wherein individuals perceive themselves as having a larger weight or body shape than is actually the case (i.e., they see themselves as fat when they are not), a fear of gaining weight or being fat, and a consistent restriction of calories (i.e., eating very little; American Psychiatric Association, 2013). BN is characterized by episodes of binge eating followed by episodes of behavior intended to compensate for the caloric intake during the binge period (e.g., vomiting, laxative use, excessive exercise; American Psychiatric Association, 2013).

These eating disorders are associated with many negative psychological and physiological outcomes (Birmingham & Treasure, 2010; Hoste & Le Grange, 2013). These include co-occurring psychological problems, such as depression, anxiety disorders, and obsessive-compulsive disorder. In terms of physiological outcomes, they include electrolyte imbalances, malnutrition, dental enamel erosion, decreased bone mass, and heart problems. Eating disorders are also associated with a greater risk of early death as a result of damage done to the body through malnutrition or purging patterns, as well as increased rates of suicide. Eating disorders are experienced by a minority of girls and women—less than 5% by most accounts (Currin, Schmidt, Treasure, & Jick, 2005; Hudson, Hiripi, Pope, & Kessler, 2007; Smink, van Hoeken, & Hoek, 2013)—but there is evidence that rates of these disorders increased throughout the 20th century (Hudson et al., 2007; Keel & Klump, 2003).

Subclinical levels of disordered eating are far more common than are diagnoses of AN and BN. These can include patterns of disordered eating that do not reach the specific diagnostic criteria for these disorders (Solmi, Hatch, Hotopf, Treasure, & Micali, 2014), but they can also include more normative patterns of disordered eating, such as commonly skipping meals, regularly restricting calories, and exercising obsessively (Tiggemann, 2011). Dieting is very common among women and girls, and this behavioral pattern is not solely connected to women's weight or body mass index, a metric calculated based on weight and height (Ackard, Croll, & Kearney-Cooke, 2002). In other words, many dieters do not "need" to lose weight.

The media are constantly providing information about the latest, greatest no-fail diets. These diets typically do not meet recommended, balanced nutrition standards and usually rely on gimmicks, such as juice fasts and high protein/no carb meal plans. Research has shown that these diets can work—at least for a short period of time—but they work because the restrictive nature of these diets results in fewer calories being consumed (Bravata et al., 2003). These very restrictive diets may result in decreased caloric intake, in part, because of a lack of interest in the foods that are allowed as part of the diet. This same lack of interest, or boredom, can lead to stopping the diet and looking for new options to lose weight or maintain thinness; thus, the weight lost is typically gained back, resulting in a yo-yo weight pattern that has been linked to negative health outcomes (Bouchard, 2002; Mann et al., 2007).

With the increased focus on a thin but toned body ideal for women, we have also seen an uptick in attention paid to possible fitness regimens that women and girls can undertake to lose weight while shaping and toning their bodies. We are no longer just dealing with *thinspiration* a term that can actually be traced to its use on pro-anorexia websites; we now have "fitspiration" media messages (Thomas & Schaefer, 2013). A quick search for these terms on Pinterest (an online scrapbooking site where users can "pin" images to virtual bulletin boards) yielded myriad images under each term. The images associated with these topics overlap a great deal, and it is difficult to sort them into distinct categories. The fitspiration movement on social media ostensibly moves beyond weight and body size or shape toward a focus on fitness regardless of body appearance. That said, the material online still largely depicts very thin, very toned young women with little to no visible body fat, and it typically includes no critique of a thin ideal (Stover, 2014). The intense and consistent pattern of physical activity necessary for most people to achieve and maintain a thin, toned body as depicted in print and online media would typically be considered excessive (Mond, Hay, Rodgers, & Owen, 2006); thus, it is nearly impossible for people with busy lives and multiple roles to manage this ideal, unlike models and other celebrities whose "job" is to look "good." This pattern also far exceeds the level of physical activity recommended for adults by the Centers for Disease Control and Prevention (i.e., 2.5 hours of brisk walking or its equivalent per week plus strength training two days per week; CDC, 2014).

PEER INFLUENCE

The media are, by no means, the only way that women and girls learn about measures they can take to try to meet the thin ideal. Other women and girls are a common source of this information. Peers can provide information about what they believe has and has not worked for them in the past. They can also provide positive reinforcement when weight is lost or one's body shape changes, thereby reinforcing and encouraging the use of the tactics used to achieve that change (Lieberman, Gauvin, Bukowski, & White, 2001). Similarly, they can convey social disapproval when weight is gained, exercise patterns are not maintained, or taboo foods are consumed. Those around us are also being influenced by social norms, including appearance norms, and they are also likely to have internalized the thin ideal. When we veer off course, we are signaling a lack of desire to fit in and conform to acceptable norms. Therefore, others who have internalized these norms and adhere, or try to adhere, to them may try to bring us back in line by encouraging us to diet, exercise, or pass up that piece of chocolate cake. They may see this as being helpful, but, at an unconscious level, it is also a way to bolster their feelings about their own choices and punish us for stepping out of line.

In our current age of virtual connection, thanks to the Internet, myriad social networks (e.g., Facebook, Twitter, Instagram), and the presence of microcomputers in our pockets through the growing presence of smartphones, we can find information and other people to support or criticize our choices very quickly and easily. Again, one can visit Pinterest to see myriad images meant to serve as either or both thinspiration or fitspiration or type the words "miracle diet" into Google and get more than one million search results. Although people may be particularly concerned about explicitly pro-anorexia (known as pro-ana) websites (Norris, Boydell, Pinhas, & Katzman, 2006), much of the information on these sites can be found in many places online. In this way, women and girls may be encountering virtual peers on a regular basis who provide them with information about what to do and not do in regard to their appearance. We know that negative comments about appearance are associated with negative body image, and that the effects of those comments on people's self-esteem can persist from childhood into adulthood (McLaren, Kuh, Hardy, & Gauvin, 2004; Murray, Touyz, & Beumont, 1995; Paxton, Schultz, Wertheim, & Muir, 1999). Peers, along with the media and parents, have been found to be a key influence on body image (Keery, van den Berg, & Thompson, 2004). Once again, it is clear that the thin ideal is inescapable—messages about it are around us at all times.

CHALLENGING THE THIN IDEAL

Despite the fact that the thin ideal is a near constant in the lives of many women, it is important to recognize that thinness itself can be problematic.

Few would argue that eating disorders are good things or that the health consequences of them are not real. Despite this, many continue to adhere to the idea that thinness is a sign of health and fitness and, therefore, is a goal to be aspired to, not for the sake of appearance but for the sake of one's physical health. However, research has not indicated a clear and consistent link between thinness and good health. In fact, research has indicated that both thinness and intentional weight loss have been related to increased mortality rates (Gaesser, 1999). Dieting, particularly with fad diets that are very restrictive or involve intermittent fasting, have been linked to negative health effects, such as vitamin deficiency, malnutrition, and muscle loss (Collier, 2013). It is true that increased physical fitness and activity can result in health gains among those who are classified as overweight, but weight loss does not need to happen to achieve these gains.

The weight-neutral Health at Every Size approach is now being recommended as a public health intervention strategy focused on nutrition and activity without a focus on appearance or weight as a key indicator of health (Bombak, 2014). The idea is to focus on what bodies can do and how they function rather than on how they look. It is possible, for example, to be thin and to have high cholesterol, high blood pressure, or diabetes. Similarly, it is possible to be classified as overweight, or even obese, and have good cardiovascular fitness. External appearance should not be considered a key marker for physical health and well-being. By shifting away from a focus on appearance, we may, subsequently, see additional shifts in individuals' attitudes toward their bodies as research has shown that people generally hold more positive attitudes about how their bodies function than about how they look (Franzoi, 1995). At the same time, this shift from form to function may make it more likely that the thin ideal can be replaced by a more diverse array of options that could be part of a healthy ideal.

For the time being, however, we still live in a culture where we are surrounded by thin ideal images and messages. We cannot sit idly by and wait for ideals to shift so that women can feel better about themselves and recognize that everyone will never fit a single appearance ideal, whether it is thin, curvy, fat, or muscled. We need to start now to help women understand that these ideals are unrealistic and to influence the media and fashion industry to shift the norms of attractiveness. That is, we need to work at both individual and cultural levels to create positive change.

Feminism has often been seen as a tool of resistance against negative social messages aimed toward women, and messages about the body are no exception to this. One study showed that, although feminist-identified women critiqued cultural messages about appearance and beauty, they still endorsed them, at least to some extent, and felt conflict that their feminist beliefs did not fully align with their appearance beliefs (Rubin, Nemeroff, & Russo, 2004). Other research has shown that feminists may experience some protection due to their lower rates of endorsement of the norm of thinness as compared to women who did not self-identify as feminists (Hurt et al., 2007). In other words, for those who can reduce the importance of thinness, the negative pattern of surveying one's body and finding it too far from the thin ideal, body shame and other negative outcomes may be reduced or removed.

Feminism can provide tools that help women to critique cultural messages about beauty and thinness; however, only 25% or fewer women identify as feminists (e.g., CBS News Monthly Poll, 2005, 2006; Swanson, 2013). Given this, it is important to consider other ways to help girls and women critique these messages about beauty and thinness. Media literacy programs have been shown to have a significant impact on internalization of the thin ideal, body dissatisfaction, and dieting among adolescents (Wilksch, Tiggemann, & Wade, 2006; Wilksch & Wade, 2009). Intervention programs where those who have internalized the thin ideal voluntarily take a stance against it have also been shown to lower rates of thin ideal internalization, body dissatisfaction, and dieting in college-aged samples (Becker, Ciao, & Smith, 2008; Stice, Chase, Stormer, & Appel, 2001). In sum, active critique of the thin ideal can help reduce its impact.

It is also important to recognize that critiquing the thin ideal is not enough to result in cultural change. We need to recognize that problems lie not just in associating thin with beautiful and beautiful with good (therefore, thin = good). Rather, the belief that thin is good also reflects a cultural belief that fat is bad, and that those who are fat, or at least are not thin, are themselves bad or are lesser in some way (e.g., have less self-control, have poorer health, are less happy; Chrisler, 2012).

Appearance ideals do shift over time; we have seen this with the rising focus on muscle tone in concert with the thin ideal over the past few decades. Just shifting to a new ideal is not enough. As long as we do that, there will always be a small group of women who conform to the ideal and a much larger group of women who do not. Those who do not fit the ideal, the cultural norm people are encouraged to strive to meet, will always be seen as less worthy. Yes, the thin ideal is dangerous in part because the thin body put forth as a goal is not one most can achieve through healthy means or without surgical intervention. It is also dangerous because it is creating inherent inequity: the haves and have-nots of body types. Replacing this ideal with another may shift some of the attention toward physical health risks associated with pursuit of the thin ideal. It will not, however, solve the underlying problem of body dissatisfaction among myriad women who do not see themselves reflected in the body type touted as ideal and desirable. Challenging the thin ideal is not just about challenging this one ideal; it is about challenging the idea that there can ever be a single ideal female body, that there is only one acceptable appearance. It is also about challenging the idea that appearance is what can make women happy. Rather, we need to work to free women from a focus on their appearance so that they can be happy with who they are and what they can accomplish. If women were not so focused on appearance, they would have more time, energy, and attention available to be better able to focus on other goals in their lives.

REFERENCES

Ackard, D. M., Croll, J. K., & Kearney-Cooke, A. (2002). Dieting frequency among college females: Association with disordered eating, body image, and related psychological problems. *Journal of Psychosomatic Research, 52,* 129–136.

American Psychiatric Association. (2013). *Diagnostic and statistical manual of mental disorders* (5th ed.). Arlington, VA: Author.

Bandura, A. (1977). *Social learning theory.* Englewood Cliffs, NJ: Prentice Hall.

Bearman, S. K., Presnell, K., Martinez, E., & Stice, E. (2006). The skinny on body dissatisfaction: A longitudinal study of adolescent girls and boys. *Journal of Youth and Adolescence, 35,* 217–229.

Becker, A. E. (2004). Television, disordered eating, and young women in Fiji: Negotiating body image and identity during rapid social change. *Culture, Medicine, and Psychiatry, 28,* 533–559.

Becker, A. E., Burwell, R. A., Herzog, D. B., Hamburg, P., & Gilman, S. E. (2002). Eating behaviours and attitudes following prolonged exposure to television among ethnic Fijian adolescent girls. *British Journal of Psychiatry, 180,* 509–514.

Becker, C. B., Ciao, A. C., & Smith, L. M. (2008). Moving from efficacy to effectiveness in eating disorders prevention: The sorority body image program. *Cognitive and Behavioral Practice, 15,* 18–27.

Birmingham, C. L., & Treasure, J. (2010). *Medical management of eating disorders* (2nd ed.). Cambridge: Cambridge University Press.

Bombak, A. (2014). Obesity, health at every size, and public health policy. *American Journal of Public Health, 104,* 60–67.

Bouchard, C. (2002). Genetic influences on body weight. In C. G. Fairburn & K. D. Brownell (Eds.), *Eating disorders and obesity: A comprehensive handbook* (pp. 16–21). New York: Guilford.

Bravata, D. M., Sanders, L., Huang, J., Krumholz, H. M., Olkin, I., Gardner, C. D., & Bravata, D. M. (2003). Efficacy and safety of low-carbohydrate diets: A systematic review. *Journal of the American Medical Association, 289,* 1837–1850.

Calogero, R. M., Boroughs, M., & Thompson, J. K. (2007). The impact of Western beauty ideals on the lives of women and men: A sociocultural perspective. In V. Swami & A. Furnham (Eds.), *Body beautiful: Evolutionary and sociocultural perspectives* (pp. 259–298). New York: Palgrave Macmillan.

Calogero, R. M., & Thompson, J. K. (2009). Sexual self-esteem in American and British college women: Relations with self-objectification and eating problems. *Sex Roles, 60*, 160–173.

Calogero, R. M., & Thompson, J. K. (2010). Gender and body image. In J. C. Chrisler & D. R. McCreary (Eds.), *Handbook of gender research in psychology* (vol. 2, pp. 153–184). New York: Springer.

Capodilupo, C. M. (2014). One size does not fit all: Using variables other than the thin ideal to understand black women's body image. *Cultural Diversity and Ethnic Minority Psychology.* in press. doi: 10.1037/a0037649.

CBS News Monthly Poll. (2005). Q60: Feminist. Retrieved from http://www.icpsr.umich.edu/icpsrweb/ICPSR/ssvd/variables/04327-0001_Q60?q=feminist.

CBS News Monthly Poll. (2006). Q27: Feminist. Retrieved from http://www.icpsr.umich.edu/icpsrweb/ICPSR/ssvd/variables/04615-0001_Q27?q=feminist.

Centers for Disease Control and Prevention (CDC). (2014). How much physical activity do adults need? Retrieved from http://www.cdc.gov/physicalactivity/everyone/guidelines/adults.html.

Chrisler, J. C. (2008). Fear of losing control: Power, perfectionism, and the psychology of women. *Psychology of Women Quarterly, 32*, 1–12.

Chrisler, J. C. (2012). "Why can't you control yourself?" Fat *should be* a feminist issue. *Sex Roles, 66*, 608–616.

Collier, R. (2013). Intermittent fasting: The next big weight loss fad. *Canadian Medical Association Journal, 185*, E321–E322.

Currin, L., Schmidt, U., Treasure, J., & Jick, H. (2005). Time trends in eating disorder incidence. *British Journal of Psychiatry, 186*, 132–135.

Dion, K. E., Berscheid, E., & Walster, E. (1972). What is beautiful is good. *Journal of Personality and Social Psychology, 24*, 285–290.

Dittmar, H., Halliwell, E., & Stirling, E. (2009). Understanding the impact of thin media models on women's body-focused affect: The roles of thin-ideal internalization and weight-related self-discrepancy activation in experimental exposure effects. *Journal of Social and Clinical Psychology, 28*, 43–72.

Engeln-Maddox, R. (2006). Buying a beauty standard or dreaming of a new life? Expectations associated with media ideals. *Psychology of Women Quarterly, 30*, 258–266.

Erchull, M. J., Liss, M., & Lichiello, S. (2013). Extending the negative consequences of media internalization and self-objectification to dissociation and self-harm. *Sex Roles, 69*, 583–593.

Ferguson, C. J. (2013). In the eye of the beholder: Thin-ideal media affects some, but not most, viewers in a meta-analytic review of body dissatisfaction in women and men. *Psychology of Popular Media Culture, 2*, 20–37.

Festinger, L. (1954). A theory of social comparison processes. *Human Relations, 7*, 117–140.

Franzoi, S. L. (1995). The body-as-object versus the body-as-process: Gender differences and gender considerations. *Sex Roles, 33*, 417–437.

Fredrickson, B. L., & Roberts, T-A. (1997). Objectification theory: Toward understanding women's lived experiences and mental health risks. *Psychology of Women Quarterly, 21*, 173–206.

Fredrickson, B. L., Roberts, T-A., Noll, S. M., Quinn, D. M., & Twenge, J. M. (1998). That swimsuit becomes you: Sex differences in self-objectification, restrained eating, and math performance. *Journal of Personality and Social Psychology, 75*, 269–284.

Gaesser, G. A. (1999). Thinness and weight loss: Beneficial or detrimental to longevity? *Medicine and Science in Sports and Exercise, 31*, 1118–1128.

Garner, D. M. (1997, February). Survey says: Body image poll results. *Psychology Today*. Retrieved from http://www.psychologytoday.com/articles/199702/survey-says-body-image-poll-results.

Gerbner, G., Gross, L., Morgan, M., & Signorielli, N. (1994). Growing up with television: The cultivation perspective. In J. Bryant & D. Zillman (Eds.), *Media effects: Advances in theory and research* (pp. 17–42). Hillsdale, NJ: Erlbaum.

Grabe, S., Ward, L. M., & Hyde, J. S. (2008). The role of the media in body image concerns among women: A meta-analysis of experimental and correlational studies. *Psychological Bulletin, 134*, 460–476.

Harrison, K. (2003). Television viewers' ideal body proportions: The case of the curvaceously thin woman. *Sex Roles, 48*, 255–264.

Harrison, K., & Cantor, J. (1997). The relationship between media consumption and eating disorders. *Journal of Communication, 47*, 40–67.

Harrison, K., Taylor, L. D., & Marske, A. L. (2006). Women's and men's eating behavior following exposure to ideal-body images and text. *Communication Research, 33*, 507–529.

Hebl, M. R., King, E. B., & Lin, J. (2004). The swimsuit becomes us all: Ethnicity, gender, and vulnerability to self-objectification. *Personality and Social Psychology Bulletin, 30*, 1322–1331.

Hoste, R. R., & Le Grange, D. (2013). Eating disorders in adolescence. In W. T. O'Donohue, L. T. Benuto, & L. W. Tolle (Eds.), *Handbook of adolescent health psychology* (pp. 495–506). New York: Springer.

Hudson, J. I., Hiripi, E., Pope Jr., H. G., & Kessler, R. C. (2007). The prevalence and correlates of eating disorders in the National Comorbidity Survey replication. *Biological Psychiatry, 61*, 348–358.

Hurt, M. M., Nelson, J. A., Turner, D. T., Haines, M. E., Ramsey, L. R., Erchull, M. J., & Liss, M. (2007). Feminism: What is it good for? Feminine norms and objectification as the link between feminist identity and clinically relevant outcomes. *Sex Roles, 57*, 355–363.

Karazsia, B. T., van Dulmen, M. H. M., Wong, K., & Crowther, J. H. (2013). Thinking meta-theoretically about the role of internalization in the development of body dissatisfaction and body change behaviors. *Body Image, 10*, 433–441.

Keel, P. K., & Klump, K. L. (2003). Are eating disorders culture-bound syndromes? Implications for conceptualizing their etiology. *Psychological Bulletin, 129*, 747–769.

Keery, H., van den Berg, P., & Thompson, J. K. (2004). An evaluation of the tripartite influence model of body dissatisfaction and eating disturbance with adolescent girls. *Body Image, 1*, 237–251.

Kelley, H. H. (1955). The two functions of reference groups. In G. E. Swanson, T. M. Newcomb, & E. L. Hartley (Eds.), *Readings in social psychology* (2nd ed., pp. 410–414). New York: Holt.

Kilbourne, J. (1999). *Can't buy my love: How advertising changes the way we think and feel*. New York: Simon & Schuster.

Langlois, J. H., Kalakanis, L., Rubenstein, A. J., Larson, A., Hallam, M., & Smoot, M. (2000). Maxims or myths of beauty? A meta-analytic and theoretical review. *Psychological Bulletin, 126*, 390–423.

Levine, M. P., & Harrison, K. (2004). Media's role in the perpetuation and prevention of negative body image and disordered eating. In J. K. Thompson (Ed.), *Handbook of eating disorders and obesity* (pp. 695–717). New York: Wiley.

Lieberman, M., Gauvin, L., Bukowski, W. M., & White, D. R. (2001). Interpersonal influence and disordered eating behaviors in adolescent girls: The role of peer modeling, social reinforcement, and body-related teasing. *Eating Behaviors, 2*, 215–236.

Lopez, E., Blix, G. G., & Blix, A. G. (1995). Body image of Latinas compared to body image of non-Latina white women. *Health Values, 19*, 3–10.

Lowes, J., & Tiggemann, M. (2003). Body dissatisfaction, dieting awareness, and the impact of parental influence in young children. *British Journal of Health Psychology, 8*, 135–147.

Mahalik, J. R., Morray, E. B., Coonerty-Femiano, A., Ludlow, L. H., Slattery, S. M., & Smiler, A. (2005). Development of the conformity to feminine norms inventory. *Sex Roles, 52*, 417–435.

Mann, T., Tomiyama, A. J., Westling, E., Lew, A., Samuels, B., & Chatman, J. (2007). Medicare's search for effective obesity treatments: Diets are not the answer. *American Psychologist, 62*, 220–233.

McCreary, D. R., & Sadava, S. W. (1999). Television viewing and self-perceived health, weight, and physical fitness: Evidence for the cultivation hypothesis. *Journal of Applied Social Psychology, 29*, 2342–2361.

McKinley, N. M., & Hyde, J. S. (1996). The objectified body consciousness scale: Development and validation. *Psychology of Women Quarterly, 20*, 181–215.

McLaren, L., Kuh, D., Hardy, R., & Gauvin, L. (2004). Positive and negative body-related comments and their relationship with body dissatisfaction in middle-aged women. *Psychology & Health, 19*, 261–272.

Mond, J. M., Hay, P. J., Rodgers, B., & Owen, C. (2006). An update on the definition of "excessive exercise" in eating disorders research. *International Journal of Eating Disorders, 39*, 147–153.

Moradi, B., & Huang, Y. P. (2008). Objectification theory and psychology of women: A decade of advances and future directions. *Psychology of Women Quarterly, 32*, 377–398.

Murray, S. H., Touyz, S. W., & Beumont, P. J. (1995). The influence of personal relationships on women's eating behavior and body satisfaction. *Eating Disorders, 3*, 243–252.

Noll, S. M., & Fredrickson, B. L. (1998). A mediational model linking self-objectification, body shame, and disordered eating. *Psychology of Women Quarterly, 22*, 623–636.

Norris, M. L., Boydell, K. M., Pinhas, L., & Katzman, D. K. (2006). Ana and the internet: A review of pro-anorexia websites. *International Journal of Eating Disorders, 39*, 443–447.

Pashler, H. (1994). Dual-task interference in simple tasks: Data and theory. *Psychological Bulletin, 116*, 220–244.

Paxton, S. J., Schutz, H. K., Wertheim, E. H., & Muir, S. L. (1999). Friendship clique and peer influences on body image concerns, dietary restraint, extreme weight-loss behaviors, and binge eating in adolescent girls. *Journal of Abnormal Psychology, 108*, 255–266.

Rodin, J., Silberstein, L. R., & Striegel-Moore, R. H. (1984). Women and weight: A normative discontent. In T. B. Sonderegger (Ed.), *Nebraska symposium on motivation: Psychology and gender* (pp. 267–307). Lincoln: University of Nebraska Press.

Rubin, L. R., Nemeroff, C. J., & Russo, N. F. (2004). Exploring feminist women's body consciousness. *Psychology of Women Quarterly, 28*, 27–37.

Smink, F. R., van Hoeken, D., & Hoek, H. W. (2013). Epidemiology, course, and outcome of eating disorders. *Current Opinion in Psychiatry, 26*, 543–548.

Smolak, L. (2012). Appearance in childhood and adolescence. In N. Rumsey & D. Harcourt (Eds.), *Oxford handbook of the psychology of appearance* (pp. 123–141). London: Oxford University Press.

Solmi, F., Hatch, S. L., Hotopf, M., Treasure, J., & Micali, N. (2014). Prevalence and correlates of disordered eating in a general population sample: The South East London Community Health (SELCoH) study. *Social Psychiatry and Psychiatric Epidemiology, 49*, 1335–1346.

Stice, E., Chase, A., Stormer, S., & Appel, A. (2001). A randomized trial of a dissonance-based eating disorder prevention program. *International Journal of Eating Disorders, 29*, 247–262.

Stover, C. (2014). "Divulging the eat deets": Postfeminist self-surveillance on women's fitness blogs. eScholarship, University of California. UCLA Center for the Study of Women. Retrieved from https://escholarship.org/uc/item/7rv4v26h.

Swanson, E. (2013, April 16). Poll: Few identify as feminists, but most believe in equality of sexes. *Huffington Post*. Retrieved from http://www.huffingtonpost.com/2013/04/16/feminism-poll_n_3094917.html.

Tantleff-Dunn, S., Barnes, R. D., & Larose, J. G. (2011). It's not just a "woman thing:" The current state of normative discontent. *Eating Disorders, 19*, 392–402.

Thomas, J. J., & Schaefer, J. (2013). *Almost anorexic: Is my (or my loved one's) relationship with food a problem?* Cambridge, MA: Harvard University Press.

Thompson, J. K., & Cafri, G. (2007). *The muscular ideal: Psychological, social, and medical perspectives*. Washington, DC: American Psychological Association.

Thompson, J. K., Heinberg, L. J., Altabe, M., & Tantleff-Dunn, S. (1999). *Exacting beauty: Theory, assessment, and treatment of body image disturbance*. Washington, DC: American Psychological Association.

Thompson, J. K., & Tantleff, S. (1992). Female and male ratings of upper torso: Actual, ideal, and stereotypical conceptions. *Journal of Social Behavior & Personality, 7*, 345–354.

Tiggemann, M. (2011). Mental health risks of self-objectification: A review of the empirical evidence for disordered eating, depressed mood, and sexual dysfunction. In R. M. Calogero, S. Tantleff-Dunn, & J. K. Thompson (Eds.), *Self-objectification in women: Causes, consequences, and counteractions* (pp. 139–159). Washington, DC: American Psychological Association.

Wilksch, S. M., Tiggemann, M., & Wade, T. D. (2006). Impact of interactive school-based media literacy lessons for reducing internalization of media ideals in young adolescent girls and boys. *International Journal of Eating Disorders, 39*, 385–393.

Wilksch, S. M., & Wade, T. D. (2009). Reduction of shape and weight concern in young adolescents: A 30-month controlled evaluation of a media literacy program. *Journal of the American Academy of Child & Adolescent Psychiatry, 48*, 652–661.

Wolf, N. (1991). *The beauty myth: How images of beauty are used against women*. New York: Random House.

Wooley, O. W., Wooley, S. C., & Dyrenforth, S. R. (1979). Obesity and women: A neglected feminist topic. *Women's Studies International Quarterly, 2*, 81–92.

Zones, J. S. (2000). Beauty myths and realities and their impacts on women's health. In M. B. Zinn, P. Hondagneu-Sotelo, & M. Messner (Eds.), *Gender through the prism of difference* (2nd ed., pp. 87–103). Boston: Allyn & Bacon.

Chapter 9

From Fat Shaming to Size Acceptance: Challenging the Medical Management of Fat Women

Ashley E. Kasardo and Maureen C. McHugh

Fat women are big losers in the current war on obesity. Many groups and individuals are invested in fat women losing weight—"for their own good." Doctors tell fat women to lose weight and frequently connect all of their health problems or symptoms to their size. Fat women may also receive advice to lose weight from their hairstylists, their dentists, their neighbors, their parents, their children, and even from complete strangers. Some of their friends and family members may hint at or encourage them to lose weight, whereas others are more direct. Coworkers engage in "fat talk" around them, discussing how much weight they themselves want to lose, or have lost, which foods they allow themselves to eat, and which foods are "bad." Well intentioned or not, such comments are misinformed and frequently serve to shame fat women.

THE WAR ON OBESITY

Entire industries have a vested interest in maintaining the war on obesity and on women's (unsuccessful) attempts to lose weight. The diet industry, with the assistance of health care professionals, continues to sell a product that has been demonstrated to be ineffective. Because dieters are almost guaranteed to regain the weight they lose, the diet industry can count on fat individuals to be lifelong customers. Advertising agencies also profit from this effort, as do researchers and clinicians in a variety of fields who have been funded to investigate the perils of obesity and to search for more effective methods of weight loss. "Our national war on fat has created a colossal health and diet industry closely enmeshed with government agencies. Profit motives for our $60 billion diet industry and fat stigma have become so entangled that it has become difficult, perhaps impossible, to even entertain the possibility that we are fighting the wrong war . . . the purpose of the diet industrial complex is to keep people dieting . . . rather than to seek health" (Farrell, 2011, p. 14).

In addition to advice to lose weight, fat women experience hostility, prejudice, and discrimination on a daily basis (Seacat, Dougal, & Roy, 2014). Farrell (2011, p. 176) tied fat stigma and the denigration of fat and fat people to the profits of the diet industrial complex: "The shame of fatness fuels our extraordinarily large weight loss industry." Fat is a stigmatized condition in many Western countries, which exposes fat women to daily indignities and humiliation. Seacat and colleagues (2014) studied the diary entries on weight-based interactions of 50 overweight women, who recorded an average of three fat-shaming moments per day. For example, a waitress asked a fat woman if she wanted a diet Coke, or just brought her a diet soda, when she had ordered a regular soda. Teenagers made mooing sounds within hearing range of a fat woman. People on public transportation laughed when a fat woman had difficulty fitting into a seat designed for smaller riders. Farrell (2011) referred to such experiences as rituals of humiliation.

There is considerable evidence of stigma and hostility toward fat people, especially women. Although it is generally seen as wrong to discriminate against people for a characteristic they cannot control, fat prejudice is accepted based on the mistaken widespread belief that fat people can become thin if they want to do so. The medicalization of fat as "obesity" and the subsequent war on obesity endorses dieting and suggests that weight can be controlled through caloric management and exercise, which gives people permission to demonstrate hostility and discrimination against fat women who appear to have refused to diet or seem to be too lazy to exercise. Contrary to popular opinion, and in many cases mistaken medical opinion, scientific evidence continues to demonstrate that, for the most part, weight is not within the control of an individual. Being fat is not in itself a disease, and dieting is not an effective intervention for being fat or obese. The war on obesity, including attempts to shame fat women into becoming thin, not only interferes with fat women's pursuit of health, but it also contributes to poor psychological and physical health. This chapter proposes alternative approaches to health for fat women, which do not involve shaming, dieting, and punitive exercise.

Weight Bias

Size acceptance advocates encourage taking back the word *fat* as a simple descriptor and not using it as a derogatory term. "Overweight" implies that there is a certain "right" weight to which everyone can be compared. However, in actuality everyone has a weight that is unique and right for them (Wann, 1998). "Obese" is a medical term that communicates society's tendency to medicalize eating behavior (Robison & Erdman, 1998). In a study of the impact of weight labels, Smith, Schmoll, Konik, and Oberlander (2007) found that women labeled as fat, overweight, or obese were perceived to be more unhealthy and fat than were women described as full figured. They concluded that weight terminology influences how women are perceived and that different weight terms "evoke varying levels of weight stigma" (p. 1001). Therefore, we recommend that the word fat be used without negative connotations (Berg, 1998; Brown, 1989; Crandall, 1994; Wann, 1998). In this chapter, the words fat or person of size are utilized as weight descriptors. Terminology such as obese, overweight, and normal size are utilized only when specific researchers have used them to describe weight in their respective studies.

Fat oppression is hatred and discrimination against fat people, especially fat women, solely because of their body size. It is the "stigmatization of being fat, the terror of fat, the rationale for a thousand diets . . . and exercise programs. . . . It is, like physical and sexual violence against women, sexism in action" (Brown & Rothblum, 1989, p. 1). Fat prejudice, which is defined as negative attitudes toward or dislike of fat people, stereotypes about fat people, or discrimination against people perceived as fat (Danielsdottir, O'Brien, & Ciao, 2010), has been widely documented, as has size oppression, which is defined as hatred of and discrimination against fat people solely because of their body size (Brownell, Puhl, Schwartz, & Rudd, 2005; Crandall, 1994; Danielsdottir et al., 2010; Fikkan & Rothblum, 2012). Fat prejudice (also known as weight bias or sizism) indicates that body size is one of the few personal attributes considered to be an acceptable target of prejudice (Puhl & Brownell, 2003; Watts & Cranney, 2009).

Puhl and Heuer (2009) explained that "weight bias translates into inequities in employment settings, health-care facilities, and educational institutions often due to widespread negative stereotypes that overweight and obese persons are lazy, unmotivated, lacking in self-discipline, less competent, non-compliant, and sloppy" (p. 941). These stereotypes are rarely challenged, and, as a result, people of size are "vulnerable to social injustice, unfair treatment, and impaired quality of life as a result of substantial disadvantages and stigma" (Puhl & Heuer, 2009, p. 941). Unlike racism, sexism, and homophobia, fat oppressive attitudes are embraced, excused, or rationalized by many, including otherwise progressive persons (Schoenfielder & Wieser, 1983). The belief that fat people ought to work harder to become thin is an expression of this prejudice.

Gender

Sizism differentially impacts men and women: It impacts women more severely than it does men (Brown, 1989; Fikkan & Rothblum, 2012; Ristovski-Slijepcevic, Bell, Chapman, & Beagan, 2010; Tiggemann & Rothblum, 1988). Weight is ranked as the third most prevalent cause of perceived discrimination among women, following gender and age (Puhl, Andreyeva, & Brownell, 2008). This is a serious problem because it results in a "reduction in opportunities in the domains of employment, education, and marital relationships" that impacts fat women's economic opportunities (Fikkan & Rothblum, 2012, p. 587).

Fikkan and Rothblum (2012, p. 575) explored the idea that "culture allows for much less deviation from aesthetic ideals for women than it does for men," which means that women are more likely to be judged harshly, to be dissatisfied with their bodies, and to engage in "corrective" action to change their weight and shape. Beauty ideals (including the ideal weight) are culturally influenced and have shifted from idealizing a full-figured body to favoring and promoting extreme thinness (Fraser, 2009). Robison, Putnam, and McKibbin (2007a) reported that weight loss promotion began in the early 20th century and "coincided with women securing the right to vote and demanding a more visible and active role in shaping society" (p. 144).

Theorists have observed or documented that issues related to body image and (dis)satisfaction are central to women's lives and are sources of distress (Bordo & Heywood, 2004; Chrisler, 2011; Rodin, Silberstein, & Striegel-Moore, 1984; Wolf, 1991). Brown (1989) asserted that fat oppression is aimed particularly at women, and she identified fat prejudice as a form of patriarchal oppression that has severely impacted women's lives. In her clinical psychology practice, Brown has observed that fat oppression divides women, prevents women from adequately feeding and nurturing themselves, and prevents them from being fed and nurtured by other women. Feminist psychologists have commented on the degree to which fat oppression drains energy and resources from women's lives; the millions of dollars spent on weight loss and diet schemes could alternatively be spent to improve the quality of women's lives (Saltzberg & Chrisler, 1995; Smith, 2004).

Cultural expectations for women equate beauty with thinness (Chrisler, 1989), and they influence body satisfaction and impact women and men differently. Men also experience body dissatisfaction, but instead of facing the thinness ideal, men face the muscular ideal; they focus on building muscle mass, whereas women focus on trying to lose weight (Bell & McNaughton, 2007). This pursuit of thinness via dieting takes a toll emotionally, physically, and also economically (see Chapter 8 in this volume). The fashion industry and the media collaborate with medicine and the diet industry to create an anti-fat bias in contemporary culture that directly affects women's well-being (Farrell, 2011).

Stigma

Weight is a stigmatizing condition. Anti-fat stigma is consistent and severe (Solovay, 2000). Crocker, Cornwell, and Major (1993) argued that "two important dimensions along which stigmatizing conditions differ are visibility and controllability" (p. 67); "overweight might be the most debilitating" (p. 60) stigma as it is both observable and perceived to be under an individual's control, therefore, individuals are often blamed for this condition. The perception that fat women can (easily) become thin through self-discipline in caloric intake and physical exercise is at the core of the stigmatization and rejection of fat women. Hilbert, Rief, and Braehler (2007) examined people's beliefs about the perceived causes of obesity; obesity was widely viewed as caused by lack of activity (82.4%) and overeating (72.8%); only one-third (34.9%) of those surveyed agreed that heredity is important. The belief that variables under the control of the fat person (i.e., diet and exercise) are the principal factors in obesity results in stigma and fat prejudice.

The belief that weight is volitionally controlled, paired with a cultural preference for thinness, leads to anti-fat attitudes (Crandall & Martinez, 1996). Crandall (1994) and others (e.g., Musher-Eizenmann, Holub, Miller, Goldstein, & Edwards-Leeper, 2004; Puhl & Brownell, 2003) believe that attribution of controllability results in the stigmatization of fat individuals, who are perceived as responsible for their condition. Thus, the medical approach, which emphasizes that fat people can lose weight by dieting, contributes significantly to the stigma attached to fat and to openly expressed disdain for fat people. Although research indicates that body weight is affected by an interaction of biological and environmental factors and that diets are ineffective, fat individuals are viewed as people who could control their weight but do not (Puhl & Brownell, 2003).

Medicalization Perpetuates Weight Bias

The medical approach is that obesity is a disease that can be remedied by weight loss and exercising willpower (Robison et al., 2007a; Solovay, 2000). The medical model assumes that weight loss results in improved health; thus, losing weight is the standard, culturally endorsed solution (Bacon & Aphramor, 2011; Erdman, 1999; Robison et al., 2007a). Discrimination against fat people and the acceptability of fat prejudice stem from the belief that fat people can become thin if they choose to do so. Contrary to popular opinion, scientific evidence over the past 25 years continues to point to the fact that weight is not fully within the control of the individual. Biological mechanisms that regulate weight loss have been identified. Current dieting and weight management strategies have been found to be ineffective; 95% of individuals who diet either do not lose weight or gain the lost weight back.

A medicalized view of body size sets up the dichotomy that fat is unhealthy and thinness is healthy. In 2002, Surgeon General Richard Carmona referred to the "obesity epidemic" as the "terror within; a threat that is every bit as real to America as the weapons of mass destruction" (Bacon & Aphramor, 2014, p. 11). However, fat as a health risk is exaggerated, and health concerns are used to stigmatize fat people (Burgard, 2009). Medical researchers have maintained that obesity is a health problem that is related to an array of chronic illnesses and even to mortality; thus, weight loss is the route to good health. In the practice of medicine, and in research generally, the body mass index (BMI) is used to determine the healthy weights for individuals. The BMI is a mathematical formula that uses height and weight to determine one's weight status on a scale that consists of several weight cutoffs (Campos, 2005). According to U.S. government standards, these weight cutoffs include classification as underweight, normal weight, overweight, or obese (Gaesser, 2002). The BMI has been critiqued as an indicator of health. Burgard (2009) described the weight cutoffs as "arbitrary dividing lines"(p. 49), and Campos (2005) asserted that the BMI is a cultural construct and not scientific fact. Studies show that the correlation between health problems and BMI is only 0.3, which means that 91% of health outcomes are not related to one's BMI (Burgard, 2009). Furthermore, research does not support the belief that weight loss will improve health status. Such research is difficult to conduct because very few people maintain weight loss over two years. Wann (1998) has concluded that the health argument against fat is actually a "big smokescreen for fat hatred" (p. 33).

CHALLENGING THE MEDICAL MODEL

Robison and colleagues (2007a) described the war on obesity as resting on claims that obesity is a cause of premature death, that excess fat is a direct cause of disease, and that weight loss results in health benefits. It is critical for health professionals and consumers to examine how valid those claims are. As it turns out, research does not support the validity of any of them.

The Paradox of Fat

In what is sometimes called the "obesity paradox," epidemiological studies show that individuals who are overweight or moderately obese live at least as long as normal weight people, and often longer (Bacon & Aphramor, 2011). This evidence is only paradoxical for individuals who believe that being fat is a disease or a health risk. Despite common myths, elevated weight is not associated with decreased longevity. Research has shown that individuals who are fat and fit have longer life spans than do individuals who are thin and sedentary (Gaesser, 2002). In addition, there are more annual deaths in the underweight category than in the overweight or obese categories (Bacon, 2008), although thinness-related deaths are rarely discussed in the media.

Although obesity is correlated with risk for many diseases, epidemiological studies typically do not control for factors such as fitness, activity, nutrient intake, weight cycling (the yo-yo effect), or socioeconomic status (Bacon & Aphramor, 2011). When these factors are controlled, the increased risk of disease for overweight individuals is reduced or disappears completely.

Diets Do Not Work

The proposed medical solution to the "obesity epidemic" is to lose weight, following the simple formula to eat less and exercise more, except that things are not that simple. This formula comes with numerous assumptions, including that people are fat through their own volition and that weight is completely controllable, both of which are fallacies. The truth is more complicated. Biology and internal bodily mechanisms explain why losing weight is not as simple, or as necessary, as is usually assumed.

The body has internal weight-regulation mechanisms that work to maintain homeostasis. The body's mechanism to maintain weight is termed the set-point (Bacon & Aphramor, 2014). This weight-regulation system can be disrupted, and even dysregulated, if repeated attempts are made to lose weight. Bacon and Aphramor (2014) noted that weight loss triggers strong responses from the body that are designed to limit weight loss or even to promote weight gain. Basically, the body is designed to hold on to weight rather than to let it go. This has evolutionary underpinnings. From an evolutionary perspective, years ago, food was not as readily available as it is in most societies today. It was advantageous for our ancestors to have genes that encouraged fat storage, which made it more likely they would survive cold winters, illnesses, and famines, and thus be able to reproduce. Clearly the environment has changed, and food is now more plentiful in most places than it once was. "The world we've created is very different than the one we were designed for" (Bacon & Aphramor, 2014, p. 67). Consider how this impacts people's attempts at weight loss. At first, a woman who is dieting might lose some weight. Given the body's weight regulatory mechanisms, however, the body "notices" this loss and, if weight loss exceeds a certain amount, the body will respond to halt or reverse the loss (Bacon & Aphramor, 2014). "Compensatory adjustments" can be made to maintain one's set-point, such as increased feelings of hunger or lowered metabolic rate caused in part by reduced amounts of leptin in the body (Bacon & Aphramor, 2014, p. 20). If a woman ignores these hunger cues to try to continue her diet, she may get into the habit of ignoring and not responding to other cues from her body that are important to good health (e.g., sleepiness, thirst, cravings for certain nutrients). Ironically dieting, like overeating, involves dismissing hunger cues from the body.

Ineffectiveness and Repercussions of Dieting

The set-point mechanisms are overworked in the case of chronic dieting, which results in even less leptin release, which could be related to why individuals with a history of dieting tend to gain weight over time and weigh more than they did when they started to diet (Bacon & Aphramor, 2014). Yo-yo dieting, or cycling from losing to gaining weight, impacts bodily functions and may even raise the body's set-point to a higher weight. Yo-yo dieting "habituates the metabolism to store extra fat as soon as the deficit ends in preparation for the next perceived shortage" (Bacon & Aphramor, 2014, pp. 68–69). Weight cycling creates stress on the body's systems, contributes to hypertension and insulin resistance, and is associated with poorer cardiovascular outcomes (Bacon & Aphramor, 2011) and kidney damage (Campos, 2005). Engaging in calorie restriction can cause inflammation, as can repeatedly losing and regaining weight, which is a risk factor for what are often termed "obesity-related diseases," including heart disease and diabetes (Bacon & Aphramor, 2014). The Iowa Women's Health Study (described by Gaesser, 2002) was initiated in 1986 to evaluate the relation between intentional weight loss and mortality. The 42,000 older women (ages 55 to 69) in the study were asked about intentional weight loss of 20 pounds or more. In no case was intentional weight loss statistically associated with lower mortality rate, but in 74% of statistical comparisons of women who lost weight with women who did not, weight loss was associated with higher mortality risk. The death rate was 260% higher for women who lost weight than for those whose weight remained stable. The results of this study indicate that, in terms of health, overweight women may be better off staying overweight.

Feelings of guilt about eating can impact metabolism and weight regulation (Bacon & Aphramor, 2014). In a recent study (Kuijer & Boyce, 2014), participants were asked if they associated eating chocolate cake with guilt or with celebration; 27% of participants associated it with the former and 73% with the latter. Participants who reported feeling guilty also reported a perceived loss of control over their eating behaviors. When the weight status of the participants was examined 18 months after the initial interviews, those who associated eating cake with guilt had gained more weight than those who associated eating cake with pleasure; the pleasure group was more likely than the guilt group to maintain a stable weight over time. Kuijer and Boyce concluded that there is not an adaptive connection between guilt and eating.

As Bacon and Aphramor (2014) pointed out, not experiencing long-term weight loss is actually a sign that the body's internal weight regulation system is successful. However, people who do not lose weight from dieting can experience shame and blame for "failing" at their goal, despite the well-documented 90% to 95% failure rate (Robison, Putnam, & McKibbin, 2007b). Health care professionals should ask themselves whether it is ethical to recommend weight loss as an intervention, given the lack of efficacy of diet-based approaches as well as the potential negative physiological and psychological consequences that can result from dieting (Bacon & Aphramor, 2011; Chrisler, 1989; Robison et al., 2007b), including feelings of guilt.

Weight Bias and Health

A medicalized perspective toward size impacts treatments that are prescribed for patients. Bacon and Aphramor (2014) cited an example of both a heavy and a thin individual seeking treatment for joint pain. Depending on the cause of the problem, the joint pain might be exacerbated by the weight of the heavier person, but that does not mean that weight loss should be the doctor's prescription. The heavier patient deserves the same treatment regimen that would be recommended for the thin patient, for example, stretching and strengthening exercises and possible surgery. There is no disease that occurs in individuals who are fat that does not also occur in individuals who are thin.

A medicalized perspective toward fat can impact individuals' health care–seeking behaviors. Research has documented that people of size face bias from doctors, nurses, dieticians, and mental health care providers (Puhl & Brownell, 2006; Sabin, Marini, & Nosek, 2012; Schwartz, Chambliss, Brownell, Blair, & Billingham, 2003). In a study of primary care physicians, Foster and colleagues (2003) found that more than 50% of physicians viewed obese patients as awkward, unattractive, ugly, and noncompliant. Approximately one-third of participants characterized obese individuals as weak willed, sloppy, or lazy. Thus, it appears physicians "share broader society's negative stereotypes about the personal attributes of obese persons" (p. 1168). Fat bias also impacts the clinical judgment of mental health clinicians, which has been shown to result in a more serious diagnosis being assigned to fat clients (Agell & Rothblum, 1991; Davis-Coelho, Waltz, & Davis-Coehlo, 2000; Young & Powell, 1985).

Hebl and Xu (2001) measured physicians' reactions to patients labeled as average weight, overweight, or obese, and they found that the weight of patients influenced how physicians reacted to and treated them. More tests were prescribed for heavier patients, physicians reported that they would spend less time with heavier patients, and they viewed heavier patients more negatively than average-weight patients. In addition, physicians had less desire to help heavier patients and judged them to be less healthy, worse at taking care of themselves, and less self-disciplined. Hebl and Xu concluded that "physicians continue to play an influential role in lowering the quality of healthcare that overweight and obese patients receive" (p. 1246). Other researchers have shown that implicit (below the level of conscious awareness) and explicit (known and reportable) fat bias is as pervasive among health professionals as it is among the general public (Sabin et al., 2012; Schwartz et al., 2003). Given this strong and often obvious bias, obese patients can become reluctant to seek health care, which can have negative consequences for their health status (Schwartz et al., 2003)

Patients of size report weight discrimination in health care settings and subsequent avoidance of preventative health care (Sabin et al., 2012; Wee, McCarthy, Davis, & Phillips, 2000). For example, in an investigation of weight stigma among overweight and obese adults, Puhl and Brownell (2006) found that physicians and family members were the most frequent sources of weight bias reported. More than one-half of participants reported having received inappropriate comments about their weight from their doctors, and their experience of stigma was positively correlated with BMI. In another study (Anderson & Wadden, 2004), overweight patients reported having been treated disrespectfully by health care professionals because of their weight.

Research has demonstrated that the negative attitudes of health care providers toward fat women can result in inadequate medical care (Puhl & Heuer, 2009; Wee, McCarthy, Davis, & Phillips, 2000). A higher BMI is associated with fewer or worse preventative health care services, including delayed clinical breast examinations, gynecologic examinations, and papanicolaou smears (Fontaine, Faith, Allison, & Cheskin, 1998; Wee et al., 2000). Fat women have also postponed seeking health care because of disrespectful treatment (Amy, Aalborg, Lyons, & Keranen, 2006). In a survey about perceived barriers to gynecological screenings, Amy and colleagues (2006) found that 68% of the overweight and obese women reported having delayed seeking health care, and 85% of respondents reported that weight was a barrier to receiving health care. Fat participants reported having perceived negative attitudes and disrespectful treatment from providers, having received unsolicited advice about losing weight, having been embarrassed about being weighed, and having found that gowns, medical equipment, and exam tables were too small for them. Olson, Schumaker, and Yawn (1994) found that women of higher BMI status were more likely than other women to state that they had delayed medical care because of embarrassment about weight or because they did not want a lecture regarding their weight.

Fat Stigma and Fat Shaming

The failure of fat people to comply with the sociocultural norms of attractiveness and thinness often results in a judgment of morality and character (e.g., lack of willpower) (Phelan, Link, & Dovidio, 2008). This then leads to repeated shaming and stigmatization, which represents an attempt to increase fat women's conformity to the existing norms of the thin ideal. Thus, for some people, stigmatizing fat individuals is viewed as a way to motivate them to engage in a healthier lifestyle, based on the assumption that fat people will try to avoid stigmatization by altering their behavior.

As discussed earlier, the process of shaming is based on the belief that fat people can become thin and attractive with the right amount of willpower and reduced calorie intake. However, research challenges that assumption, as researchers have documented numerous negative consequences of weight stigma. Puhl and Heuer (2010) reviewed a number of studies that show that perceived stigmatization and discrimination results in unhealthy eating behavior, eating disorders, and lower levels of physical activity, all of which can result in further weight gain.

Fat shaming and teasing about weight do not result in weight loss; even if the targets of the shaming are motivated to diet, it is unlikely that they will lose enough weight to become thin or that the diet will enhance their health status. In a recent study (Seacat et al., 2014), researchers reviewed 50 overweight women's diary entries about weight-based interactions. They found that the negative feelings associated with fatness can lead to reduced psychological and physical health and well-being.

The experience of weight-based teasing is prevalent, especially in the United States and Canada. Girls classified as both normal weight and overweight reported higher prevalence of weight-based teasing than did boys of the same size (Goldfield et al., 2010). A landmark study by Eisenberg, Neumark-Sztainer, and Story (2003) showed that weight-based teasing was consistently associated with body dissatisfaction, low self-esteem, depressive symptoms, and even suicidal ideation. They reported that teasing about body weight was consistently associated with anxiety, psychological distress, and disordered eating, that these associations held for both boys and girls, and that they were independent of weight status. In another study (Grilo, Wilfley, Brownell, & Rodin, 1994), the frequency of having been teased about weight and size during childhood was negatively correlated with adult participants' evaluation of their appearance and positively correlated with their body dissatisfaction. The findings suggest that teasing about weight or size during childhood and adolescence is a risk factor for the development of negative body image. Moreover, weight-based teasing by family members has also been associated with unhealthy weight-control behaviors and poorer psychological functioning (Fulkerson, Strauss, Neumark-Sztainer, Story, & Boutelle, 2007).

Shame and self-blame are often responses to failure to lose weight; preoccupation with food and body dissatisfaction can also result (Bacon & Aphramor, 2014). Dieting itself negatively impacts psychological well-being (McFarlane, Polivy, & McCabe, 1999), and it is associated with weight preoccupation, food preoccupation, body dissatisfaction, overeating, and binge eating (Bacon & Aphramor, 2011; Brady, Gingras, & Aphramor, 2013; Robison et al., 2007a). Dieting can have other negative psychological repercussions, including depression, disordered eating, and low self-esteem (Wooley & Garner, 1994).

Size discrimination is pervasive, and the stress related to discrimination is a risk factor for most obesity-related diseases, including cardiovascular disease and diabetes (Bacon & Aphramor, 2014). In fact, research has demonstrated that once one's basic needs are met, responses to life circumstances are the key determinants to health; "social differences actually account for most of society's stark health differences" (Bacon & Aphramor, 2014, p. 22). The perceived unfairness model (Jackson, Kubzansky, & Wright, 2006) proposed that the experience of discrimination sets off "a cascade of psychological and physiological processes" that, if experienced repeatedly, can contribute to poor health. Unfairness makes people feel hostile, and research has demonstrated direct effects of hostility on heart and lung function (Jackson et al., 2006). Other research has shown that experiencing oppression or discrimination leads to worse health outcomes than those of individuals who experience greater privilege, and these disparities are not necessarily related to health behaviors (Bacon & Aphramor, 2014; Klonoff & Landrine, 1995; Landrine & Klonoff, 1996; Moody, Brown, Matthews, & Bromberger, 2014). Individuals living with various threats (e.g., poverty, racism, sexism, sizism) can experience stress responses that actually reduce bodily resilience. This chronic stress can impact one's cardiovascular and immune systems. Chronic stress can make a "person vulnerable to wide range of poor health outcomes, including infections, diabetes, high blood pressure, heart attack, stroke, and depression" (Bacon & Aphramor, 2014, p. 25). Thus, it is possible that health concerns that have been blamed on fat are actually related to the fat-shaming environments that people of size inhabit.

AN ALTERNATIVE TO MEDICALIZATION: HEALTH AT EVERY SIZE

An alternative to weight-management treatments is the Health at Every Size (HAES) approach, which focuses, not on losing weight, but instead on promoting self-acceptance, appreciation of size diversity, and engagement in self-care strategies. HAES prioritizes a person's emotional, physical, and spiritual well-being without weight loss as a goal. It encourages physical activities for pleasure rather than as regimented exercise routines. HAES also seeks to end weight bias by recognizing that someone's size or weight does not reflect the way a person eats, what a person's physical activity level is, or whether a person has any particular psychological issues.

This compassionate and empirically supported approach is respectful and health centered, and it encourages people to become attuned to bodily cues rather than attempt to ignore them (Bacon & Aphramor, 2014). HAES takes a holistic view of health and urges people to appreciate the bodies they have and to find compassionate ways to engage in self-care (e.g., getting sufficient sleep, nutrition, exercise, and relaxation). This approach does not assert that everyone is at a "healthy" weight, but instead asks people to shift their focus from changing their size to enhancing self-care and letting their weight fall where it would naturally according to their set-point (Bacon & Aphramor, 2014). Healthy bodies come in a variety of shapes and sizes, and they maintain a stable weight (Bacon & Aphramor, 2014).

It is worth noting the additional ways that HAES's view of health differs from a medicalized paradigm. A medicalized perspective of health and weight considers activity and nutrition as primary markers of health, whereas HAES takes a "life-course approach to health" (Bacon & Aphramor, 2014, p. 104). A life-course approach means considering people's life-world (i.e., the reality of their life). Lifestyle is but one factor in a multifaceted system (including structural, political, economic, psychosocial, developmental, and genetic factors) (Bacon & Aphramor, 2014). HAES recognizes that bodily responses occur in the context of people's social environment, and the cumulative impact of various factors, including discrimination, can foster health or disease (Bacon & Aphramor, 2014). If a disease model of health is utilized, its myopic focus on weight, diet, and exercise decreases attention to other factors that impact metabolism, including "lived realities of inequality" (Bacon & Aphramor, 2014, p. 173).

Update on Health at Every Size

From 2003 to 2013, the Association for Size Diversity and Health described five principles of HAES on their web page, which included accepting and respecting diversity of body shape and size; recognizing that health and well-being are multidimensional; promoting health and well-being for people of all sizes; promoting eating that balances nutritional need, hunger, satiety, appetite, and pleasure; and promoting enjoyable physical activity without the goal of weight loss. These principles were updated and expanded in early 2014 to reflect social determinants of health. HAES principles still include weight inclusivity (accepting and respecting diversity of body shapes and rejecting pathologizing specific weights), eating for well-being (promoting eating based on internal cues and pleasure instead of an externalized eating plan), and life-enhancing movement (supporting physical activities that allow people of all sizes, abilities, and interests to engage in enjoyable movement).

Principles expanded upon in the revision include health enhancement (supporting health policies that equalize access to information and services that improve well-being and personal practices that improve human well-being) and respectful care (acknowledging biases and working to end weight discrimination, stigma, and bias; providing information and services with an understanding of other diversity dimensions, such as socioeconomic status, race, gender, and sexual orientation, that impact weight stigma and supporting environments that address these inequalities) (ASDAH, 2014). The tenets of HAES have been expanded to reflect the intersectionality of people's identities as well as to promote the need for application of its principles not only to the health and well-being of individuals but also to the way we understand public health in general.

An HAES approach promotes body acceptance, but it does so in a realistic way. Being ambivalent about one's body is normal and to be expected; true acceptance takes time, and it cannot occur overnight (Bacon & Aphramor, 2014). A body acceptance approach encourages challenging judgments other people make about their bodies. "Judgment evokes despair as you believe there is something wrong with you, meaning you are not entitled to the food that you want, and you need to deprive yourself as punishment or remedy" for your weight (Bacon & Aphramor, 2014, p. 156). Although it can be a lengthy process to work toward body acceptance given all of the negative messages from culture and society (see Chapter 8, this volume), being compassionate toward oneself has more positive health benefits than engaging in self-loathing (Bacon & Aphramor, 2011; Robison et al., 2007a).

Research supports HAES and demonstrates that improvements in various markers in health can occur in individuals of all sizes, irrespective of whether weight change occurs (Bacon & Aphramor, 2014). For instance, blood pressure, cholesterol, and glucose levels can be normalized without weight loss (Bacon et al., 2002; Bacon, Stern, Van Loan, & Keim, 2005). The HAES approach (sometimes termed the non-diet or intuitive eating approach) has been associated in a number of studies with statistically significant improvements in physiological measures, health behaviors, and psychosocial outcomes. For instance, participants in HAES treatment groups showed improvements in blood pressure, lipid levels, cardiorespiratory health, eating and activity habits, self-esteem, body image, and mood (Bacon, 2008; Bacon & Aphramor, 2011; Bacon et al., 2002; Bacon et al., 2005; Schaefer & Magnuson, 2014). Follow-up studies show that these positive health changes have been maintained for up to two years (Bacon et al., 2005; Schafer & Magnuson, 2014). HAES interventions can develop the ability to be conscious of physical signs of hunger and satiety (Provencher et al., 2007), which have been found to have a long-term beneficial impact on eating behaviors (Provencher et al., 2009). In a review of interventions that promote a non-diet approach to health, Schaefer and Magnuson (2014) documented that these approaches have positive long-term health benefits and lower dropout rates than traditional dieting programs.

The feminist slogan "the personal is political" is relevant to body image and body satisfaction, and size equality is a social justice issue (Bacon & Aphramor, 2014). "Blaming illness on behaviors stops us from addressing the policies and systems that shape our lives in unequal and unhealthy ways" (Bacon & Aphramor, 2014, p. 97). It is beneficial to encourage individuals to engage in improved self-care, but it is also important to acknowledge that social and structural change is needed to improve health equality (Bacon & Aphramor, 2014). Thus, we encourage patients and health care professionals to promote an HAES perspective, but we also recognize and support the importance of collective efforts to promote this health paradigm and to decrease oppression of all types that leads to health disparities.

Suggestions for Health Care Professionals

A HAES paradigm shift may be required for appropriate ethical practice (Bacon & Aphramor, 2011), and health care professionals are encouraged to become educated about and adopt the HAES paradigm of health and wellness into their practice. As Bacon and Aphramor (2014) noted, "HAES puts health and caring back at the heart of health care" (p. 29). It is important for health care professionals to become knowledgeable about the HAES model and the evidence that supports it (Bacon & Aphramor, 2011), including the physiology of fat, the ineffectiveness of dieting, and the risks of weight cycling. Patients should be disabused of myths about dieting and presented with research that shows that diets do not work (Chrisler, 1989). As Burgard (2009) noted, it is "hypocritical to prescribe practices for heavier people that we would diagnose as eating disordered in thin ones" (p. 42).

We encourage health care practitioners to challenge their beliefs about size and assumptions regarding weight and health (Bacon & Aphramor, 2011; Robison et al., 2007b). Health cannot be determined simply by looking at a patient's size. Do not assume that you know the eating habits or activity level of a patient. Deep introspection could be useful to health care professionals to examine their personal biases and their own relationships with food, eating, and their bodies (Brady et al., 2013; Robison et al., 2007b).

Patients must never be shamed and blamed for their size. No matter what their size is, patients deserve to be treated with dignity, respect, and compassion. It is important to acknowledge sizism and be sensitive to the amount and range of stigmatizing experiences a patient may experience and to provide empathy and support. Both medical and mental health practitioners should acknowledge that stigma and oppression impact health (Bacon & Aphramor, 2011; Jackson et al., 2006). Psychotherapists should assess how clients of size cope with this stigma (Bacon & Aphramor, 2014; Puhl & Brownell, 2006) and help them to develop additional coping strategies. Weight-based stigma should be avoided, such as using as the terms *overweight* and *obese* to describe patients (Bacon & Aphramor, 2011; Smith et al., 2007). The word *fat* should be transformed from a condition or disease to simply a description (McHugh & Kasardo, 2012).

Interventions for medical problems should be the same for patients of all sizes (Robison et al., 2007b); they should always meet ethical standards and focus on health, not weight (Bacon & Aphramor, 2011). Interventions should be holistic, including a client's physical, emotional, social, occupational, intellectual, and spiritual health. Body satisfaction and respect for size diversity should be promoted. In addition, interventions involving physical activity and eating should encourage self-care rather than external guidelines or criteria (Bacon & Aphramor, 2011).

Brady and colleagues' (2013) analysis of HAES through a relational-cultural lens also provides guidelines for health care professionals. According to relational-cultural theory, problems arise through disconnection in relationships, and this disconnection can result from abuses of power that prevent mutual empowerment (Brady et al., 2013). These power imbalances are often present in relationships between practitioners and patients, which might be referred to as "power-over" relationships, as compared to "power-with" relationships, in which individuals create change together (Brady et al., 2013). It could be helpful for dieticians and other health care professionals to promote connection with their patients instead of a relationship in which the professional is viewed as the expert. More egalitarian relationships with patients, where their lived experience and perspective about their bodies is respected and honored, could help practitioners to develop rapport and engage in effective treatment with their patients. Patients will be able to find more allies in the health care community if an HAES paradigm is applied (Bacon & Aphramor, 2014). It could change the face of health care if patients could engage with medical professionals as allies instead of finding doctor–patient interactions to be a barrier to seeking appropriate health care.

Empowerment for Patients

An HAES paradigm will help people to improve their resilience, enhance their self-care, and advocate for themselves (Bacon & Aphramor, 2014). This is so important, given the difficulties that can emerge when women try to get respectful health care in a realm that is known to be biased against people of size. Although systemic change within the public health care system and individual changes among health care professionals are essential to a paradigm shift, patients' increased self-efficacy is important to combat the medicalization of fat. Fat patients deserve the same respect and treatment plans given to thin patients, and this section is dedicated to them.

It is important to be knowledgeable about HAES and the truth about weight, health, size stigma, and the oppressive cultural beauty ideal. You do not have to feel ashamed about your body. You are not a failure because you did not lose weight when you dieted. Diets do not work; *the diets are the failure*. Realize that eating is not a moral activity; you are not good or bad because of what you eat. Reflect on forms of activity that could be enjoyable for you and engage in them, rather than in activities others have "prescribed" for you. Active living contributes to health (Bacon & Aphramor, 2014); this refers to regular movement as part of everyday life, which could include activities such as vacuuming, doing laundry, gardening, and playing with children or pets. Given the pervasiveness of size stigma, it could be helpful to reflect on your emotions regarding your size and the treatment you receive, including how you respond to discrimination. A size acceptance community exists, including online resources; engaging in this community and receiving support from them could be helpful to you. Ultimately, your worth does not have to be dictated by your weight! Neither does your health. It is not acceptable or ethical if a doctor immediately prescribes weight loss when you talk about your concerns.

Clinical psychologist Stacey Nye (2014) recently blogged about her experience with seeing a new physician, whose first suggestion for lowering her risk of breast cancer was to lose weight. Her physician specifically recommended beginning a no-wheat diet. When she mentioned that she has food allergies and does not currently consume wheat, he asked, "If you don't eat wheat, then why aren't you thin?" She vowed that the next time she met with the doctor, she would discuss HAES with him. She would ask for evidence-based treatment recommendations, as opposed to weight loss, or recommendations that he might also give to a thin patient. She said that if her doctor is not responsive to her needs, she would find a size-friendly doctor. She wrote: "Everyone is entitled to shame free, blame free, and compassionate health care." If health care professionals persist in promoting a weight-centered paradigm of health or are not communicating respectfully or listening to you, please remember that changing doctors is almost always an option (Eating Disorder Law Blog, 2013). When health care professionals mention weight as problematic, you should speak up and inquire if the problem could be caused by anything other than weight (Eating Disorder Law Blog, 2013). Trusting your instincts is of the utmost importance. As you become more attuned to your body, you will know when you do not feel well and need medical attention. You deserve to have your voice heard.

Imagine going to a physician and receiving treatment that is health centered instead of weight focused. Visualize a doctor who discusses coming into sync with your bodily cues of satiety and hunger instead of discussing how to calculate calories. Imagine treatment goals to enhance health, including self-esteem and quality of life, instead of dieting and weight loss. Envision a doctor who respects a variety of body sizes instead of one who chastises patients who "eat too much" and do not "exercise enough" (Miller & Jacob, 2001; Robison, 2005). What might sound like a fantasy visit to a physician's office can actually be reality if the medicalization of weight is replaced with the body-respecting HAES approach.

CONCLUSION

Medicalization promotes the thin ideal and the belief that one must be thin to be healthy. However, research does not support this. Dieting and weight loss are promoted as the solution to "fat," but not only is dieting ineffective in sustaining weight loss, but negative repercussions, including negative physical and psychological consequences, can also ensue. The assertion that fat always equates to ill health is simply untrue. Research has demonstrated that the experience of size stigma and yo-yo dieting can result in negative health consequences that are then attributed to being fat. HAES provides a health-centered approach geared toward compassionate and respectful care. It acknowledges the social determinants of health and illness, and it recognizes that facing discrimination impacts one's health. It is imperative for health care professionals to utilize this approach both for the well-being of patients and to maintain ethical practice standards. Fat is not a disease. Prescribing weight loss is not a cure. Let us work to move away from size stigma toward size acceptance, from body shame to body pride, from a model of disease to a model of well-being. In doing so, we will improve women's physical and mental health and their quality of life.

REFERENCES

Agell, G., & Rothblum, E. D. (1991). Effects of clients' obesity and gender on the therapy judgments of psychologists. *Professional Psychology: Research and Practice, 22*, 223–229.

Amy, N. K., Aalborg, A., Lyons, P., & Keranen, L. (2006). Barriers to routine gynecological cancer screenings for white and African-American obese women. *International Journal of Obesity, 30,* 147–155.

Anderson, D. A., & Wadden, T. A. (2004). Bariatric surgery patients' view of their physicians' weight-related attitudes and practices. *Obesity Research, 12,* 1587–1595.

Association for Size Diversity and Acceptance (ASDAH). (2014). HAES principles. *Association for Size Diversity and Health.* Retrieved from https://www.sizedi versityandhealth.org/content.asp?id=152.

Bacon, L. (2008). *Health at Every Size: The surprising truth about your weight.* Dallas, TX: BenBella Books.

Bacon, L., & Aphramor, L. (2011). Weight science: Evaluating the evidence for a paradigm shift. *Nutrition Journal, 10,* 1–13.

Bacon, L., & Aphramor, L. (2014). *Body respect: What conventional health books get wrong, leave out, and just plain fail to understand about weight.* Dallas, TX: BenBella Books.

Bacon, L., Keim, N. L., Van Loan, M. D., Derricote, M., Gale, B., Kazaks, A., & Stern, J. S. (2002). Evaluating a non-diet wellness intervention for improvement of metabolic fitness, psychological well-being and eating and activity behaviors. *International Journal of Obesity, 26,* 854–865.

Bacon, L., Stern, J. S., Van Loan, M. D., & Keim, N. L. (2005). Size acceptance and intuitive eating improve health for obese, female chronic dieters. *Journal of the American Dietetic Association, 105,* 929–936.

Bell, K., & McNaughton, D. (2007). Feminism and the invisible fat man. *Body and Society, 13,* 108–132

Berg, M. (1998). Choose sensitive, accurate terms. *Healthy Weight Journal, 12,* 12–13.

Bordo, S., & Heywood, L. (2004). *Unbearable weight: Feminism, Western culture, and the body.* (tenth anniv. ed.). Los Angeles: California University Press.

Brady, J., Gingras, J., & Aphramor, L. (2013). Theorizing health at every size as a relational-cultural endeavor. *Critical Public Health, 23,* 345–355.

Brown, L. S. (1989). Fat-oppressive attitudes and the feminist therapist: Directions for change. In L. S. Brown & E. D. Rothblum (Eds.), *Overcoming fear of fat* (pp. 19–30). Binghamton, NY: Harrington Park Press.

Brown, L. S., & Rothblum, E. D. (1989). *Overcoming fear of fat.* Binghamton, NY: Harrington Park Press.

Brownell, K. D., Puhl, R. M., Schwartz, M. B., & Rudd, L. (Eds.). (2005). *Weight bias: Nature, consequences, and remedies.* New York: Guildford.

Burgard, D. (2009). What is health at every size? In E. D. Rothblum & S. Solovay (Eds.), *The fat studies reader* (pp. 42–53). New York: New York University Press.

Campos, P. (2005). *The diet myth: Why America's obsession with weight is hazardous to your health.* New York: Gotham Books.

Chrisler, J. C. (1989). Should feminist therapist do weight loss counseling. In L. S. Brown & E. D. Rothblum (Eds.), *Overcoming fear of fat* (pp. 31–38). Binghamton, NY: Harrington Park Press.

Chrisler, J. C. (2011). Leaks, lumps, and lines: Stigma and women's bodies. *Psychology of Women Quarterly, 35*, 202–214.

Crandall, C. S. (1994). Prejudice against fat people: Ideology and self-interest. *Journal of Personality and Social Psychology, 66*, 882–894.

Crandall, C. S., & Martinez, R. (1996). Culture, ideology, and antifat attitudes. *Personality and Social Psychology Bulletin, 22*, 1165–1176.

Crocker, J., Cornwell, B., & Major, B. (1993). The stigma of overweight: Affective consequences of attributional ambiguity. *Journal of Personality and Social Psychology, 64*, 60–70.

Danielsdottir, S., O'Brien, K. S., & Ciao, A. (2010). Anti-fat prejudice reduction: A review of published studies. *Obesity Facts, 3*, 47–58.

Davis-Coelho, K., Waltz, J., & Davis-Coelho, B. (2000). Awareness and prevention of bias against fat clients in psychotherapy. *Professional Psychology: Research and Practice, 31*, 682–684.

Eating Disorder Law Blog. (2013). Weight bias in our doctor's office: The problem and action steps you can take to solve it. Kantor & Kantor, LLP. Retrieved from http://www.kantorlaw.net/Eating_Disorder_Blog/2013/May/Weight_Bias_in_Your_Doctors_Office_The_Problem_a.aspx.

Eisenberg M. E., Neumark-Sztainer D., & Story, M. (2003). Associations of weight-based teasing and emotional well-being among adolescents. *Archives of Pediatric and Adolescent Medicine, 157*, 733–738.

Erdman, C. K. (1999). *Fat as a therapeutic issue: Raising awareness in ourselves and our clients.* Retrieved from www.nedic.ca/knowthefacts.

Farrell, A. E. (2011). *Fat shame: Stigma and the fat body in American culture.* New York: New York University Press.

Fikkan, J. L., & Rothblum, E. D. (2012). Is fat a feminist issue? Exploring the gendered nature of weight bias. *Sex Roles, 66*, 575–592.

Fontaine, K. R., Faith, M. S., Allison, D. B., & Cheskin, L. J. (1998). Body weight and health care among women in the general population. *Archives Family Medicine, 7*, 381–384.

Foster, G. D., Wadden, T. A., Makris, A. P., Davidson, D., Sanderson, R. S., Allison, D. B., & Kessler, A. (2003). Primary care physicians' attitudes about obesity and its treatment. *Obesity Research, 11*, 1168–1177.

Fraser, L. (2009). The inner corset: A brief history of fat in the United States. In E. D. Rothblum & S. Solovay (Eds.), *The fat studies reader* (pp. 11–14). New York: New York University Press.

Fulkerson, J. A., Strauss, J., Neumark-Sztainer, D., Story, M., & Boutelle, K. (2007). Correlates of psychosocial well-being among overweight adolescents: The role of the family. *Journal of Consulting and Clinical Psychology, 75*, 181–186.

Gaesser, G. A. (2002). *Big fat lies: The truth about your weight and your health.* Carlsbad, CA: Gurze Books.

Goldfield, G., Moore, C., Henderson, K., Buchholz, A., Obied, N., & Flament, M. (2010). The relation between weight-based teasing and psychological adjustment in adolescents. *Paediatric Child Health, 15*, 283–288.

Grilo, C. M., Wilfley, D. E., Brownell, K. D., & Rodin, J. (1994). Teasing, body image, and self-esteem in a clinical sample of obese women. *Addictive Behavior, 19*, 443–450.

Hebl, M. R., & Xu, J. (2001). Weighing the care: Physicians' reactions to the size of a patient. *International Journal of Obesity, 25*, 1246–1252.

Hilbert, A., Rief, W., & Braehler, E. (2007). What determines public support of obesity intervention? *Journal of Epidemiology and Community Health, 61*, 585–590.

Jackson, B., Kubzansky, L. D., & Wright, R. J. (2006). Linking perceived unfairness to physical health: The perceived unfairness model. *Review of General Psychology, 10*, 21–40.

Klonoff, E. A., & Landrine, H. (1995). The schedule of sexist events: A measure of lifetime and recent sexist discrimination in women's lives. *Psychology of Women Quarterly, 19*, 439–472.

Kuijer, R. G., & Boyce, J. A. (2014). Chocolate cake. Guilt or celebration? Associations with healthy eating attitudes, perceived behavioral control, intentions, and weight loss. *Appetite, 74*, 48–54.

Landrine, H., & Klonoff, E. A. (1996). The schedule of racist vents: A measure of racial discrimination and a study of its negative physical and mental health consequences. *Journal of Black Psychology, 22*, 144–168.

McFarlane, T., Polivy, J., & McCabe, R. E. (1999). Help, not harm: Psychological foundation for a nondieting approach toward health. *Journal of Social Issues, 55*, 261–276.

McHugh, M. C., & Kasardo, A. E. (2012). Anti-fat prejudice: The role of psychology in explication, education, and eradication. *Sex Roles, 66*, 617–627.

Miller, W. C., & Jacob, A. V. (2001). The health at any size paradigm for obesity treatment: The scientific evidence. *Obesity Reviews, 2*, 37–45.

Moody, D. L. B., Brown, C., Matthews, K. A., & Bromberger, J. T. (2014). Everyday discrimination prospectively predicts inflammation across 7-years in racially diverse midlife women: Study of women's health across the nation. *Journal of Social Issues, 70*, 298–314.

Musher-Eizenmann, D. M., Holub, S. C., Miller, A. B., Goldstein, S. E., & Edwards-Leeper, L. (2004). Body size stigmatization in preschool children: The role of control attributions. *Journal of Psychiatric Psychology, 29*, 613–620.

Nye, S. (2014). If you don't eat wheat, then why aren't you thin? Association for Size Diversity and Health HAES Blog. Retrieved from http://healthatevery sizeblog.org/page/4/.

Olson, C. L., Schumaker, H. D., & Yawn, B. P. (1994). Overweight women delay medical care. *Archives Family Medicine, 3*, 888–892.

Phelan, J. C., Link, B. G., & Dovidio, J. F. (2008). Stigma and prejudice: One animal or two? *Social Science and Medicine, 67*, 358–367.

Provencher, V., Begin, C., Tremblay, A., Mongeau, L., Boivin, S., & Lemieux, S. (2007). Short-term effects of a health-at-every-size approach on eating behaviors and appetite ratings. *Obesity, 15,* 957–966.

Provencher, V., Begin, C., Tremblay, A., Mongeau, L., Corneau, L., Dodin, S., . . . Lemieux, S. (2009). Health-at-every-size and eating behaviors: 1-year follow-up results of a size acceptance intervention. *American Dietetic Association, 103,* 1854–1861.

Puhl, R. M., Andreyeva, T., & Brownell, K. D. (2008). Perceptions of weight discrimination: Prevalence and comparison to race and gender discrimination in America. *International Journal of Obesity, 32,* 1–9.

Puhl, R. M., & Brownell, K. D. (2003). Psychosocial origins of obesity stigma: Toward changing a powerful and pervasive bias. *Obesity Reviews, 4,* 213–227.

Puhl, R. M., & Brownell, K. D. (2006). Confronting and coping with weight stigma: An investigation of overweight and obese adults. *Obesity, 14,* 1802–1815.

Puhl, R. M., & Heuer, C. A. (2009). The stigma of obesity: A review and update. *Obesity, 17,* 941–964.

Puhl, R. M., & Heuer, C. A. (2010). Obesity stigma: Important considerations for public health. *American Journal of Public Health, 100,* 1019–1028.

Ristovski-Slijepcevic, S., Bell, K., Chapman, G., & Beagan, B. L. (2010). Being thick indicates you are eating, you are healthy and you have an attractive body shape: Perspectives on fatness and food choice amongst Black and White men and women in Canada. *Health Sociology Review, 19,* 317–329.

Robison, J. (2005). Health at every size: Toward a new paradigm of weight and health. *Medscape General Medicine, 7,* 13.

Robison, J., & Erdman, C. (1998). Needed: New terminology for the new paradigm. *Healthy Weight Journal, 12,* 58–59.

Robison, J., Putnam, K., & McKibbin, L. (2007a). Health at every size: A compassionate, effective approach for helping individuals with weight-related concern (Part I). *American Association of Occupational Health Nurses Journal, 55,* 143–150.

Robison, J., Putnam, K., & McKibbin, L. (2007b). Health at every size: A compassionate, effective approach for helping individuals with weight-related concerns (Part II). *American Association of Occupational Health Nurses Journal, 55,* 185–192.

Rodin, J., Silberstein, L., & Striegel-Moore, R. (1984). Women and weight: A normative discontent. *Nebraska Symposium on Motivation, 32,* 267–307.

Sabin, J.A., Marini, M., & Nosek, B.A. (2012). Implicit and explicit anti-fat bias among a large sample of medical doctors by BMI, race/ethnicity, and gender. *PLoS ONE, 7*(11), e48448.

Saltzberg, E. A., & Chrisler, J. C. (1995). Beauty is the beast: Psychological effects of the pursuit of the perfect female body. In J. Freeman (Ed.), *Women: A feminist perspective* (5th ed., pp. 306–315). Mountain View, CA: Mayfield.

Schaefer, J. T., & Magnuson, A. B. (2014). A review of interventions that promote eating by internal cues. *Journal of the Academy of Nutrition and Dietetics, 114,* 734–760.

Schoenfielder, L., & Wieser, B. (Eds.). (1983). *Shadow on a tightrope: Writings by women on fat oppression.* Iowa City, IA: Aunt Luke Books.

Schwartz, M. B., Chambliss, H. O., Brownell, K. D., Blair, S. N., & Billington, C. (2003). Weight bias among health professionals specializing in obesity. *Obesity Research, 11,* 1033–1039.

Seacat, J. D., Dougal, S. C., & Roy, D. (2014). A daily diary assessment of female weight stigmatization. *Journal of Health Psychology* (in press)

Smith, C. (2004). Women, weight and body image. In J. C. Chrisler, P. D. Rozee, & C. Golden (Eds.), *Lectures on the psychology of women* (3rd ed.). New York: McGraw Hill.

Smith, C. A., Schmoll, K., Konik, J., & Oberlander, S. (2007). Carrying weight for the world: Influence of weight descriptors on judgments of large-sized women. *Journal of Applied Social Psychology, 37,* 989–1006.

Solovay, S. (2000). *Tipping the scales of justice: Fighting weight-based discrimination.* Amherst, NY: Prometheus Books.

Tiggemann, M., & Rothblum, E. D. (1988). Gender differences in social consequences of perceived overweight in the United States and Australia. *Sex Roles, 18,* 75–86.

Wann, M. (1998). *Fat! So?* Berkeley, CA: Ten Speed Press.

Watts, K., & Cranney, J. (2009). The nature and implications of implicit weight bias. *Current Psychiatry Reviews, 5,* 110–126.

Wee, C. C., McCarthy, E. P., Davis, R. B., & Phillips, R. S. (2000). Screening for cervical and breast cancer: Is obesity an unrecognized barrier to preventive care? *Annals of Internal Medicine, 132,* 697–704.

Wolf, N. (1991). *The beauty myth: How images of beauty are used against women.* New York: Morrow.

Wooley, S. C., & Garner, D. M. (1994). Controversies in management: Should obesity be treated? Dietary treatments for obesity are ineffective. *British Medical Journal, 309,* 655–656.

Young, L. M., & Powell, B. (1985). The effects of obesity on the clinical judgments of mental health professionals. *Journal of Health and Social Behavior, 26,* 233–246.

Chapter 10

Medicalizing Women's Weight: Bariatric Surgery and Weight-Loss Drugs

Julie Konik and Christine A. Smith

The equating of fat with illness has been used as a threat against individuals of all sizes, as it creates an unwarranted fear of fat. As Chiolero and Paccaud noted (2009), "the increasing prevalence of obesity[1] during the last decades has been reported as a 'major public health issue,' a '21st century epidemic,' up to an apocalyptic 'obesity tsunami'" (p. 568). They added that, in response to these dire warnings, a variety of agencies have launched programs to fight obesity. Furthermore, the U.S. diet industry has expanded to generate $61 billion in yearly sales (Marketdata Enterprises, 2014). However, few voices have questioned whether this "war on obesity," often promoted in both scholarly and popular media, is a fruitless, if not deleterious, endeavor. This "war" is not predicated on solid empirical evidence. Furthermore, it suggests that fat people are "the enemy" and implicitly (if not explicitly) justifies prejudice against them (Chrisler, 2012).

The research on obesity tends to be divided into two epistemological poles: a "realistic" one that takes an essentialist view of obesity as a biomedical "fact" and a "constructionist" view that situates the "obesity epidemic" within a cultural context (Patterson & Johnston, 2012). Boero (2007) expanded the constructionist approach by positing that "the 'obesity epidemic' is what I call a 'post-modern epidemic' in which the ostensible concern for public health is diverted from structural forces and the focus in turn squarely on the individual" (p. 58). We propose that a constructionist lens is the most beneficial one through which to view obesity. A key point of our analysis is that women's weight has become medicalized or in "need" of intervention to obtain "ideal" levels. However, before we begin our analysis, it is necessary to provide an overview of some key concepts that have become gendered in the research on overweight and obesity. These include standards, rates, and correlates of these constructs.

CONCEPTUALIZING OBESITY

The body mass index (BMI) is the benchmark for the nosology of overweight and obesity, and it is calculated by dividing one's weight in kilograms by the square of one's height in meters. The U.S. National Institutes of Health's National Heart, Lung, and Blood Institute's (1998) guidelines delineated a BMI between 25.0 and 29.9 as "overweight" and 30.0 or greater as "obese." Obesity is further categorized as grade 1 (30 to <35), grade 2 (35 to <40), and grade 3 (40 and greater) (Flegal, Graubard, Williamson, & Gail, 2005). The 1998 guidelines were revised from earlier categorizations with 29.0 as the minimum threshold for "overweight" (Nicholls, 2013). The guidelines were not lowered because of evidence that showed that higher BMIs are related to poor health, but in response to pressure by outside forces, including pharmaceutical companies that manufacture weight-loss drugs (Bacon, 2008). As a result of the revised guidelines, literally overnight, many more people were deemed "obese," which meant a lot more potential prescriptions for weight-loss drugs and referrals for bariatric surgery.

The BMI has been criticized for obfuscating the heterogeneity within weight classifications, which, in turn, has allowed it to become a key pillar on which the "obesity epidemic" rests (Nicholls, 2013). One reason for this is that BMI is not only correlated with fat, but also with bone density and mass (Nicholls, 2013). Furthermore, as Charo and LaCoursiere (2014) noted, "BMI as a measure of adiposity is limited in that it examines solely the height and weight of an individual, without accounting for muscle density, body fat percentage, and body fat distribution of the individual or those differences within the population" (p. 434). For example, different ethnic groups may possess different amounts of fat within the same BMI level (Nicholls, 2013), and healthy, fit athletes (with lots of muscle) have high BMIs. Thus, BMI fails to provide a precise measure of fat; instead it is a "muddy" measure of body composition. Although BMI is correlated with hypertension, diabetes, asthma, and arthritis, use of the BMI to sort people into risk groups for these illnesses appears to be arbitrary (Stommel & Schoenborn, 2010). For example, risk does not significantly differ from a BMI of 24 ("normal") to a BMI of 25 ("overweight").

Distributions and Implications of BMI

According to the World Health Organization (2014), worldwide obesity rates have almost doubled since 1980. Further, among adults worldwide who were age 20 or older in 2008, more than 1.4 billion could be classified as overweight. A gender difference emerged in these findings, as nearly 300 million women, but only 200 million men, were classified as obese. In the United States, researchers (Ogden, Carroll, Kit, & Flegal, 2014) estimated that 69% of the population could be labeled overweight or obese, but they found no statistically significant gender differences in these rates.

However, important differences do exist among women by race or ethnicity, as several researchers have reported that African American women and Latinas tend to have higher BMIs than European American and Asian American women. For example, Charo and LaCoursiere (2014) found that African American, Latina, and European American women had obesity rates of 56.6%, 44.4%, and 32.8%, respectively. Other research shows that Latinas and African American women tend to weigh more than European American women, yet they are more satisfied with their bodies (see Fikkan & Rothblum, 2012, for a review). The trends are similar among children: 22% of Latinas/Latinos and 20% of African American children are classified as obese in the United States, compared to 14% and 9% of their European American and Asian American counterparts, respectively (Ogden et al., 2014).

To add socioeconomic class to the analysis, Ailshire and House (2011) reported that from 1986 to 2002, working-class African American women had the largest BMI increase, whereas the smallest increase occurred with upper-class European American men. Furthermore, Charo and LaCoursiere (2014) found that 42% of women living in households at less than 130% of the U.S. poverty level were considered obese, whereas this rate was only 29% for women living in households with incomes greater than 350% of the poverty level.

Class is a major contextual factor for disparities in BMIs, and many studies have shown that income negatively correlates with obesity (Visscher, Snijder, & Seidell, 2010). According to a report issued by the U.S. government (White House, 2014), women are poorer than men in the United States for a variety of reasons, including pay inequity and pressures of bearing the financial responsibility for children and other dependents. If we combine this with the economic effects of racial discrimination, we find that women of color are most likely to experience intersectionality of financial oppression and obesity.

The relation between income and obesity may be bidirectional. Not only might obesity rates increase as a result of economic inequity, but individuals who are fatter may also face more work-related discrimination due to anti-fat stigma (Mason, 2012). There is also compelling evidence that fat women face greater weight-related discrimination than fat men do (see Fikkan & Rothblum, 2012, for a review). For example, in a nationally representative U.S. sample, women with a BMI between 30 and 35 were three times more likely than their male counterparts to report weight-based job discrimination (Puhl, Andreyeva, & Brownell, 2008). Furthermore, fat women are more likely than fat men to remain single, obtain lower levels of education, and live in poverty (Heitmann, 2010). Smith (2012) proposed that this gender disparity may be undergirded by the mandate that women be physically attractive, a mandate unachievable for fat women because the beauty ideal is very thin. This effect is particularly magnified for women in the workplace, and more research is necessary to study the ways in which body size and weight-based discrimination intersect, especially in women's lives.

LINKS BETWEEN OBESITY AND HEALTH: THE "OBESITY PARADOX"

The relation between weight and health has received copious attention in both scholarly and popular media. However, the news media emphasize more "alarmist" and "individual-blaming" scientific studies, which propose that obesity causes disease and thus fuels fears of an "obesity epidemic" (Saguy & Almeling, 2008, p. 53). Often ignored is the research that demonstrates the "obesity paradox," which is the finding that people with a high BMI have lower mortality or more positive health outcomes than those of average or lower weight (Bacon & Aphramor, 2011; Hainer & Aldhoon-Hainerová, 2013). Of course, the obesity paradox would not be a paradox at all if not for the firmly held belief that fat is always dangerous to health.

The obesity paradox has been found for pneumonia (Nie et al., 2014), renal cell carcinoma (Hakimi et al., 2013), coronary heart disease, chronic heart failure, stroke, thromboembolism, peripheral arterial disease, type 2 diabetes, chronic obstructive pulmonary disease, osteoporosis, hemodialysis patients, and mortality related to surgery (Hainer & Alhood-Hainerová, 2013). Flegal, Kit, Orpana, and Graubard (2013) reviewed 97 published studies that examined the link between BMI and mortality. They found that being classified as overweight (BMI 25 to <30) is linked to lower mortality than being classified as "normal" weight. They found no effect on mortality for obesity grade 1 (30 to <35) and grade 2 (35 to <40); only grade 3 (BMI 40 or greater) was linked to higher mortality. The researchers suggested that possible explanations for lower mortality among overweight and grades 1 and 2 obese patients may include a "greater likelihood of receiving optimal medical treatment, the cardioprotective metabolic effects of increased body fat, and benefits of higher metabolic reserves" (p. 77). In summary, the obesity paradox demonstrates that being "overweight" offers protective benefits not conferred upon those who are of "normal" weight or "underweight."

In addition to overlooking the obesity paradox, biomedical researchers have rarely examined possible confounding factors in the relation between obesity and disease. The correlations between disease and obesity may actually be attributable to unmeasured variables, such as genetics, poverty, education, yo-yo dieting, fitness level, and amount of physical activity (Bacon & Aphramor, 2011; Chiolero & Paccaud, 2009). In addition, the stigma of fat, which causes stress for those who are teased, harassed, and discriminated against, may also contribute to negative health outcomes. In summary, as Bacon (2008) pointed out, for most diseases, there is little or no evidence that weight is the primary cause.

The trend to medicalize obesity began in the United States after World War II (Boero, 2007). One example of how this trend has continued can be seen in the U.S. Food and Drug Administration's (FDA's) Working Group on Obesity (2004), which noted in a report that obese people are "likely to need medical intervention to reduce weight and mitigate associated diseases and other adverse health effects" (C. Therapeutics, 4. OWG Therapeutics Recommendations section, para. 1). Three major "treatments" for overweight and obesity have emerged: lifestyle modification, bariatric surgery, and pharmacotherapy (i.e., weight-loss medications; Burke & Wang, 2011). These interventions have typically been marketed to women, who are held to a more stringent weight standard than are men (Boero, 2007). We now turn to a discussion of how bariatric surgery and weight-loss pharmacotherapy have been practiced to the detriment of women. We conclude by proposing alternatives to "reshape" the way women's weight is viewed by society.

BARIATRIC SURGERY

It is estimated that at least 36,000 bariatric surgeries were performed in 2000, and at least 220,000 in 2009, which represents a sixfold increase (Elliott, 2012). The vast majority of those (81% to 86%) who have had the surgery are women and girls (Gelinas, Delparte, Hart, & Wright, 2013), although overall obesity prevalence rates are equal across genders. The number of children and adolescents, as young as five years old, referred for weight-loss surgery has also been increasing (Black, White, Viner, & Simmons, 2013).

Weight-loss surgery has generally been recommended for those with a BMI of 40 or greater, or with a BMI of 35 or greater and a serious medical condition that is obesity related (National Institutes of Health, 2000). Many medical researchers tout bariatric surgery as the best treatment for severe obesity and maintain that the surgery results in long-term weight loss and improved quality of life for a majority of patients (Buchwald et al., 2004; Deitel & Shikora, 2002; Encinosa, Du, & Bernard, 2011; Karlsson, Taft, Ryden, Sjostrom, & Sullivan, 2007). Benefits are reported to include reductions in diabetes, hypertension, and sleep apnea (Buchwald et al., 2004), improved memory (Alosco et al., 2014), improved appearance satisfaction (Wysoker, 2005), reduction in depression and anxiety (Wnuk, 2013), and improvement in polycystic ovary syndrome, gastroesophageal reflux, and degenerative joint disease (Maggard et al., 2005).

According to the American Society for Metabolic and Bariatric Surgery (2014), there are three types of weight-loss surgeries: laparoscopic gastric bypass, laparoscopic adjustable gastric band, and sleeve gastrectomy. Each reduces the size of the stomach using a saline band (laparoscopic adjustable gastric band) or surgical procedure that amputates either part of the stomach (sleeve gastrectomy) or amputates the stomach and attaches it to the middle of the small intestine to limit the amount of calories and nutrients absorbed (laparoscopic gastric bypass). This latter procedure is also referred to as Roux-en-Y and is currently the most commonly used because of its lower cost and complication rate (Sussenbach et al., 2014).

The amount of weight lost with bariatric surgery varies, and the loss may not be maintained. Gelinas et al. (2013) reported that, at six months postsurgery, 42.2% of women and 45.3% of men had lost more than 10% of their "excess" body weight, whereas 16.3% of women and 3.8% of men had actually gained weight. Many patients lose weight during the first two years postsurgery, and then they lose little additional weight or even begin to gain weight (Buchwald et al., 2004; Magro et al., 2008). Buchwald and colleagues (2004) reported an average decrease in BMI of 14.2 and a decrease in actual weight of 39.7 kilograms. A meta-analysis conducted by Maggard et al. (2005) showed an average weight loss of over 30 kilograms three years postsurgery, but a long-term study showed only a 10% weight loss over 10 years (Karlsson et al., 2007). Thus, most patients continue to be classified as clinically overweight or obese postsurgery (Magro et al., 2008).

The side effects that may arise from bariatric surgery are often downplayed in the medical literature or seen as minor compared to the benefits (Erdely, 2008; Groven, Raheim, & Engelsrud, 2010). However, complication rates range from 2.5% to 41.7% among bariatric patients postsurgery, and commonly reported side effects include infections, alcoholism and substance abuse, malnutrition, eating disorders, internal bleeding, tremors, pain, pulmonary embolism, deep vein thrombosis, and intestinal and digestive problems (Buchwald et al., 2004; Encinosa et al., 2011; Ertelt et al., 2008; Ivezaj, Saules, & Weidemann, 2012; Maggard et al., 2005; Meany, Conceicao, & Mitchell, 2013; Stein & Malta, 2013). Ziegler, Sirveaux, Brunaud, Reibel, and Quilliot (2009) found that one-third to two-thirds of bariatric patients report vomiting when feeling full or when food was lodged in the gastric pouch or upper digestive tract; cold intolerance, hair loss, and fatigue were also common complaints.

One side effect of bariatric surgery that is particularly notable is "dumping syndrome," which is marked by diarrhea, vomiting, sweating, and dizziness about 30 to 60 minutes after eating (Maggard et al., 2005), as well as nausea, gas, burping, and other intestinal noises. Ziegler et al. (2009) reported that dumping syndrome is common and occurs in about 70% of patients. Although this may seem like a serious and uncomfortable concern, it has actually been praised by both medical professionals and bariatric patients. For example, Fosberg, Engstrom, and Soderberg (2013) wrote:

> The fear of dumping was described as similar to an antabuse effect and helped them refrain from eating too much or wrong foods. Participants described a new sense of control because they knew that their changed anatomy limited their previous overeating. (p. 97)

Perhaps most disturbing, a number of studies have shown increased mortality after weight-loss surgery. Adams and colleagues (2012) found that deaths from accidents and suicide were 58% higher in a postsurgical group than in a control group. Similarly, Omalu et al. (2007) reported death rates substantially higher for those who had bariatric surgery than in an age- and gender-matched control population. In addition, Smith, Goodman, and Edwards (1995) noted a surgical mortality rate of 3.4% over a 7-year period, and Flum, Salem, Elrod, Dellinger, and Cheadle (2005) found that bariatric patients aged 65 and older had a threefold increase in their risk of mortality.

Groven et al. (2010) interviewed 22 women who had had weight-loss surgery. Many of these women reported ambivalence, struggles with food and eating, and continued difficulties with "dumping syndrome." It is interesting that several mentioned they had had no health concerns before the surgery. Five women specifically noted chronic problems and regret regarding the procedure. These women reported few health problems before the surgery, but they had feared future risk because of their weight. Although each had lost a considerable amount of weight, they reported constant pain and fatigue, as well as nutritional deficiencies and gastrointestinal problems.

Why would individuals risk their lives to lose weight? Fat people are continually given the message that they are deficient and lack self-control (Chrisler, 2012). After years of attempting to lose weight, suffering health problems, and delaying life goals until they become thin, many may believe that weight-loss surgery is their last resort (Wysoker, 2005). Wee, Jones, Davis, Bourland, and Hamel (2006) found that 84% of patients about to have bariatric surgery ranked health concerns as their number one reason for having had the surgery. Yet, 77% of those same patients rated their current health as good or very good. Groven and colleagues (2010) found that many reported having surgery not because of health problems but because of fear of future problems after having received constant messages that they are ticking time bombs about to explode with illness.

Groven and colleagues (2010) also noted that many of the women in their study reported having had surgery because they were ashamed of their appearance and were stigmatized due to their weight. In focus groups of women and men who were at least two years postsurgery, women who had had bariatric surgery reported feeling "normal" and no longer being stigmatized because of their weight (Stolzenberger, Meany, Marteka, Korpak, & Morello, 2013). The data from the groups reflect experiences of bias, ostracism, and criticism that contributed to a poor quality of life before the surgery. Respondents noted a heightened awareness of how they had been ostracized at work and in social settings as obese persons. However, Gilmartin (2013) interviewed individuals who experienced massive weight loss (through bariatric surgery or other means) and found that they felt depressed, suicidal, socially marginalized, and ugly because of their postweight-loss bodies' loose and hanging skin. Thus, even a "very successful" weight loss may not improve women's well-being.

The International Diabetes Federation (IDF, 2011) has proposed that bariatric surgery be an "accepted option" for individuals with type 2 diabetes who have a BMI of 35 or more and that the surgery be "considered" for those with a BMI between 30 and 35 if their diabetes is not controlled (p. 1). Others (Schauer et al., 2014) have proposed bariatric surgery for diabetics with a BMI of 27 or higher, a criterion significantly lower than that recommended for people who do not have diabetes. Given the IDF's warning that "diabetes is looming as one of the greatest public health threats of the 21st century" (p. 3) and the general fear aroused by the "war on obesity," it is no wonder that many people with diabetes have turned to bariatric surgery in the belief that it will be the cure-all for their medical worries.

However, the available research is not conclusive about the efficacy of bariatric surgery as a long-term treatment for diabetes (Hinneburg, 2012; IDF, 2011; Yamaguchi, Faintuch, Hayashi, Faintuch, & Cecconello, 2012). Although some patients' type 2 diabetes appears to have been "cured" after bariatric surgery, others' conditions have not changed or not changed significantly. Not enough time has passed for researchers to follow up with those patients whose diabetes appears to have been cleared up in order to see whether the positive effects were maintained (IDF, 2011), and little is known about the metabolic and psychiatric implications for diabetic patients who choose surgery (Hinneburg, 2012). More research is needed on the effects of bariatric surgery on diabetic patients and on all patients with a BMI under 35 (IDF, 2011).

The overall number of bariatric patients who regret their decision to have surgery or who seek to have it reversed is difficult to estimate because of the emphasis on success and the need to justify the effort involved. Many of those who have problems postsurgery have reported being silenced by other bariatric patients or told to emphasize the positives (Groven et al., 2010). A recent Google search turned up a number of entries for "weight loss surgery regret," but the only published study to date that addresses this issue is the one by Groven et al. (2010).

WEIGHT-LOSS DRUGS

The standard recommended for weight-loss pharmacotherapy is a BMI of at least 30 kg/m^2 or at least 27 kg/mg^2 for those with weight-related comorbidities (Bray & Greenway, 2007; Gadde, 2014). In addition, a variety of weight-loss pills are available over the counter to anyone. The frequent use of pharmaceutical weight-loss interventions has occurred despite several high-profile drugs having been pulled from the market due to adverse effects. Since 1997, four major antiobesity drugs have been withdrawn: fenfluramine/dexfenfluramine with or without phentermine (i.e., fen-phen, Redux) and sibutramine, both due to cardiovascular complications; phenylpropanolamine due to stroke; and rimonabant due to psychiatric disorders, including depression and suicidal ideation (Manning, Pucci, & Finer, 2014).

Currently, three weight-loss drugs are approved by the FDA for long-term use (Gadde, 2014). These are Xenical (orlistat; approved in 1999), Belviq (lorcaserin, approved in 2012), and Qsymia, also known as Qnexa (phentermine and topiramate; approved in 2012). Orlistat has been on the market for the longest time and thus has the most documentation of negative effects. Orlistat is available in both prescription and over-the-counter (OTC) forms (the OTC is marketed as Alli), which makes it widely available. The adverse effects of orlistat include flatulence, oily anal discharge, fecal incontinence, and vitamin malabsorption (Woo, 2009). Consumer information for Alli implies that the drug may serve as an aversive conditioner; that is, patients link consuming fatty foods with the gastrointestinal effects associated with taking the drug. Similar to "dumping syndrome," previously discussed in relation to bariatric surgery, any weight loss may be due to eating a lower-fat diet rather than to orlistat itself.

A number of other drugs are also used off-label for weight loss. These include Byetta, Symlin, and Victoza (which were designed to treat diabetes), Topamax (an epilepsy drug), Pristiq, Wellbutrin, and Zyban (antidepressants), and amphetamines (prescribed primarily for attention deficit/hyperactivity disorder; Kim, Lin, Blomain, & Waldman, 2014). All result in minimal weight loss and significant side effects. At least two, Pristiq and amphetamines, have anorexia as a potential side effect (Kim et al., 2014).

One over-the-counter drug that is currently marketed to promote weight loss is ephedra. Because it is an herbal substance, individuals seeking weight loss may see it as a healthier, nonmedical alternative (Fleming, 2007). However, a clinical study showed that ephedra use resulted in a very small weight loss (about two pounds) and increased the risk of psychiatric symptoms, heart palpitations, and gastrointestinal problems (Shekelle et al., 2003). Ephedra has also been linked to a number of deaths (Campos, 2004). Thus, it is not a safe or healthy alternative.

Although an increasing number of weight-loss drugs have gone on the market in the United States in recent years, rates of obesity have not declined significantly during this time period. In other words, weight loss associated with antiobesity drugs "is not as dramatic as one might expect . . . (and) they do not appear to be the definitive weight loss interventions" (Avena, Murray, & Gold, 2013, p. 1). For example, one review showed that, after 12 months, the average weight loss from orlistat was four pounds (Dombrowski, Knittle, Avenell, Araujo-Soares, & Sniehotta, 2014). Although often marketed as a panacea, weight-loss medications are recommended by pharmaceutical companies as one component of a comprehensive lifestyle modification. However, in practice, they are often prescribed in isolation (Burke & Wang, 2011).

Weight-loss pills, like fad diets, are especially ineffective in the long term. The current FDA system of drug approval does not require antiobesity pharmacotherapy to demonstrate sustained weight loss (Manning et al., 2014). In an attempt to curtail their deleterious side effects, many patients discontinue the drugs (Encinosa, Bernard, Steiner, & Chen, 2005; Encinosa et al., 2011). However, according to one researcher (Bray, 2010), the only way to maintain weight loss with pharmacotherapy is to remain on the medication for life. He wrote:

> Obesity is a chronic disease that has many causes. Cure, however, is rare, and treatment is thus aimed at palliation, i.e., producing and maintaining weight loss. Physicians do not expect to cure diseases such as hypertension or hypercholesterolemia with medications. Rather, they expect to palliate them. When the medications for any of these chronic diseases are discontinued, the disease is expected to recur. This means that medications only work when they are used. The same argument applies for medications used to treat obesity. (p. 327)

In light of their inefficacy in maintaining long-term weight loss, why are weight-loss pills prescribed so often? One possible answer to this question comes from Bacon (2008), who posited that pharmaceutical companies and obesity researchers have had questionable, even unethical, relationships. For example, makers of Xenical and Meridia funded the International Obesity Task Force, which helped establish the threshold of "overweight" at a BMI of 25. Others have also written about the associations between obesity researchers and the pharmaceutical industry (Campos, 2004; Oliver, 2006).

RESHAPING "OBESITY" AS A MEDICAL EPIDEMIC

Although some scientists and physicians tout the improved health of those who have undergone medical weight-loss interventions and argue that they are the most effective way for fat people to lose weight and become healthy, others have suggested that health and well-being can be achieved without these interventions. Furthermore, fat stigma needs to be challenged as the discrimination suffered by fat people can serve as a contributor to poor health. However, one reason why fat stigma is such a difficult problem to address is because the biomedical perspective that fat is in and of itself unhealthy is so entrenched.

The Health at Every Size (HAES) movement is an alternative to weight-focused health initiatives (Bacon & Aphramor, 2011). A key assumption of HAES is that stigmatizing fat is detrimental to fat people's physical and mental health (Burgard, 2009). The real problem is not fat, but the focus on dieting and weight loss as a proxy for health (Saguy, 2013). There are several core tenets that undergird HAES programs (Bacon & Aphramor, 2011): accepting one's body, monitoring internal regulatory states (e.g., eating intuitively, learning to identify hunger and satiety cues), and engaging in intrinsically enjoyable physical activity. HAES promotes acceptance of size diversity and prioritizes healthy behaviors rather than weight loss. It is discussed in more depth in Chapter 9 in this volume.

CONCLUSION

In this chapter, we reviewed current weight-loss treatments that are marketed as lifesavers to fat individuals. However, these interventions have not demonstrated long-term efficacy, can have serious complications and side effects, and they may even be fatal. Moreover, they are rooted in the erroneous assumption that fat is always unhealthy, whereas a growing body of research supports the obesity paradox and promotes ways that people can be healthy at any size. We are optimistic that the growing scholarship on the social context of fat (known as "fat studies") can work to ameliorate the negative effects of fat stigma and reshape the "obesity" debates.

NOTE

1. We utilize the terms *obese* and *overweight* when they refer to clinical classifications of weight in the research literature. Otherwise, we refer to *fat*, the term used by fat activists and by fat studies scholars to challenge questionable weight classifications and transcend the stigmatization engendered by the terms obese and overweight (see Wann, 2009).

REFERENCES

Adams, T. D., Davidson, L. E., Litwin, S. E., Kolotkin, R. L., LaMonte, M. J., Pendleton, R. C., . . . Hunt, S. C. (2012). Health benefits of gastric bypass surgery after 6 years. *Journal of the American Medical Association, 308,* 1122–1131.

Ailshire, J. A., & House, J. S. (2011). The unequal burden of weight gain: An intersectional approach to understanding social disparities in BMI trajectories from 1986 to 2001/2002. *Social Forces, 90,* 397–423.

Alosco, M. L., Spitznagel, M., Strain, G., Devlin, M., Cohen, R. Paul, R., . . . Gunstad, J. (2014). Improved memory function two years after bariatric surgery. *Obesity, 22,* 32–38.

American Society for Metabolic and Bariatric Surgery (2014). Overview. Retrieved from http://asmbs.org/resources/metabolic-and-bariatric-surgery.

Avena, N., Murray, S., & Gold, M. (2013). The next generation of obesity treatments: Beyond suppressing appetite. *Frontiers in Psychology, 4,* 1–3.

Bacon, L. (2008). *Health at every size: The surprising truth about your weight.* Dallas, TX: BenBella Books.

Bacon, L., & Aphramor, L. (2011). Weight science: Evaluating the evidence for a paradigm shift. *Nutrition Journal, 10,* 9.

Black, J. A., White, B., Viner, R. M., & Simmons, R. K. (2013). Bariatric surgery for obese children and adolescents: A systemic review and meta-analysis. *Obesity Review, 14,* 634–644.

Boero, N. (2007). All the news that's fat to print: The American "obesity epidemic" and the media. *Qualitative Sociology, 30,* 41–60.

Bray, G. A. (2010). Drugs used clinically to reduce body weight. In P. G. Kopelman, I. D. Caterson, & W. H. Dietz (Eds.), *Clinical obesity in adults and children* (3rd ed., pp. 327–338). Hoboken, NJ: Wiley-Blackwell.

Bray, G., & Greenway, F. (2007). Pharmacological treatment of the overweight patient. *Pharmacological Reviews, 59,* 151–184.

Buchwald, H., Avidor, Y., Braunwald, E., Jensen, M. D., Pories, W, Fahrbach, K., & Schoelles, K. (2004). Bariatric surgery: A systematic review and meta-analysis. *Journal of the American Medical Association, 292,* 1724–1737.

Burgard, D. (2009). What is "Health at Every Size"? In E. R. Rothblum & S. Solovay (Eds.), *The fat studies reader* (pp. 42–53). New York: New York University Press.

Burke, L. E., & Wang, J. (2011). Treatment strategies for overweight and obesity. *Journal of Nursing Scholarship, 43,* 368–375.

Campos, P. (2004). *The obesity myth: Why America's obsession with weight is hazardous to your health.* New York: Gotham Books.

Charo, L., & LaCoursiere, D. Y. (2014). Obesity and lifestyle issues in women. *Clinical Obstetrics and Gynecology, 57,* 433–445.

Chiolero, A., & Paccaud, R. (2009). An obesity epidemic booga booga? *European Journal of Public Health, 19,* 568–569.

Chrisler, J. C. (2012). "Why can't you control yourself?" Fat should be a feminist issue. *Sex Roles, 66,* 608–616.

Deitel, M., & Shikora, S. (2002). The development of the surgical treatment of morbid obesity. *Journal of the American College of Nutrition, 21,* 365–371.

Dombrowski, S. U., Knittle, K., Avenell, A., Araujo-Soares, V., & Sniehotta, F. F. (2014). Long term maintenance of weight loss with non-surgical interventions in obese adults: Systematic review and meta-analyses of randomized controlled trials. *British Medical Journal.* Retrieved from http://dx.doi.org/10.1136/bmj.g2646.

Elliott, V. S. (2012). Bariatric surgery maintains, doesn't gain. *American Medical News.* Retrieved from http://www.amednews.com/article/20120423/business/304239976/4/.

Encinosa, W., Bernard, D., Steiner, C., & Chen, C. (2005). Use and costs of bariatric surgery and prescription weight-loss medications. *Health Affairs, 24,* 1039–1046.

Encinosa, W., Du, D., & Bernard, D. (2011). Anti-obesity drugs and bariatric surgery. In J. Cawley (Ed.), *The Oxford handbook of the social science of obesity* (pp. 792–807). New York: Oxford University Press.

Erdely, S. R. (2008). *The miracle weight loss that isn't.* Retrieved from http://www.nbcnews.com/id/26076054/ns/health-diet_and_nutrition/t/miracle-weight-loss-isnt/#.U7y5JfldXD8.

Ertelt, T. W., Mitchell, J. E., Lancaster, K., Crosby, R., Steffen, K. J., & Marino, J. M. (2008). Alcohol abuse and dependence before and after bariatric surgery: A review of the literature and a report of a new data set. *Surgery for Obesity and Related Diseases, 4,* 647–650.

Fikkan, J. L., & Rothblum, E. D. (2012). Is fat a feminist issue? Exploring the gendered nature of weight bias. *Sex Roles, 66,* 575–592.

Flegal, K. M., Graubard, B. J., Williamson, D. F., & Gail, M. H. (2005). Excess deaths associated with underweight, overweight, and obesity. *Journal of the American Medical Association, 293,* 1861–1867.

Flegal, K. M., Kit, B. K., Orpana, H., & Graubard, B. I. (2013). Association of all-cause mortality with overweight and obesity using standard body mass

216 The Wrong Prescription for Women

index categories: A systematic review and meta-analysis. *Journal of the American Medical Association, 309,* 71–82.

Fleming, R. M. (2007). The effects of ephedra and high-fat dieting: A cause for concern! *Angiology, 58,* 102–105.

Flum, D. R., Salem, L., Elrod, J. A. B., Dellinger, P., & Cheadle, A. (2005). Early mortality among Medicare beneficiaries undergoing bariatric surgery procedures. *Journal of the American Medical Association, 294,* 1903–1908.

Fosberg, A., Engstrom, A., & Soderberg, S. (2013). From reaching the end of the road to a new lighter life: People's experiences of undergoing bariatric surgery. *Intensive and Critical Care Nursing, 30,* 93–100.

Gadde, K. (2014). Current pharmacotherapy for obesity: Extrapolation of clinical trials data to practice. *Expert Opinion on Pharmacotherapy, 15,* 809–822.

Gelinas, B. L., Delparte, C. A., Hart, R., & Wright, K. D. (2013). Unrealistic weight loss goals and expectations among bariatric surgery candidates: The impact on pre- and postsurgical weight outcomes. *Bariatric Surgical Patient Care, 8,* 12–17.

Gilmartin, J. (2013). Body image concerns amongst massive weight loss patients. *Journal of Clinical Nursing, 22,* 1299–1309.

Groven, K. S., Raheim, M., & Engelsrud, G. (2010). "My quality of life is worse compared to my earlier life": Living with chronic problems after weight loss surgery. *International Journal of Qualitative Studies on Health & Well-Being, 5,* 1–15.

Hainer, V., & Aldhoon-Hainerová, I. (2013). Obesity paradox does exist. *Diabetes Care, 36*(Suppl. 2), S276–S281.

Hakimi, A. A., Furberg, H., Zabor, E. C., Jacobson, A., Schultz, N., & Ciriello, G. (2013). An epidemiologic and genomic investigation into the obesity paradox in renal cell carcinoma. *Journal of the National Cancer Institute, 13,* 1862–1870.

Heitmann, B. L. (2010). Obesity and gender. In P. G. Kopelman, I. D. Caterson, & W. H. Dietz (Eds.), *Clinical obesity in adults and children* (3rd ed., pp. 58–64). Hoboken, NJ: Wiley-Blackwell.

Hinneburg, I. (2012). Surgery against diabetes? *Medizinische Monatsschrift für Pharmazeuten, 35,* 410–415.

International Diabetes Federation Task Force on Epidemiology and Prevention [IDF]. (2011). *Bariatric surgical and procedural interventions in the treatment of obese patients with type 2 diabetes: A position statement from the International Diabetes Federation Task Force on Epidemiology and Prevention.* Retrieved from https://www.idf.org/webdata/docs/IDF-Position-Statement-Bariatric-Surgery.pdf.

Ivezaj, V., Saules, K. K., & Weidemann, A. A. (2012). "I didn't see this coming": Why are post-bariatric patients in substance abuse treatment? Patients' perceptions of etiology and future recommendations. *Obesity Surgery, 22,* 1308–1314.

Karlsson, J., Taft, D., Ryden, A., Sjostrom. L., & Sullivan, M. (2007). Ten-year trends in in health-related quality of life after surgical and conventional treatment for severe obesity: The SOS Intervention study. *International Journal of Obesity, 11*, 1248–1261.

Kim, G. W., Lin, J. E., Blomain, E. S., & Waldman, S. A. (2014). Antiobesity pharmacotherapy: New drugs and emerging targets. *Clinical Pharmacology and Therapeutics, 95*, 53–66.

Maggard, M. A., Shugarman, L. R., Suttorp, M., Maglione, M., Sugarman, H. J., Livingston, E. H., . . . Shekelle, P. G. (2005). Meta-analysis: Surgical treatment of obesity. *Annals of Internal Medicine, 142*, 547–559.

Magro, D. O., Gelonez, B, Delfini, R., Pareja, B. C., Callejas, F., & Pareja, J. C. (2008). Long-term weight regain after gastric bypass: A 5-year retrospective study. *Obesity Surgery, 18*, 648–651.

Manning, S., Pucci, A., & Finer, N. (2014). Pharmacotherapy for obesity: Novel agents and paradigms. *Therapeutic Advances in Chronic Disease, 5*, 135–148.

Marketdata Enterprises. (2014). *Market research reports*. Retrieved from http://www.dietbusinesswatch.com/Market_Research_Reports.html.

Mason, K. (2012). The unequal weight of discrimination: Gender, body size, and income inequality. *Social Problems, 59*, 411–435.

Meany, G., Conceicao, E., & Mitchell, J. E. (2013). Binge eating, binge eating disorder and loss of control eating: Effects of weight outcomes after bariatric surgery. *European Eating Disorders Review, 22*, 87–91.

National Institutes of Health. (2000). *The practical guide: Identification, evaluation, and treatment of overweight and obesity in adults*. Retrieved from http://www.nhlbi.nih.gov/guidelines/obesity/prctgd_b.pdf.

National Institutes of Health, National Heart, Lung, and Blood Institute. (1998). Clinical guidelines on the identification, evaluation, and treatment of overweight and obesity in adults: The evidence report. *Obesity Research, 6*(Suppl. 2), 51S–209S.

Nicholls, S. G. (2013). Standards and classification: A perspective on the "obesity epidemic." *Social Science & Medicine, 87*, 9–15.

Nie, W., Zhang, Y., Jee, S. H., Jung, K. J., Li, B., & Xiu, Q. (2014). Obesity survival paradox in pneumonia: A meta-analysis. *BMC Medicine, 12*, 661.

Ogden, C., Carroll, M., Kit, B., & Flegal, K. (2014). Prevalence of childhood and adult obesity in the United States, 2011–2012. *Journal of the American Medical Association, 311*, 806–814.

Oliver, J. E. (2006). *Fat politics: The real story behind America's obesity epidemic*. New York: Oxford University Press.

Omalu, B. I., Ives, D. G., Buhari, A. M., Lindner, J. L., Schauer, P. R., Wecht, C. H., & Kuller, J. H. (2007). Death rates and causes of death after bariatric surgery for Pennsylvania residents, 1995 to 2004. *Archives of Surgery, 42*, 923–928.

Patterson, M., & Johnston, J. (2012). Theorizing the obesity epidemic: Health crisis, moral panic and emerging hybrids. *Social Theory & Health, 10*, 265–291.

Puhl, R. M., Andreyeva, T. T., & Brownell, K. D. (2008). Perceptions of weight discrimination: Prevalence and comparison to race and gender discrimination in America. *International Journal of Obesity, 32*, 992–1000.

Saguy, A. C. (2013). *What's wrong with fat?* New York: Oxford University Press.

Saguy, A. C., & Almeling, R. (2008). Fat in the fire? Science, the news media, and the "obesity epidemic." *Sociological Forum, 23,* 53–83.

Schauer, P., Bhatt, D., Kirwan, J., Wolski, K., Brethauer, S., Navaneethan, S. D., . . . STAMPEDE Investigators. (2014). Bariatric surgery versus intensive medical therapy for diabetes: 3-year outcomes. *New England Journal of Medicine, 370,* 2002–2013.

Shekelle, P. G., Hardy, M. L., Morton, S. C., Maglione, M., Mojika, W. A., Suttorp, M. J., . . . Gagné, J. (2003). Efficacy and safety of ephedra for weight loss and athletic performance: A meta-analysis. *Journal of the American Medical Association, 289,* 1537–1545.

Smith, C. A. (2012). The confounding of fat, control, and physical attractiveness for women. *Sex Roles, 66,* 628–631.

Smith, S. C., Goodman, G. N., & Edwards, C. B. (1995). Roux-en-Y gastric bypass: A 7-year retrospective review of 3855 patients. *Obesity Surgery, 5,* 314–318.

Stein, P. D., & Malta, F. (2013). Pulmonary embolism and deep venous thrombosis following bariatric surgery. *Obesity Surgery, 23,* 663–668.

Stolzenberger, K. M., Meany, C. A., Marteka, P., Korpak, S., & Morello, K. (2013). Long-term quality of life following bariatric surgery: A descriptive study. *Bariatric Surgical Patient Care, 8,* 29–38.

Stommel, M., & Schoenborn, C. A. (2010). Variations in BMI and presence of health risk in diverse racial and ethnic populations. *Epidemiology, 18,* 1821–1826.

Sussenbach, S. P., Silva, E. N., Pufal, M. A., Casagrande, D. S., Padoin, A. V., & Motton, C. C. (2014). Systematic review of economic evaluation of laparotomy versus laparoscopy for patients submitted to Roux-en-Y gastric bypass. *Plos One, 9,* e99976.

U.S. Food and Drug Administration. (2004). *Calories count: Report of the Working Group on Obesity.* Retrieved from http://www.fda.gov/food/foodscience research/consumerbehaviorresearch/ucm081696.htm.

Visscher, T. S., Snijder, M. B., & Seidell, J. C. (2010). Epidemiology: Definition and classification of obesity. In P. G. Kopelman, I. D. Caterson, & W. H. Dietz (Eds.), *Clinical obesity in adults and children* (3rd ed., pp. 3–14). Hoboken, NJ: Wiley-Blackwell.

Wann, M. (2009). Fat studies: An invitation to the revolution. In E. R. Rothblum & S. Solovay (Eds.), *The fat studies reader* (pp. ix–xxv). New York: New York University Press.

Wee, C. C., Jones, D. B., Davis, R. B., Bourland, A. C., & Hamel, M. B. (2006). Understanding patients' value of weight loss and expectations for bariatric surgery. *Obesity Surgery, 16,* 496–500.

White House. (2011). *Women in America.* Retrieved from http://www.whitehouse .gov/administration/eop/cwg/data-on-women.

Wnuk, S. (2013). Psychological treatment of obesity: Bariatric surgery as one solution to obesity—Psychosocial considerations. *Journal of Psychosomatic Research, 74,* 561–562.

Woo, T. (2009). Pharmacotherapy and surgery treatment for the severely obese adolescent. *Journal of Pediatric Health Care, 23*, 206–212.

World Health Organization. (2014). *Obesity and overweight.* Retrieved from http://www.who.int/mediacentre/factsheets/fs311/en/.

Wysoker, A. (2005). The lived experience of choosing bariatric surgery to lose weight. *Journal of the American Psychiatric Nurses Association, 11*, 26–34.

Yamaguchi, C., Faintuch, J., Hayashi, S., Faintuch, J., & Cecconello, I. (2012). Refractory and new-onset diabetes more than 5 years after gastric bypass for morbid obesity. *Surgical Endoscopy, 26*, 2843–2847.

Ziegler, O., Sirveaux, M. A., Brunaud, L., Reibel, N., & Quilliot, D. (2009). Medical follow-up after bariatric surgery: Nutritional and drug issues. *Diabetes & Metabolism, 35*, 544–557.

Chapter 11

Can Women's Body Image Be "Fixed"? Women's Bodies, Well-Being, and Cosmetic Surgery

Charlotte N. Markey and Patrick M. Markey

According to the American Society of Plastic Surgeons (2014a), 15.1 million cosmetic surgery procedures were performed in the United States in 2013, a 104% increase since 2000. Ninety-one percent of these procedures were performed on women, and 51% of the patients were "repeat customers." This surge includes increases in surgical, nonsurgical, and reconstructive cosmetic procedures. In 2013, breast augmentation was the top elective surgical procedure in the United States (290,000 patients) and botulinum toxin type A injections (botox; 6.3 million patients) was the top nonsurgical procedure.

Data from the International Society of Aesthetic Plastic Surgeons (ISAPS, 2013) suggest that, although the United States ranks highest in the number of cosmetic surgeries performed (21% worldwide), many other countries boast a growing number of procedures. Approximately 29% of all procedures performed annually take place in Brazil, China, Japan, Mexico, Italy, and South Korea. A recent survey in Korea showed that 80% of Korean women desired cosmetic surgery, and 50% had even undergone cosmetic surgery at least once (Tam, Ng, Kim, Yeung, &

Cheung, 2012). Although breast augmentation procedures (arguably, elective procedures unless following a mastectomy) are among the top procedures performed worldwide, there has been a recent rise in cosmetic surgeries focused on different parts of the body. These range from nonsurgical procedures, such as botox injections, to surgical procedures, such as implants for the calves and buttocks and even labiaplasty (i.e., the plumping or reduction of the labia minora or majora; Braun, 2010; Eriksen & Goering, 2011). These statistics suggest that the 21st century represents an era of acceptance of aesthetic cosmetic surgery, particularly for women.

Even though cosmetic surgery and related nonsurgical procedures are relatively new, they hardly represent the first time the human body has been reshaped for aesthetic purposes (Brumberg, 1997). Forerunners to cosmetic surgery date back thousands of years and include practices that range from foot binding to the wearing of corsets. Women's bodies in particular have been reshaped and altered to meet changing cultural ideals of beauty and fashion; however, until recently, these procedures were not typically performed by medical professionals. As Eriksen and Goering (2011, p. 889) suggested, not only is cosmetic surgery increasingly viewed as acceptable, but it also has achieved a "complicated moral positioning as a 'health care' enterprise."

Early cosmetic surgery procedures grew out of a need for reconstructive procedures in the early 20th century following World War I. Most of the first patients were wounded male soldiers (Gilman, 1999; Haiken, 1997), and the pursuit was much less about beautifying than it was about normalizing and repairing injuries. Formal training in plastic surgery began in the 1920s at Johns Hopkins University, and the need to treat wounded soldiers once again popularized these procedures following World War II. In the 1950s, board certification programs were introduced, and plastic surgery became an integrated component of medical training (ASPS, 2014b). Organ transplants and breast implants were being performed by plastic surgeons in the 1950s and 1960s. By the 1990s, plastic surgeons in the United States alone were performing more than 1.2 million reconstructive procedures and more than 1 million cosmetic procedures annually.

The sheer number of plastic surgery procedures performed each year means that cosmetic surgery is no longer the purview of the rich and famous; men, women, old, and young are partaking in it (Sarwer, Gibbons et al., 2005). Advances in surgical medicine, reduction of risks, lower cost of procedures, and higher disposable incomes among patients make surgery both more desirable and more attainable for a growing number of people (Sarwer, Crerand, & Gibbons, 2007; Swami, 2009). One of the most important areas of body image research in the 21st century is aimed at determining attitudes toward body modification via cosmetic surgery and understanding who does and does not pursue surgery.

PREDICTORS OF COSMETIC SURGERY
INTEREST AND ATTAINMENT

Most people view surgery as a last-resort treatment option for medical conditions. It is not only expensive but also has inherent risks that most people wish to avoid. However, each year a growing number of people elect to undergo surgery in order to enhance their appearance. Why do people elect to obtain expensive and potentially dangerous surgeries for cosmetic purposes? There are a variety of demographic predictors of interest in cosmetic surgery, and gender is the most obvious one.

Due to the greater sociocultural pressure on women to attain ideals of physical and sexual attractiveness (Swami, 2007; Swami & Furnham, 2008), women report a greater willingness than men do to undergo various cosmetic procedures (Brown, Furnham, Glanville, & Swami, 2007; Swami, Arteche et al., 2008; Swami, Chamorro-Premuzic, Bridges, & Furnham, 2009). The difference between women's and men's interest in cosmetic surgery is so extreme that some have called cosmetic surgery a "gendered activity" (Dull & West, 1991). Much in the same way that society expects little girls to play with dolls or play dress up, it is increasingly accepted that women may consider cosmetic surgery in order to enhance their appearance.

Given that a number of cosmetic surgical procedures are designed to "correct" the effects of aging (e.g., a "facelift"), it is not surprising that age is a powerful predictor of pursuit of cosmetic surgery. Cultural emphasis on youth as integral to attractiveness, especially for women, has unquestionably led many women to consider cosmetic surgery. Some research even suggests that an association between interest in cosmetic surgery and "aging anxiety" exists; as women age and become more concerned about their appearance, interest in cosmetic surgery is more likely to translate into pursuit of the surgery (Slevec & Tiggemann, 2010). Interest in surgery peaks in midlife. Women 40 to 54 years of age comprise approximately one-half of all cosmetic surgery patients, and they are its largest consumer group in the United States (ASPS, 2014a; Eriksen & Goering, 2011). In recent years, this age effect has appeared to grow stronger; in 2013, the rate was 54% and 6.8 million procedures were performed on this age group of women (ASPS, 2014a).

Familiarity with cosmetic surgery and knowing someone who has had surgery make it more likely that a woman will also pursue surgery (Erikson & Goering, 2011). The majority of young adult women report knowing someone who has undergone cosmetic surgery, and, in nearly one-half of these cases, the person they know is a family member (Sarwer, Cash et al., 2005). Data from both the United States and Europe have consistently indicated strong positive correlations between knowing someone who has had surgery and women's pursuit of surgery for themselves (von

Soest, Kvalem, Skolleborg, & Roald, 2006). Familiarity with surgery might make the risks associated with a procedure seem less prohibitive when women know someone who has had a successful surgery experience.

Not only are demographic characteristics important predictors of interest in and pursuit of surgery, but other individual differences, such as personality traits and general mental health, also seem to be relevant. In one study (Swami et al., 2009), individuals who were more conscientious, less agreeable, and less open to new experiences were most likely to consider cosmetic surgery. This constellation of traits suggests that those who are especially conventional are more likely to conform to sociocultural norms and therefore more attracted to cosmetic surgery than those who are more individualistic. Perhaps not surprising is a related research finding that women who have low self-esteem tend to desire surgery more than those who have higher self-evaluations (Swami et al., 2009).

Women's mental health has been examined more generally as a possible predictor of interest in cosmetic surgery. Research by Sarwer and colleagues (Sarwer, Brown, & Evans, 2007; Sarwer, Wadden, Pertschuk, & Whitaker, 1998) showed that a higher prevalence of body dysmorphic disorder (i.e., a clinical diagnosis characterized by a persistent preoccupation with one's appearance that interferes with well-being and daily functioning) exists among cosmetic surgery patients than among the general population. The mental well-being of breast augmentation patients, in particular, has been of interest given some reports of higher-than-expected suicide rates among this subpopulation, which might be indicative of preexisting mental illness (Sarwer et al., 2003; these findings are reviewed in more detail below).

Perhaps the most substantiated predictor of interest in and pursuit of cosmetic surgery is body dissatisfaction (Brown et al., 2007; Swami et al., 2009). In general, people undergo elective surgery when they are unhappy with some element of their body. However, this does not mean that all or even most women who are dissatisfied with their appearance are interested in pursuing surgery. Sarwer and colleagues (2007) have stressed that it is essential to consider not only individuals' evaluation of their own bodies (i.e., their body dissatisfaction), but also the extent to which their appearance is important to them (i.e., their investment in their appearance). Thus, a woman who believes that her appearance is an important part of her self-worth *and* who is not satisfied with her appearance is most likely to consider and, ultimately, to pursue cosmetic surgery (Sarwer et al., 2007). Women who are dissatisfied with their bodies or appearance more generally may aim to "fix" themselves via surgery, but this dissatisfaction is a result of subjective self-evaluation, not necessarily related to objective body size or attractiveness (Slevec & Tiggemann, 2010).

In addition to women's *intrapersonal* qualities that predict their pursuit of cosmetic surgery, women's *interpersonal* experiences are also relevant.

Girls' and women's formation of body ideals take place in the contexts of families, friendships, romantic relationships, peer networks, and an increasingly pervasive world of media influence (Markey, 2010). It is within these contexts that women come to value their bodies and develop ideas about the extent to which they should accept versus "fix" their physical selves (Gillen & Markey, 2014).

The media, in particular, have been implicated in girls' and women's development of body dissatisfaction with the presentation of an endless barrage of unrealistic, digitally altered, beauty ideals (Markey, 2014). However, the explicit feedback women get from others about their bodies appears to be especially salient in shaping their views of their bodies. For example, research suggests that women who have been teased about their bodies or appearance are vulnerable to the pursuit of surgery to remedy the body part about which they were teased (Markey & Markey, 2009; Park, Calogero, Harwin, & DiRaddo, 2009). Further, women sometimes report having obtained cosmetic surgery due to a desire to secure others' attention or acceptance (Sherry, Hewitt, Lee-Baggley, Flett, & Besser, 2004) or even to get or keep a job (Tam et al., 2012). Swami, Hwang, and Jung (2012) suggested that romantic partners are likely to contribute to an individual's sense of self-worth and that surgery may be viewed as a means of improving not only one's appearance, but also one's current (or potential) romantic relationships. Breast augmentation patients in particular have indicated a desire to feel more attractive to potential or current romantic partners, and they report believing that their breast surgery will improve their sex lives, body image, marital satisfaction, and even overall quality of life (Sarwer, 2007).

Social experiences beyond women's immediate relationships are also implicated in their consideration, and pursuit, of cosmetic surgery. Sociocultural norms concerning appearance have been shown to influence not only women's dissatisfaction with their bodies but also their behavioral means of coping with this dissatisfaction. This is especially true for women who are inclined to internalize sociocultural messages regarding appearance issues and who are prone to materialism (Henderson-King & Brooks, 2009). In one study, young adults' inclination toward "celebrity worship" (i.e., the formation of parasocial relationships with celebrity icons) predicted their obtainment of cosmetic surgery within an eight-month period (Maltby & Day, 2011). However, women who experience greater media influence in general (typically assessed via television and magazine consumption) are more likely than their peers with less media experience to consider cosmetic surgery (Slevec & Tiggemann 2010; Swami, 2009). In some of our own research, we have found that women who view television shows featuring cosmetic surgery are more likely than a control group to indicate an interest in pursuing surgery (Markey & Markey, 2010). Swami and colleagues (2012) concurred with our findings and suggested that increased media coverage of cosmetic surgery and greater awareness of cosmetic procedures have normalized these procedures and reduced women's concerns about the risks associated with them.

Although research has accumulated to implicate media influences as a primary source of women's interest in and pursuit of cosmetic surgery, it is important that the link between the media and cosmetic surgery not be oversimplified. As Chrisler, Gorman, Serra, and Chapman (2012) pointed out, women are faced with a double standard as they navigate a media environment that makes body dissatisfaction a "normative discontent" and then touts products and procedures to remedy this discontent. It can feel like a no-win situation for women as media messages expound the virtues of achieving a youthful, attractive appearance and present images and ideals that are unlikely to be obtainable for the average woman without considerable cosmetic intervention. This sentiment is reflected in a recent study that showed that women can be both critical of media messages about aging, yet regularly use antiaging products (Muise & Desmarais, 2010). Women may think they should ignore conventional values placed on attractiveness but still use cosmetic products and procedures, even if they wish they were not using them. Feminist theory and research help to elucidate this conundrum, including both the philosophical and practical concerns that have been raised about cosmetic procedures and surgery.

THEORETICAL AND FEMINIST PERSPECTIVES ON WOMEN'S PURSUIT OF COSMETIC SURGERY

Many theories have been developed to account for contributors to girls' and women's body image and their interest in changing their bodies. Perhaps most relevant to a feminist appreciation of women's interest in cosmetic surgery is *objectification theory*. Fredrickson and Roberts (1997) developed objectification theory to describe how girls and women experience their own bodies as a result of others' perceptions of them. Because society values women's bodies for their appearance (more than their function, e.g., athletic skills) and because women are constantly subjected to evaluations of their appearance, they come to appreciate their own bodies based on their appearance. According to this perspective, the female body is an object to evaluate, admire, or disparage. Girls and women monitor and engage in surveillance of their own bodies because others do, and their surveillance often results in shame, anxiety, and body dissatisfaction (Henderson-King & Brooks, 2009). According to Brumberg (1997), given this sociocultural context, a woman's body risks being not merely an object but also a "project" that women are expected to work on throughout their lives.

Women's "body work" is fueled by a multibillion-dollar industry that provides a growing number of products and procedures presented as capable of improving appearance. These improvements are seen as "necessary," and women are thus encouraged to purchase goods and services that they hope will transform their bodies to match the omnipresent Western beauty ideal. Although the beauty industry advertises products and procedures under the guise of helping women to achieve their beauty potential, critics have argued that the actual outcome of these advertisements is for women to feel deficient and in constant need of improvement (Henderson-King & Brooks, 2009). Thus, self-objectification is difficult to abandon, and women pursue all kinds of body work from hair coloring and makeup to cosmetic surgery.

A feminist understanding of women's experience of objectification must not only consider the gendered nature of "the body project" (Brumberg, 1997), but also the intersection of age and gender. According to Chrisler and colleagues (2012), women's desire to maintain a youthful appearance and the social status that accompanies this youth is a primary contributor to women's pursuit of surgery. Indeed, Western society often has more favorable opinions of the appearance of older men than that of older women. Whereas older men's graying hair and facial lines are viewed as "distinguished," women are socialized to believe that they should erase signs of aging, which make them look "old." To this end, older women often pursue both superficial and invasive procedures to pass as younger than they are, and doing so is reinforced by society (Chrisler et al., 2012).

The notion that older women remain at risk for body image concerns and the experience of objectification is supported by research that we and others have conducted (Schulz, Bowler, & Markey, 2014; Tiggemann, 2004). Midlife women experience body dissatisfaction and interest in improving their appearance via surgery, even as they are enjoying a phase of their lives that typically involves more independence and freedom from gendered responsibilities, such as child care (Chrisler et al., 2012). Perhaps many of these women think that it is reasonable for them to enjoy their midlife years and to spend more time and effort on themselves and their appearance than they were able to in the decades of their twenties and thirties. Further, some feminist scholars have suggested that a choice to pursue appearance-enhancing procedures, including surgery, is not an unreasonable choice in a sexist society that makes it impossible for women to make fully autonomous decisions (Erikson & Goering, 2011).

The suggestion that cosmetic enhancement might actually increase women's sense of agency and empower them to achieve in an appearance-focused society is in stark contrast to the traditional feminist view that describes women's attempt to adhere to sociocultural prescriptions for appearance enhancement as relinquishments of their autonomy and "power" to others—often men—who dictate these norms (Bordo, 1993; Brumberg, 1997). In fact, it seems that there is no longer a clear consensus among feminist scholars regarding the meaning or potential impact of appearance-enhancing procedures or treatments on women.

Some feminist scholars have argued, consistent with objectification theory, that women's "buying into" the beauty culture is an unfortunate artifact of the current cultural norms, which coerce women into trying to change their appearance (Bordo, 1993). Others have proposed that appearance enhancement increases women's sense of agency and empowers them to achieve in an appearance-focused society (Davis, 1995). Although research does not conclusively resolve this debate, it does offer important questions and considerations about what it means, from a feminist perspective, to obtain cosmetic surgery.

Central to the debate about whether pursuing cosmetic surgery can be construed as a feminist act is the agency hypothesis. According to Davis (1995, 2003), women may choose cosmetic surgery freely in order to fight back in an unjust world. In other words, women are actively engaged in this choice, and it should be viewed as an act of agency. Consistent with the agency hypothesis, many women who seek cosmetic surgery label themselves as feminists and are aware of the cultural tendency to prioritize women's beauty over their other assets (Davis, 1995, 2003; Erikson & Goering, 2011). Davis (1995, 2003) argued that, by pursuing surgery instead of "suffering in silence" with bodies that are not culturally ideal, women are triumphing over feelings of powerlessness. Cosmetic procedures, such as liposuction, breast augmentation, or facelift, allow these women to believe they are seizing control of their lives. According to this reasoning, these actions require confidence, esteem, and a general belief among women that they "are doing it [surgery] for themselves" (Gagné & McGaughey, 2002; Gimlin, 2000).

Erikson and Goering (2011) provided an empirical test of the agency hypothesis in a study of adult women that compared cosmetic surgery patients to nonpatients. The two groups were similar in many ways, including their level of education, ethnic distribution, age, and media usage. However, in contrast to the ideas proposed by the agency hypothesis, women who underwent cosmetic surgery had lower levels of self-esteem than women who had not undergone surgery. Indeed, as opposed to a triumph of agency, women who underwent surgery were likely to have done so because they had covert sexist beliefs, were wealthy, had friends who also had undergone surgery, and felt influenced by images in the media. The researchers concluded that their findings challenge claims of the pursuit of cosmetic surgery as an act of agency, as women who pursued surgery exhibited differences in gender ideology from those who did not pursue surgery. Additional research that emerges from feminist theory is still needed to examine these different perspectives on women's pursuit of surgery and to provide context for women's experiences of the outcomes of cosmetic surgery.

OUTCOMES OF COSMETIC SURGERY

The consequences associated with poor body dissatisfaction are deleterious and range from disordered eating to impaired social relationships (Markey & Markey, 2010, 2011). Thus, ameliorating women's body image is a worthy goal. Some researchers have even referred to cosmetic surgery as "body image surgery" (Pruzinsky & Edgerton, 1990). However, before advising women to pursue surgery in an attempt to improve their body image, it is critical to evaluate the effects of cosmetic surgery on body image. Does cosmetic surgery "work" to improve women's body image and appearance satisfaction?

Research clearly indicates that most women undergo cosmetic surgery with the aim of improving not only their appearance, but also their general sense of self. For example, Cash, Duel, and Perkins (2002) examined patients from 24 U.S. clinical sites and reported that the majority anticipated improvements in their self-esteem as a result of surgery. Although most women expect surgery to improve their self-esteem, research is less clear on the actual consequences of surgery for women's self-esteem (Eriksen & Goering, 2011). At least one study showed postoperative increases in self-esteem at six months following surgery (Klassen, Fitzpatrick, Jenkinson, & Goodacre, 1996), but other research indicates no significant increase in self-esteem 12 months postoperatively (Sarwer, Gibbons et al., 2005).

Data on women's preoperative and postoperative body image and appearance satisfaction also provide inconclusive evidence for the efficacy of cosmetic surgery in improving women's body satisfaction. Research has accumulated to suggest that women are typically satisfied with postoperative outcomes in terms of the feature(s) altered by surgery (Sarwer, Gibbons et al., 2005). For example, if a woman pursues rhinoplasty (i.e., a "nose job"), she is likely to prefer her nose after surgery more than her nose before surgery. Some patients even report a reduction in overall negative body image–related emotions and more general body image improvements following surgery (Sarwer, Gibbons et al., 2005). However, other studies (Sarwer, 1998) suggest that women's general body image does not improve following cosmetic surgery, and that women's investment in their appearance does not decrease as a result of the surgery.

One way to assess women's satisfaction with cosmetic surgery is to examine their behaviors following surgery. Fifty-one percent of cosmetic surgery patients are "repeat customers" (ASPS, 2014a). This may be evidence that patients tend to be satisfied with their initial procedure and thus pursue another procedure. However, it may also be the case that the initial procedure failed to increase the patient's general body image sufficiently. That is, if rhinoplasty improves a woman's perception not only of her nose but also of her overall body image, then she would not desire additional procedures. Perhaps "fixing" one body part puts women at risk of realizing that they are dissatisfied with another part, and thus they pursue another surgery. Future researchers should help shed light on the reasons why so many women undergo multiple cosmetic surgery procedures. This repeated pursuit of surgery hardly seems to be evidence that cosmetic surgery increases overall body satisfaction.

For women with certain preexisting dispositions, body dissatisfaction tends to worsen following surgery (Sarwer, 2007). This is especially true of women with body dysmorphic disorder. Body dysmorphic disorder is characterized by extreme body dissatisfaction and often a willingness to undergo extreme procedures to remedy this dissatisfaction. Research suggests that 3% to 15% of cosmetic surgery patients have some form of body dysmorphic disorder, but, despite this subpopulation's investment in and concern about their appearance, cosmetic surgery has been found to lead either to worse body image or no improvement for 90% of patients with body dysmorphic disorder (Sarwer, 2007).

Many women pursue surgery with the hopes of improving their social relationships. However, recent research suggests that cosmetic surgery might actually have a negative impact on social relationships. For example, Tam and colleagues (2012) found that others often view women who undergo surgery negatively, and there is often a certain degree of stigma attached to cosmetic surgery recipients. It seems that, although attractiveness is valued, it is "natural beauty" that is idealized. This has even been found in the case of women's breasts. Research suggests that, when men are interested in large breasts, they prefer natural to enhanced breasts (Latteier, 1998, as cited by Chrisler, 1999). Further, the cultural context and the type of surgery may be relevant to its impact on interpersonal relationships. For example, women who have undergone surgery due to breast cancer (i.e., breast excision) report decreases in the quality of their partner relationships and a decrease in their sexual contact (Andrzejczak, Markocka-Maczka, & Lewandowski, 2013), but the extent to which this is a result of the surgery or other aspects of cancer treatment is unclear. In contrast, when breast augmentation surgery is pursued electively, there is no evidence to suggest that overall relationship quality is altered (either positively or negatively) following surgery (Kalaaji, Bjertness, Nordahl, & Olafsen, 2013).

Various mental health consequences have been associated with cosmetic surgery, which may include severe depression and other forms of psychopathology. Some evidence for this comes from research with women who have undergone breast augmentation surgery. Across several studies, the suicide rate of breast augmentation patients has been found to be double the expected rate based on population estimates (Brinton, Lubin, Burich, Colton, & Hoover, 2001; Sarwer, 2007; Sarwer, Brown et al. 2007). However, this association needs to be interpreted with extreme caution as it is possible that it was not the surgery per se that was responsible for these unfortunate outcomes, but rather that women who pursue breast augmentation appear to be at greater risk for suicide (e.g., they are more likely than other women to be psychotherapy patients and more likely to be hospitalized for psychiatric reasons; Brinton et al., 2001; Sarwer, 2007). It appears that these women may pursue breast augmentation surgery with the hope that it will improve their life circumstances and interpersonal relationships. However, when their (perhaps unrealistic) expectations are not met, their mental health may further deteriorate. The high rate of complications associated with breast augmentation surgery (up to 25% of women experience complications) may also exacerbate any mental health concerns that women already experience and can contribute to physical pain as well.

In summary, the evidence to date suggests that cosmetic surgery has the potential to improve women's satisfaction with particular body parts, but it is less likely to improve their overall appearance evaluation and body image. Further, a single cosmetic surgery procedure may increase women's interest in additional surgery and their investment in their appearance. Women's interpersonal relationships do not appear to improve as a result of cosmetic surgery, and women with mental health problems may experience some deterioration of their well-being if their experience of cosmetic surgery does not meet their (often unrealistic) expectations. Thus, it is hard to argue, especially given the financial investment and risks involved in *any* surgical procedure, that cosmetic surgery results in inevitable improvements in body image.

ALTERNATIVES TO SURGERY AND CONCLUDING THOUGHTS

With over 15 million cosmetic surgery procedures performed in the United States in 2013 and over 90% of them performed on women, it is clear that there is significant interest in these procedures that is unlikely to wane in the near future. Some have suggested that cosmetic surgery represents a medicalization of the human body in a quick-fix culture that favors medical prescriptions over behavioral or psychological approaches to well-being (Bordo, 1993). Although women often seek surgery to improve their body image and self-esteem, the psychological benefits of cosmetic surgery are unclear. Some research (Klassen et al., 1996) suggests that cosmetic surgery may enhance body image (in particular, in regard to the particular feature that was altered), but other studies (Sarwer, 1998) have shown that cosmetic surgery has little long-term effect on self-esteem or body image.

In addition to the fact that the psychological benefits of cosmetic surgery are questionable, there are serious medical risks associated with these elective procedures. Often these risks are minimized in popular and media discourse about cosmetic surgery (Chrisler, 2007), but they are a factor that warrants consideration. The Mayo Clinic (2014) delineated the general risks associated with cosmetic surgery (i.e., not unique to any particular surgery) as including complications related to the use of anesthesia (e.g., blood clots, pneumonia, and rarely, death), infection at the incision site, fluid buildup under the skin, bleeding (which, may require additional procedures or even a transfusion), obvious scarring or skin breakdown, and nerve damage (which may be permanent). With this list of risks in mind, it becomes clear why women may want to consider alternatives to surgery, especially when surgery is pursued with the intent of improving something other than a woman's physical appearance (e.g., her social life, her self-esteem, her overall happiness).

When women believe that their appearance is integral to their self-worth, they are inclined to alter their appearance to improve their self-worth (Slevec & Tiggemann, 2010). This is common sense, of course, but it highlights the importance of deriving self-worth from avenues other than physical appearance (e.g., talents, skills, social activism, spirituality). Although there is arguably nothing wrong with women deriving some of their sense of self from their perceptions of their physical appearance, deriving more of their identity from their body's functionality and from nonphysical qualities is adaptive and beneficial. In order to obtain this goal, Chrisler and colleagues (2012) suggested that feminist therapy might be a valuable option for women considering cosmetic surgery because it can help women to reject cultural messages about beauty and instead center their self-worth on other facets of their lives, such as their meaningful relationships with friends and family. In other words, one option for women seeking to improve their sense of self-worth is to alter their (and others') ideals of female beauty to be more similar to a realistic female body instead of altering their bodies to match an unrealistic cultural ideal.

Unfortunately, research does not (yet) offer clear mechanisms to "counteract" Western culture's influence on body idealization and women's desire for cosmetic surgery. Ideally, the sociocultural climate would shift in such a way that girls and women can make informed choices about their bodies and not feel required to modify their bodies to meet beauty ideals (Henderson-King & Brooks, 2009). However, campaigns to prevent girls from internalizing these beauty ideals (e.g., media literacy campaigns) have been shown to have limited effectiveness (Henderson-King & Brooks, 2009). Instead of focusing on changing cultural norms of the female ideal or warning girls and women against such norms (both of which may prove impossible or extremely difficult to achieve given the extent of media influence today), some have argued for the importance of emphasizing the value of psychological qualities and nonmaterialistic aspirations (Bordo, 1993; Burmberg, 2000). Encouraging girls and women to focus on the importance of qualities (e.g., intellect, athleticism, interpersonal skills) and intrinsic aspirations (e.g., life goals) may prove to be an effective strategy to buffer them from the risks associated with internalizing unrealistic sociocultural ideals of female beauty.

The use of cosmetic surgery to improve appearance has been compared to fashion accessorizing by some (Bordo, 1993; Swami & Mammadova, 2012). However, the body is not merely a fashion statement but an essential part of women's functional selves. It is a disservice to women to minimize the female body to nothing more than a fashion accessory, and it is an oversimplification to assume that reshaping the body will reshape women's lives in meaningful ways. Approaching the body as easily changeable and believing such changes to have vast (positive) consequences represents a deeply ingrained cultural myth. This myth suggests that one's life is easily improved through physical transformation. However, this myth can be dangerous, especially for young women who may focus on concerns about their physical bodies, when they really have deeper self-esteem or sociorelational concerns to address as they negotiate the transition to adulthood (Brumberg, 2000; Swami, 2012). When the female body is viewed as a "project" and women's body images as inherently broken and in need of fixing, time and energy are diverted from arguably more meaningful pursuits than cosmetic alteration of the body. Perhaps the question that should be asked, though, is not whether women's body images can be "fixed" via cosmetic surgery, but why they are broken in the first place.

REFERENCES

American Society of Plastic Surgeons (ASPS). (2014a). *2013 plastic surgery statistics report*. Retrieved from http://www.plasticsurgery.org/Documents/news-resources/statistics/2013-statistics/plastic-surgery-statistics-full-report-2013.pdf.

American Society of Plastic Surgeons (ASPS). (2014b). *History of plastic surgery*. Retrieved from: http://www.plasticsurgery.org/articles-and-galleries/history-of-plastic-surgery.html.

Andrzejczak, E., Markocka-Maczka, K., & Lewandowski, A. (2013). Partner relationships after mastectomy in women not offered breast reconstruction. *Psycho-Oncology, 22*, 1653–1657.

Bordo, S. (1993). *Unbearable weight: Feminism, Western culture, and the body*. Berkeley: University of California Press.

Braun, V. (2010). Female genital cosmetic surgery: A critical review of current knowledge and contemporary debates. *Journal of Women's Health, 19*, 1393–1407.

Brinton, L. A., Lubin, J. H., Burich, M. C., Colton, T., & Hoover, R. N. (2001). Mortality among augmentation mammoplasty patients. *Epidemiology, 12*, 321–326.

Brown, A., Furnham, A., Glanville, L., & Swami, V. (2007). Factors that affect the likelihood of undergoing cosmetic surgery. *Aesthetic Surgery Journal, 27,* 501–508.

Brumberg, J. J. (1997). *The body project: An intimate history of American girls.* New York: Random House.

Brumberg, J. J. (2000). *Fasting girls: The history of anorexia nervosa.* New York: Random House.

Cash, T. F., Duel, L. A., & Perkins, L. L. (2002). Women's psychosocial outcomes of breast augmentation with silicone gel-filled implants: A 2-year prospective study. *Plastic and Reconstructive Surgery, 109*(6), 2112–2121.

Chrisler, J. C. (1999). Review of "Breasts: The women's perspective on an American obsession." *Women & Therapy, 22*(44), 107–121.

Chrisler, J. C. (2007). Body image issues of women over 50. In V. Muhlbauer & J. C. Chrisler (Eds.), *Women over 50: Psychological perspectives* (pp. 6–25). New York: Springer.

Chrisler, J. C., Gorman, J. A., Serra, K. E., & Chapman, K. R. (2012). Facing up to aging: Mid-life women's attitudes toward cosmetic procedures. *Women & Therapy, 35,* 193–206.

Davis, K. (1995). *Reshaping the female body: The dilemma of cosmetic surgery.* New York: Routledge.

Davis, K. (2003). *Dubious equalities and embodied differences: Cultural studies on cosmetic surgery.* Lanham, MD: Rowman & Littlefield.

Dull, D., & West, C. (1991). Accounting for cosmetic surgery: The accomplishment of gender. *Social Problems, 38,* 54–70.

Eriksen, S., & Goering, S. (2011). A test of the agency hypothesis in women's cosmetic surgery usage. *Sex Roles, 64,* 888–901.

Fredrickson, B. L., & Roberts, T. A. (1997). Objectification theory. *Psychology of Women Quarterly, 21,* 173–206.

Gagné, P., & McGaughey, D. (2002). Designing women: Cultural hegemony and exercise of power among women who have undergone elective mammoplasty. *Gender & Society, 16,* 814–838.

Gillen, M. M., & Markey, C. N. (2014). Body image and mental health. In H. S. Friedman (Ed.), *Encyclopedia of mental health* (2nd ed.). New York: Elsevier.

Gilman, S. L. (1999). *Making the body beautiful: A cultural history of aesthetic surgery.* Princeton, NJ: Princeton University Press.

Gimlin, D. (2000). Cosmetic surgery: beauty as a commodity. *Qualitative Sociology, 23*(1), 77–98.

Haiken, E. (1997). *Venus envy: A history of cosmetic surgery.* Baltimore, MD: Johns Hopkins University Press.

Henderson-King, D., & Brooks, K. D. (2009). Materialism, sociocultural appearance messages, and paternal attitudes predict college women's attitudes about cosmetic surgery. *Psychology of Women Quarterly, 33,* 133–142.

International Society of Aesthetic Plastic Surgeons (ISAPS). (2013). *ISAPS international survey on aesthetic/cosmetic procedures performed in 2011.* Retrieved from http://www.isaps.org/Media/Default/global-statistics/ISAPS-Results-Procedures-2011.pdf.

Kalaaji, A., Bjertness, C. B., Nordahl, C., & Olafsen, K. (2013). Survey of breast implant patient's characteristics, depression rate, and quality of life. *Aesthetic Surgery Journal, 33*(2), 252–257.

Klassen, A., Fitzpatrick, R., Jenkinson, C., & Goodacre, T. (1996). Should breast reduction surgery be rationed? A comparison of the health status of patients before and after treatment: Postal questionnaire survey. *British Medical Journal, 313*, 454–457.

Maltby, J., & Day, L. (2011). Celebrity worship and incidence of elective cosmetic surgery: Evidence of a link among young adults. *Journal of Adolescent Health, 49*, 483–489.

Markey, C. N. (2010). Invited commentary: Why body image is important to adolescent development. *Journal of Youth and Adolescence, 39*, 1387–1391.

Markey, C. N. (2014). *Smart people don't diet: How psychology, common sense, and the latest science can help you lose weight permanently.* New York: Da Capo Press.

Markey, C. N., & Markey, P. M. (2009). Correlates of young women's interest in obtaining cosmetic surgery. *Sex Roles, 61*, 158–166.

Markey, C. N., & Markey, P. M. (2010). A correlational and experimental examination of reality television viewing and interest in cosmetic surgery. *Body Image, 7*, 165–171.

Markey, C. N., & Markey, P. M. (2011). Body image. In. R. J. Levesque (Ed.), *Encyclopedia of adolescence* (pp. 310–320). New York: Springer.

Mayo Clinic. (2014). *Cosmetic surgery risks.* Retrieved from http://www.mayoclinic.org/tests-procedures/cosmetic-surgery/basics/risks/prc-20022389.

Muise, A., & Desmarais, S. (2010). Women's perceptions and use of anti-aging products. *Sex Roles, 63*, 126–137.

Park, L. E., Calogero, R. M., Harwin, M. J., & DiRaddo, A. M. (2009). Predicting interest in cosmetic surgery: Interactive effects of appearance-based rejection sensitivity and negative appearance comments. *Body Image, 6*, 186–193.

Pruzinsky, T., & Edgerton, M. T. (1990). *Body image change in cosmetic plastic surgery. Body images: Development, deviance and change.* New York: Guilford.

Sarwer, D. B. (1998). Re: Psychological characteristics of women who undergo single and multiple cosmetic surgeries. *Annals of Plastic Surgery, 40*, 309.

Sarwer, D. B. (2007). The psychological aspects of cosmetic breast augmentation. *Plastic and Reconstructive Surgery, 120*, 110S–117S.

Sarwer, D. B., Brown, G., & Evans, D. (2007). Cosmetic breast augmentation and suicide. *American Journal of Psychiatry, 164*, 1006–1013.

Sarwer, D. B., Cash, T. F., Magee, L., Williams, E. F., Thompson, J. K., Roehrig, M., . . . Romanofski, M. (2005). Female college students and cosmetic surgery: An investigation of experiences, attitudes, and body image. *Plastic and Reconstructive Surgery, 115*, 931–983.

Sarwer, D. B., Crerand, C. E., & Gibbons, L. M. (2007). Cosmetic surgery to enhance body shape. In J. K. Thompson & G. Cafri (Eds.), *The muscular ideal: Psychological, social, and medical perspectives* (pp. 183–198). Washington, DC: American Psychological Association.

Sarwer, D. B., Gibbons, L. M., Magee, L., Baker, J. L., Casas, L. A., Glat, P. M., . . . Young, V. L. (2005). A prospective, multi-site investigation of patient satisfaction and psychosocial status following cosmetic surgery. *Aesthetic Surgery Journal, 25,* 263–269.

Sarwer, D. B., LaRossa, D., Bartlett, S. P., Low, D. W., Bucky, L. P., & Whitaker, L. A. (2003). Body image concerns of breast augmentation. *Plastic Reconstructive Surgery, 112,* 83–90.

Sarwer, D. B., Wadden, T. A., Pertschuk, M. J., & Whitaker, L. A. (1998). Body image dissatisfaction and body dysmorphic disorder in 100 cosmetic surgery patients. *Plastic and Reconstructive Surgery, 101,* 1644–1649.

Schulz, J., Bowler, G., & Markey, C. N. (2014). *Preserving the positive: Body image and interest in cosmetic surgery among emerging and mid-life adults.* Manuscript in progress.

Sherry, S. B., Hewitt, P. L., Lee-Baggley, D. L., Flett, G. L., & Besser, A. (2004). Perfectionism and thoughts about having cosmetic surgery performed. *Journal of Applied Biobehavioral Research, 9,* 244–257.

Slevec, J., & Tiggemann, M. (2010). Attitudes toward cosmetic surgery in middle-aged women: Body image, aging, anxiety, and the media. *Psychology of Women Quarterly, 34,* 65–74.

Swami, V. (2007). *The missing arms of Venus de Milo: Reflections on the science of physical attractiveness.* Brighton, UK: Book Guild.

Swami, V. (2009). Body appreciation, media influence, and weight status predict consideration of cosmetic surgery among female undergraduates. *Body Image, 6,* 315–317.

Swami, V., Arteche, A., Chamorro-Premuzic, T., Furnham, A., Stieger, S., Haubner, T., & Voracek, M. (2008). Looking good: Factors affecting the likelihood of having cosmetic surgery. *European Journal of Plastic Surgery, 30,* 211–218.

Swami, V., Chamorro-Premuzic, T., Bridges, S., & Furnham, A. (2009). Acceptance of cosmetic surgery: Personality and individual difference predictors. *Body Image, 6,* 7–13.

Swami, V., & Furnham, A. (2008). *The psychology of physical attraction.* London: Routledge.

Swami, V., Hwang, C. S., & Jung, J. (2012). Factor structure and correlates of the acceptance of Cosmetic Surgery Scale among South Korean university students. *Aesthetic Surgery Journal, 32,* 220–229.

Swami, V., & Mammadova, A. (2012). Associations between consideration of cosmetic surgery, perfectionism dimensions, appearance schemas, relationship satisfaction, excessive reassurance-seeking, and love styles. *Individual Differences Research, 10,* 81–94.

Tam, K. P., Ng, H. K-S., Kim, Y-H., Yeung, V. W-L., & Cheung, F. Y-L. (2012). Attitudes toward cosmetic surgery patients: The role of culture and social contact. *Journal of Social Psychology, 152,* 458–479.

Tiggemann, M. (2004). Body image across the adult life span: Stability and change. *Body Image, 1*(1), 29–41

von Soest, T., Kvalem, I. L., Skolleborg, K. C., & Roald, H. E. (2006). Psychosocial factors predicting the motivation to undergo cosmetic surgery. *Plastic and Reconstructive Surgery, 117*(1), 51–62

Chapter 12

Women's Loss of Self through Antidepressants: The Depression Diagnosis as a Form of Social Control

Alisha Ali

I have come to know that my sadness is not a problem to be solved. It is my humanity.

Melissa Febos (2013, p. 31)

After several decades of research on depression, scientists have amassed a wealth of data that can inform our understanding of risk factors for depression and corresponding models of treatment. These data show us trends, averages, and the most likely outcomes of various treatment approaches that we can use to predict the course of depressive episodes for people in the general population. What these data do not show is the degree of suffering a woman diagnosed with depression experiences when the advice she is given and the treatments she is offered are grossly incompatible with her needs and with her own understanding of her distress.

This chapter explores the fundamental incompatibility between what is "known" by those who claim expertise in the field of depression and what is lived by women who are diagnosed as depressed. I approach this exploration as one who has a foot in two different worlds: I am a research psychologist who has spent decades studying depression in some of the world's most respected medical schools, psychiatric institutes, and psychology departments. At the same time, I am a feminist scholar who has taken as my life's work the goal of exposing the damage that occurs when women are diagnosed with depression and then led (or misled) on a path of treatment that, in my estimation, often results in more harm than help.

Most women who experience the constellation of symptoms known as depression do not seek professional help for those symptoms. However, those who choose to seek help do so based on a generally high level of trust in their care providers. I pose the question: To what extent is that trust justified? Well-trained, well-intentioned professionals (including psychiatrists, psychologists, counselors, and social workers) have been taught to follow models of conceptualization and treatment that reflect the current state-of-the-art scientific knowledge about depression. However, the processes involved in the creation and dissemination of this knowledge can be flawed and result in misleading information. I argue that women as empowered consumers must learn to trust their *own* knowledge about themselves and their bodies, and—equally important—they must educate themselves about the risks associated with the common treatments for depression.

My beliefs underlying this argument are as follows. The societal view of the depressed woman is of a "weak female" whose moods and thoughts are governed by her hormones and malfunctioning neurochemicals. A central notion in this view is that the depressed woman must be medicated and remain medicated in order to function properly in the service of society, her family, and her social image. Consideration of the assumptions underlying this belief can reveal the host of ways in which the idea of women's depression has been deliberately constructed to create a helpless and numbed population of lifelong consumers of antidepressants. This chapter will look critically at the machines of "progress" from which the current constructions of depression are derived. I also discuss the need to explore and understand the roots of sadness, the belief that women's anger and dissatisfaction must be chemically neutralized, and the medical industry's insistence on ignoring the broad range of adverse outcomes and placebo findings connected to antidepressants.

Depression has long been understood by feminist scholars to arise, at least in part, from traumatic experiences and from long-term life circumstances such as poverty, discrimination, subordinate status, devaluation, and marginalization. However, the dominant professional literature does not represent the reality that the experience of depression can be precipitated and exacerbated by women's treatment within the medical and psychiatric systems. This is an area of research and activism that has only recently begun to emerge, and—as we would expect—there has been tremendous backlash from the mainstream medical establishment in an attempt to counter these viewpoints. This backlash is bolstered by a large investment in advertising and outreach (often in the form of public awareness campaigns) created through collaboration between pharmaceutical companies and those identified as psychiatric experts. Their collaboration creates an uphill battle for those who seek to know and understand the real outcome data on antidepressants. Feminist scientists (Ali, Caplan, & Fagnant, 2010; Caplan, 1995; Caplan & Cosgrove, 2004; Cosgrove & Wheeler, 2013; Smith, 2010; Worell & Remer, 2002) hope that our work can begin to level the field in this battle by spreading key information about depression and alternatives to mainstream treatment to the public.

There is much that we know about depression—but much more that we *do not* know—including whether it is all that useful to use "depression" as a single label to cover the varied sorts of suffering and distress encountered by those who are deeply unhappy (Cohen & Jacobs, 2007). My goal here is to explore the complexities and biases involved in the generation of knowledge about depression. This understanding requires an openness to holding two seemingly inconsistent ideas in mind. One is the idea that mental health professionals care greatly about providing the best treatment possible to their clients and patients. The other is that this treatment often causes damage to women diagnosed as depressed. I ask you as a reader to be open to the possibility that what we call "excellent clinical care" is often harmful, and that the current scientific knowledge is often predicated on assumptions and motivations that are at odds with the needs of women who experience emotional distress.

DEFINING DEPRESSION: THE CONSTRUCTION OF DISTRESS AS ILLNESS

Depression has received a tremendous amount of attention in clinical, empirical, and popular writing for decades. It is rare to find an article in a women's magazine about life stress, juggling career and home, or lack of sleep that does not also discuss depression. This attention is welcomed by many depression experts because it is assumed to mark an increase in public awareness about the prevalence of depression in American society, especially among women. Indeed, the epidemiological and clinical data do show increasing rates of depression in the United States as well as globally. The World Health Organization now ranks depression as producing a higher burden than any other disease with respect to disability years among those in midlife. It is estimated that approximately 20% of Americans will experience depression at some point in their lives, a rate that has increased steadily over recent decades (CDC, 2010). Most researchers have reported that women are at far greater risk of depression than men are; estimates of women's depression risk are approximately twice that of men (Galambos, Leadbeater, & Barker, 2004; Kessler et al.,

2003). Although the gender difference in rates of depression is found across numerous clinical and epidemiological studies, the underlying cause of this difference remains a point of contentious debate among scholars, clinicians, and theorists in the mental health field and beyond.

According to the *Diagnostic and Statistical Manual of Mental Disorders* (*DSM-5*; American Psychiatric Association, 2013), depression is defined as extreme sadness and/or a loss of interest in life or activities that persists for two weeks or more. Additional symptoms include sleep disturbance, irritability, restlessness, feelings of guilt and worthlessness, changes in appetite, difficulty with concentration, and suicidal thoughts. Evidence from longitudinal research has repeatedly documented that most depressive episodes are precipitated by major life stress, either in the form of a single severe stressor or ongoing, chronic stressful life conditions (e.g., Ali, Oatley, & Toner, 2002; Astbury, 2010; Brown, 1998; Patten, 2003). Evidence has also shown that most people who experience depression once will go on to experience repeated episodes; data show recurrence of episodes in approximately 75% of those diagnosed with depression (Boland & Keller, 2009). The recurring nature of depression is taken by some as a sign that depression is primarily a biological disease; however, depression's chronicity may equally be attributed to the chronic nature of disempowering and threatening circumstances encountered on a regular basis by those at high risk (including such circumstances as violence, poverty, and homelessness).

To understand the diagnostic label of "depression," it is important to situate the notion of diagnosis itself in a broader context. In psychology and psychiatry, students are taught that diagnosis is an essential step in providing help for those who suffer from mental distress because a diagnosis confers on the suffering an agreed-upon definition and accepted language that can be used as a shorthand to capture a specific category of illness. It is generally assumed that this shorthand label does the following: (a) it represents a scientifically supported category that has been defined systematically through meticulous, thorough consideration of the available data concerning what the given category of mental illness is and how it is experienced by sufferers; (b) it is consistently and reliably applied in the same manner across all appropriate patients by all appropriately trained clinicians; and (c) the systematic, consistent application of diagnosis leads to far better treatment outcomes for sufferers than would be possible without the label.

Each of those three assumptions has been convincingly challenged by scientists and clinicians. For instance, psychologist Paula Caplan (1995), psychiatrist Daniel Carlat (2010), and sociologists Herb Kutchins and Stuart Kirk (1997) described the process used to create various diagnostic categories in the *DSM*. The categories were chosen and defined by a simplistic consensus process that involved relatively small groups of individuals, many of whom had known financial ties to pharmaceutical companies that produce drugs specifically for the conditions those groups supported for inclusion in the manual (Cosgrove, 2013). Regarding the reliability of the diagnoses themselves, data show that variables such as the gender of the patient influence which diagnoses are applied, even when clinicians are presented with identical symptom profiles for women and men (Belitsky et al., 1996; Hamilton, Rothbart, & Dawes, 1986). Moreover, as I discuss in the next section, the treatment outcomes that result from the diagnosis of depression are often not what patients expect or need.

Despite the biases and inconsistencies inherent in diagnosis, I have found that many women labeled as depressed are grateful for the label. There are understandable reasons for this. For one thing, it is assumed that a proper diagnosis is an essential first step on the path to successful treatment. In addition, an official diagnostic label confers an air of legitimacy on a woman's suffering and shows it to be a medical illness. It is of concern, of course, that a woman feels the need to turn to the medical establishment in order to convince family and friends—as well as herself—that her suffering is valid and real.

The search for the etiological factors underlying depression has in some crucial ways created two camps of researchers who study gender and depression. Simplistically stated, the first camp consists of researchers who aim to find a biological cause (i.e., a hormonal cause) for women's depression. These researchers cite evidence that women's rates of depression rise at precisely the times that women's hormones are changing (e.g., puberty, menopause, and the postpartum period) (Galambos et al., 2004; Hankin et al., 1998). The other camp consists of more sociologically oriented or feminist researchers who view women's depression as a result of social and contextual factors that put them at greater risk than men of becoming depressed. These researchers focus on empirical demonstrations of the causal effects of such factors as sexual assault, workplace harassment, and poverty, all of which are more likely to affect women than men.

Feminist researchers also point out that the phases of hormonal change identified as risk periods for depression are also times of social and interpersonal stress for girls and women. Such stressors occur commonly across diverse populations. During puberty, girls see their bodies becoming more womanlike, and the accompanying changes (including larger hips and curves) are often unwelcome. Similarly, menopause carries unwelcome bodily changes for many women (based partly on the cultural imperative that women must act and look young regardless of their age); menopause can also coincide with times of stress over one's physical health and the health of significant others, such as a spouse or parent. During the postpartum period as well, women undergo life changes that involve stressful adaptation to new responsibilities and pressures as well as insufficient sleep. Also, despite portrayals in the media and in the public consciousness of postpartum depression as caused solely by women's hormones (Martinez, Johnston-Robledo, Ulsh, & Chrisler, 2000), there are no consistent scientific data that demonstrate a direct association between postpartum depression and women's hormone levels (Whiffen, 2004, 2006). There is evidence, however, showing that new fathers also report elevated rates of depression (Ballard, Davis, Cullen, Mohan, & Dean, 1994; Vandell, Hyde, Plant, & Essex, 1997), which has prompted debate over the very nature of what is considered to be postpartum depression (Whiffen, 2004).

ANTIDEPRESSANTS: THE ANSWER OR THE PROBLEM?

My first job in psychology was as a volunteer research assistant on an inpatient adolescent ward at a prominent teaching hospital. I was an undergraduate psychology student, only a teenager myself and thus only a couple of years older than most of the teens living on the ward. I was struck by the many ways that these teens seemed to have *lived* and experienced a life outside of the confines of school and family, unlike the safe and relatively protected life I had known while in high school. However, now their movements were monitored and only a few were allowed any off-ward privileges unless accompanied by hospital staff. One girl on that ward—I'll call her Christa—at first spoke very little to me or to anyone else. However, as weeks passed, Christa began speaking more and more, mostly during the free time that the patients were allowed to spend in the art room. As she worked her fingers into large slabs of clay, she would talk about the struggles she had had in school and her sense that she was an outsider among her peers. She was eloquent and funny, and I was fascinated by her insights into the ways that all people attempt to maintain a feeling of individuality while also trying to be accepted and to belong. She knew she was different from other people, but she embraced that difference as something she valued in herself.

Gradually, I noticed changes in Christa: she became withdrawn and quiet and seemed increasingly lonely. She seemed to have lost the excitement she had shown in reflecting on people, feelings, and ideas. Shortly after these changes began, the nurses and psychiatrists reported in our weekly staff meeting that they were very encouraged by Christa's recent progress. They stated that she finally seemed to be "more subdued, less troubled, and more easily managed." The use of that phrase to describe a once-vibrant, insightful girl has stayed with me over the past decades and has informed my understanding of depression. The ward staff attributed the changes in Christa to the effectiveness of antidepressants. However, I wondered—and still continue to wonder—was it necessary for Christa to lose her vibrancy in order to become less "depressed"? Christa was the first of thousands of depressed girls and women whom I have encountered in my years as a psychologist, and I asked myself then a question similar to questions I have asked about others who have been medicated for depression: How did Christa come to unlearn what she had once deeply known about herself?

The number of women who take antidepressants has grown exponentially in recent decades in the United States. According to the Centers for Disease Control (2010), women are 2.5 times more likely than men to be prescribed antidepressants; 23% of women between the ages of 40 and 59 now take them. Although the likelihood of being on an antidepressant increases with the severity of diagnosed depression for both men and women, at the most severe levels, 40% of women, but only 20% of men, are on antidepressants. In addition, over one-third of women, but less than one-fifth of men, diagnosed with moderate depression take antidepressants. Overall, more than 1 in 10 Americans age 12 and older take antidepressants.

Despite the public's general trust in antidepressant medication, many researchers and clinicians have begun to write about their growing suspicions regarding the risks and benefits of these drugs. Carlat (2010) described such suspicions, not only in relation to antidepressants but also in relation to the very enterprise of psychiatric diagnosis and treatment. He described how psychiatry has shed its previous identity of providing talk therapy and instead now focuses on the chemical factors rather than the human factors in mental suffering. In addition to the dramatic shift in psychiatry toward prescribing rather than talking, there are also concerns that patients who are prescribed antidepressants are not given the opportunity to arrive at an informed decision about whether to start on antidepressants. Many health care providers who prescribe antidepressants to their patients are general practitioners with little specific training in psychiatry. Furthermore, many doctors and nurses receive ongoing "training" about psychiatric medications primarily from drug company representatives who are paid to increase the number of prescriptions written for their antidepressants and other drugs (Carlat, 2010). Also of concern is the fact that over two-thirds of all people in the United States who are taking antidepressants have not seen a mental health provider of any kind within the past year (CDC, 2010). Taken together, these facts illustrate that significant numbers of the U.S. population take these drugs regularly but are not supported in their decision to do so through knowledge about the drugs or their side effects.

Regarding "side effects," many researchers and clinicians have focused in recent years on the damaging effects of taking antidepressants, and several have noted that "side effects" is far too benign a term to use given the seriousness of the effects of these drugs. The model that has emerged from the data on the detrimental workings of antidepressants—known as the "disease-centered model" of drug action (Moncrieff & Cohen, 2006)—lays out the many ways in which antidepressants alter brain functions, which in turn creates cognitive and emotional impairment. Participants who have been asked to describe the effects of antidepressants in various studies (including participants given only a single dose) report feelings of sedation, slowing of motor functions, severe sleep disruption, dizziness, memory impairment, headaches, difficulties with sexual functioning, and extreme drowsiness (Chrisler & Caplan, 2002; Gartlehner et al., 2008; Healy, 2004; Knegtering, Eijck, & Huijsman, 1994; Mayers & Baldwin, 2005; Tranter, Healy, Cattell, & Healy, 2002; Wingen, Bothmer, Langer, & Ramarkers, 2005). Participants who take antidepressants also report feelings of flat affect, blunted emotional response, and a general feeling of not caring about things that are happening to themselves or to others in their lives (Moncrieff & Cohen, 2006).

Even worse is the series of scientific studies that demonstrate that taking antidepressants can itself lead to a severe, chronic, treatment-resistant form of depression known as *tardive dysphoria* (Fava, 1994). Antidepressant-induced depression has been found in research studies across various samples, including previously nondepressed patients who were given antidepressants for anxiety or panic disorder, patients who had initially been only mildly depressed but then took the antidepressant imipramine for long periods, and normal control research participants who were given antidepressants in study protocols (Aronson, 1989; Fava, Bernardi, Tomba, & Rafanelli, 2007; Fux, Taub, & Zohar, 1993; Healy, 2000). Tardive dysphoria is also thought to account in part for the common finding that patients who take antidepressants over the long term develop a tolerance to the drug and, therefore, experience more and more severe depression at higher and higher antidepressant doses (Sharma, 2001; Solomon, Leon, & Mueller, 2005).

Researchers have also identified a condition now officially known as *serotonin syndrome*, a syndrome induced by selective serotonin reuptake inhibitors (SSRIs) and other antidepressants. Also known as serotonin toxicity, this life-threatening condition is characterized by neuromuscular abnormalities, extreme hyperactivity, and damage to a range of mental faculties (Buckley, Dawson, & Isbister, 2014; Shruti & Liebelt, 2012). In a recently published report on the prevalence and course of serotonin syndrome, the team of authors (all toxicologists) stated the following:

> Serotonin syndrome is a potentially fatal and largely avoidable adverse drug reaction caused by serotonergic drugs. The steady increase in the use of such drugs means all doctors need to be aware of what drugs increase serotonin and how to promptly recognize the syndrome and determine if it is potentially life threatening. (Buckley et al., 2014, p. 348)

Most recently, evidence has come to light that suggests a link between antidepressant use—most commonly SSRIs (e.g., Prozac, Paxil, Zoloft, Celexa)—and suicide, primarily among individuals younger than age 25 (Mann et al., 2006). Pharmaceutical companies have invested greatly in countering these research claims (Whitaker, 2011), but the U.S. Food and Drug Administration (FDA) in 2004 began requiring manufacturers of antidepressants to include a black box warning to inform consumers of the risk of suicide in youths who take antidepressants (Newman, 2004). Furthermore, and of particular relevance to the high rates of antidepressant use among women, there is growing evidence that antidepressants— particularly SSRIs—cause birth defects. Studies have documented that babies born to antidepressant-using mothers are at a significantly increased risk of such birth defects as cardiovascular abnormalities, seizures, feeding difficulties, low birth weight, and respiratory distress (Diav-Citrin et al., 2008; Oberlander, Warburton, Misri, Aghajanian, & Hertzman, 2006; Suri et al., 2002). In their study of birth abnormalities with a sample of 2,191 women, Diav-Citrin and colleagues (2008) found that the only significant predictors of cardiovascular anomalies in newborns were when the expectant mother smoked 10 or more cigarettes per day or took antidepressants.

In addition to the wealth of evidence that shows the damage that antidepressants can do, Moncrieff and Cohen (2006) concluded from their systematic examination of available data on antidepressant use that "no evidence shows that antidepressants or any other drugs produce long-term elevation of mood or other effects that are particularly useful in treating depression" (p. 961). These numerous cautionary reports raise the question: Why do the public and many mental health professionals still favor the use of antidepressants? The answer lies largely in the fact that drug trials of antidepressants often represent a highly skewed and biased picture of the overall data collected on the effects of these drugs. One reason for this is the simple fact that studies that show positive and significant effects are more likely to be accepted for publication in a scientific journal than are studies that do not show significant results, partly because positive findings are considered more noteworthy than negative or insignificant findings.

However, there are large numbers of unpublished studies that show antidepressants to function no better than placebos in reducing depressive symptoms (Carlat, 2010; Kirsch, 2009). In a recent article in the *New England Journal of Medicine* (Turner, Matthews, Linardatos, Tell, & Rosenthall, 2008), psychiatrist Erick Turner and his colleagues reported on their examination of reviews of antidepressant trials by the FDA and compared those findings to the effects reported in published studies. They found that 94% of the published studies showed positive effects for antidepressant use, whereas only 51% of the overall FDA studies showed positive results for antidepressants.

Another more sinister reason for the misrepresentation of the effects of antidepressants in reports is the active control of information by pharmaceutical companies that have a clear interest in propagating the conception of antidepressants as helpful, not harmful. In his book *Anatomy of an Epidemic*, Whitaker (2010) reported on the numerous examples of editors of psychiatry journals who were also paid large sums from pharmaceutical companies to support prescriptions of their antidepressants. The concerns run even deeper than those conflicts. As Carlat (2010) stated:

> In order to provide prescribers with evidence to use their products, companies have brought their marketing departments front and center into the research business. When they have had trouble finding legitimate independent researchers to test treatments, they have designed and funded those tests themselves. When they haven't been able to fund academics to write up the results, they have hired ghost writers, and then pay academics to simply put their names on the articles. And when, heaven forbid, they have conducted studies that haven't shown their drugs to be effective, they have slipped the studies into file drawers, hoping that nobody would ever find out they were conducted. (p. 101)

Such cover-ups have contributed to the public's belief that antidepressants are the effective, safe solution to a problem that lies *within* the depressed person. The depressed woman is constructed as a psychologically defective being, governed by emotions that need to be controlled.

DEPRESSION DIAGNOSIS AND TREATMENT AS SOCIAL CONTROL

Mental health professionals and the public at large are led to believe that the diagnosis and treatment of depression are based firmly in scientific evidence and that drug treatment is the most effective and useful approach in helping a person to overcome depression. This widespread perception has shaped our very understanding of depression as an illness and has caused us to ignore the broader social implications of having such a large percentage of the U.S. female population on antidepressants of some kind. In conducting research in this area for nearly three decades—and interviewing hundreds of women diagnosed as depressed—I have witnessed a trend that worries me: Women on antidepressants, although they often report an improvement in self-destructive thoughts, frequently also report feelings of apathy and disconnection from the social world. This trend is disturbing because it highlights the role that antidepressants can play as a source of women's oppression.

Oppression can be viewed as the forces at play any time a group or groups of people are threatened in their ability to enact their fundamental human rights. Oppression often begins with an insidious process of marginalization, such as the case of sanctions against women's political participation at the turn of the past century when women were barred from taking part in activities (e.g., voting, running for office) that were considered out of their realm of interest and comprehension. So, how does psychiatric diagnosis relate to social oppression? Oppression is a form of social control that involves actively limiting the ability of an individual or group to fulfill their desired roles or activities in society. The process of psychiatric labeling (as in labeling a person as a "depressive" or as "bipolar") is a form of social control that is based on marginalization. This marginalization functions through a process that social-science scholars refer to as *othering*. Othering involves dehumanizing individuals by deeming them different from or "other than" the consensually accepted norm. In the process of othering, "different from" is equated with "worse than" or "less than." Othering also reinforces the power of those in privileged positions; the process of dehumanizing one group and privileging another is a key mechanism of social control. In the case of psychiatric diagnosis, this control is exerted by medical experts against those who are deemed mentally ill.

The treatment that follows the label of "depressed" essentially takes the depressed woman out of society in many cases—either through the disengaged, numbing effects of antidepressants or through hospitalization. The absence of these women from public life should be a cause of concern for a number of reasons. For one thing, being socially engaged and connected to those around us is a central element of selfhood for all of us, and no person should have to choose between that and psychological wellness. Second, it is not only women's sadness that is neutralized by antidepressants; anger is also often neutralized and replaced with apathy. I contend that many women who are the most prone to depression—those who are disadvantaged and disempowered—represent the very voices that are most needed for progressive social change in society. Theirs are the experiences and insights that must be told and spread widely so that the rest of society can learn the realities and effects of suffering economically, socially, and personally. Saving one woman from the possible aftermath of the depression diagnosis can represent a course of action that can lead to social change and mobilize others to fight against oppression. Therefore, finding alternatives to antidepressant treatment is not only necessary to help individual women, but it can also be a step toward invigorating social movements that help disenfranchised women and other oppressed groups.

FINDING ALTERNATIVES IN THE TREATMENT OF DEPRESSION

Given all of the disturbing evidence on the effects of antidepressants, how are we to make decisions about treatment options for ourselves or for a loved one who has been diagnosed with depression? One factor we must be aware of concerns the limits of aggregated scientific data when it comes to predicting outcomes for a single individual case. As scientists, we must collect data from sufficiently large numbers of research participants within any given study in order for the data to be considered valid. This is the requisite of attaining an adequate sample size: a certain number of participants is needed in order for scientists to feel confident that the data make sense and that the results are reliable and generalizable beyond that particular sample. This is partly why reports of single case studies are often considered by mental health researchers to be speculative. However, even intimate knowledge about the data on depression cannot ever tell us how a person diagnosed with depression will respond to any given treatment. So this is the challenge: If a person is suffering emotionally—unable to get out of bed, or even having suicidal thoughts—what is the best course of action?

The problem is that no amount of data collected from *other people* can truly tell a woman about herself. So the treatment decision is always essentially a gamble: We play the odds of predicting what might happen based on what we know. This means a given woman could be one of the people who can be helped—at least in the short-term—by taking antidepressants. However, it would be preferable first to consider options that do not carry with them a likelihood of altering a person's physical and mental health in detrimental ways. This preference has led practitioners and researchers to search for viable treatment alternatives that could help those who suffer from extreme sadness and emotional anguish.

One popular approach to help individuals diagnosed with depression is cognitive behavioral therapy (CBT). CBT can be used in individual or group therapy, and it can be used as therapist-facilitated self-help for individuals who cannot (or do not wish to) attend weekly therapy sessions (Coull & Morris, 2011). In CBT, the therapist works with the client to identify specific patterns of thought and behavior associated with the client's depression. For example, negative self-attributions can lead to negative mood states. Reframing such thoughts and trying new, more positive thought patterns can reduce the likelihood of feeling depressed. The helpful patterns of thoughts and behaviors eventually, with practice, become integrated into the client's daily life and transform her or his self-perceptions in a positive way. Some research has shown that CBT is more effective than antidepressant medication in helping people to recover from depression (Butler, Chapman, Forman, & Beck, 2006; Rohde et al., 2008).

A promising area of research is the use of CBT specifically to address insomnia. Insomnia is a key symptom of depression for many women, but it is also a factor that drives depression by keeping individuals from functioning in their day-to-day lives. Eliminating insomnia can be extremely useful in preventing full-blown depression for many women. Similarly, exercise—even very mild, nonstrenuous, regular exercise, such as walking or jogging—has been shown to be effective in reducing depression. Both of these alternatives are not only approaches that can be maintained over the long term without dangerous side effects, but they also carry other health benefits that can contribute to overall wellness.

My research team members and I have begun exploring other approaches that seem to hold possibilities for prevention of depression in high-risk groups. One approach is a model of antioppression advocacy (Ali, McFarlane, Hawkins, & Udo-Inyang, 2011) in which we support low-income and homeless women to engage in community activism regarding such issues as affordable housing and access to mental health care. In addition, in a recent study with women and men living below the poverty line, we found that participating in a poverty transition program that uses a microlending business model to support clients' entrepreneurial ventures produced reductions in depressive symptoms at rates comparable to many of the published rates for antidepressants (Ali, Hawkins, & Chambers, 2010).

Another promising alternative to mainstream approaches to depression is Dana Jack's model based on the theory of self-silencing (Jack, 1991; Jack & Ali, 2010), which posits that women's depression arises from a loss of voice and a progressive self-devaluation that stems from sociocultural pressures for women to be kind and giving and always please others. This devaluation leads to a loss of sense of self in which women place greater value on others and less and less value on themselves, thereby precipitating feelings of worthlessness that, in turn, lead to depression. There is evidence that self-silencing can be reduced through narrative and arts-based interventions that in turn could reduce depressive symptoms (Jack & Ali, 2010). A fruitful avenue for treatment alternatives is the use of this model to inform the development of interventions in clinical care and community settings to encourage girls and women to find and express their voices through group processes, creative arts therapies, and empowerment-based collective action (Worell & Remer, 2002).

CONCLUSION

The various alternatives discussed in this chapter demonstrate that innovative models can be generated if we look beyond the usual medical practice in conceptualizing and preventing depression. By enacting and empirically testing alternative approaches, we can arrive at a contextualized understanding of depression that is based on sound science and on the need for ethical care. Part of an ethical stance includes an active insistence that women must be provided adequate and accurate information about the risks of antidepressant medication before they start taking these drugs. Such education begins with the dissemination to health care providers—including general practitioners—of information about the full range of scientific evidence on risks and adverse effects. By partnering with scientists and editors of both professional journals and popular magazines, we can begin the process of revealing more of the truth that antidepressants are often not the most helpful solution to counteracting the widespread problem of women's unhappiness and despair. Moreover, alternative conceptualizations of women's emotional suffering can lead us to cast a critical gaze on the sociocultural problems that can precipitate such suffering, thereby contributing to social change rather than to social oppression.

REFERENCES

Ali, A., Caplan, P. J., & Fagnant, R. (2010). Gender stereotypes in diagnostic criteria. In J. C. Chrisler & D. R. McCreay (Eds.), *Handbook of gender research in psychology* (vol. 2, pp. 91–109). New York: Springer.

Ali, A., Hawkins, R. L., & Chambers, D. A. (2010). Recovery from depression among clients transitioning out of poverty. *American Journal of Orthopsychiatry, 80,* 26–33.

Ali, A., McFarlane, E., Hawkins, R., & Udo-Inyang, I. (2011). Social justice revisited: Psychological recolonization and the challenge of anti-oppression advocacy. *Race, Gender, and Class, 19,* 322–335.

Ali, A., Oatley, K., & Toner, B. B. (2002). Life stress, self-silencing, and domains of meaning in unipolar depression: An investigation of an outpatient sample of women. *Journal of Social and Clinical Psychology, 21,* 669–685.

American Psychiatric Association. (2013). *Diagnostic and statistical manual of mental disorders* (5th ed.). Washington, DC: Author.

Aronson, T. A. (1989). Treatment emergent depression with antidepressants in panic disorder. *Comprehensive Psychiatry, 30,* 267–271.

Astbury, J. (2010). The social causes of women's depression: A question of rights violated. In D. C. Jack & A. Ali (Eds.), *Silencing the self across cultures: Depression and gender in the social world* (pp. 19–46). New York: Oxford University Press.

Ballard, C. G., Davis, R., Cullen, P. C., Mohan, R. N., & Dean, C. (1994). Prevalence of postnatal psychiatric morbidity in mothers and fathers. *British Journal of Psychiatry, 164,* 782–788.

Belitsky, C. A., Toner, B. B., Ali, A., Yu, B., Osborne, S. L., & deRooy, E. (1996). Sex-role attitudes and clinical appraisal in psychiatry residents. *Canadian Journal of Psychiatry, 41,* 503–508.

Boland, R. J., & Keller, M. B. (2009). Course and outcome of depression. In I. H. Gotlib & C. L. Hammen (Eds.), *Handbook of depression* (pp. 23–43). New York: Guilford.

Brown, G. W. (1998). Genetic and population perspectives on life events and depression. *Social Psychiatry and Psychiatric Epidemiology, 33,* 363–372.

Buckley, N. A., Dawson, A. H., & Isbister, G. K. (2014). Serotonin syndrome. *British Medical Journal, 348*, 1–4.

Butler, A. C., Chapman, J. E., Forman, E. M., & Beck, A. T. (2006). The empirical status of cognitive-behavior therapy: A review of meta-analyses. *Clinical Psychology Review, 26*, 17–31.

Caplan, P. J. (1995). *They say you're crazy: How the world's most powerful psychiatrists decide who's normal.* Reading, MA: Addison-Wesley.

Caplan, P. J., & Cosgrove, L. (2004). Is this really necessary? In P. J. Caplan & L. Cosgrove (Eds.), *Bias in psychiatric diagnosis* (pp. xiii–xv). Lanham, MD: Jason Aronson.

Carlat, D. (2010). *Unhinged: The trouble with psychiatry—a doctor's revelation about a profession in crisis.* New York: Free Press.

Centers for Disease Control and Prevention (CDC). (2010). *Current depression among adults.* Retrieved from http://www.cdc.gov/mmwr/preview/mm wrhtml/mm5938a2.htm.

Chrisler J. C., & Caplan, P. J. (2002). The strange case of Dr. Jekyll and Ms. Hyde: How PMS became a cultural phenomenon and a psychiatric disorder. *Annual Review of Sex Research, 13*, 274–306.

Cohen, D., & Jacobs, D. H. (2007). Randomized controlled trials of antidepressants: Clinically and scientifically irrelevant. *Debates in Neuroscience, 1*, 44–54.

Cosgrove, L. (2013). Industry's colonization of psychiatry: Ethical and practical implications of financial conflicts of interest in the *DSM-5. Feminism & Psychology, 23*, 92–106.

Cosgrove, L., & Wheeler, E. E. (2013). Drug firms, the codification of diagnostic categories, and bias in clinical guidelines. *Journal of Law, Medicine and Ethics, 41*, 644–653.

Coull, G., & Morris, P. G. (2011). The clinical effectiveness of CBT-based self-help interventions for anxiety and depressive disorders: A systematic review. *Psychological Medicine, 41*, 2239–2252.

Diav-Citrin, O., Shechtman, S., Weinbaum, D., Wajnberg, R., Avgil, M., Di Gianantonio E., . . . Omoy, A. (2008). Paroxetine and fluoxetine in pregnancy: A prospective, multicenter, controlled observational study. *British Journal of Clinical Pharmacology, 66*, 695–705.

Fava, G. A. (1994). Do antidepressant and antianxiety drugs increase chronicity in affective disorders? *Psychotherapy and Psychosomatics, 61*(3–4), 125–131.

Fava, G. A., Bernardi, M., Tomba, E., & Rafanelli, C. (2007). Effects of gradual discontinuation of selective serotonin reuptake inhibitors in panic disorder with agoraphobia. *International Journal of Neuropsychopharmacology, 10*, 835–838.

Febos, M. (2013). Home. In S. Botton (Ed.), *Goodbye to all that* (pp. 19–31). Berkeley, CA: Seal Press.

Fux, M., Taub, M., & Zohar, J. (1993). Emergence of depressive symptoms during treatment for panic disorder with specific 5-hydroxytryptophan reuptake inhibitors. *Acta Psychiatrica Scandinavica, 88*, 235–237.

Galambos, N. L., Leadbeater, B. J., & Barker, E. T. (2004). Gender differences in and risk factors for depression in adolescence: A 4-year longitudinal study. *International Journal of Behavior Development, 28*, 16–25.

Gartlehner, G., Gaynes, B. N., Hansen, R. A., Thieda, P., DeVeaugh-Geiss, A., Krebs, E. E., . . . Lohr, K. N. (2008). Comparative benefits and harms of second-generation antidepressants. *Annals of Internal Medicine, 149*, 734–750.

Hamilton, S., Rothbart, M., & Dawes, R. M. (1986). Sex bias, diagnosis, and *DSM-III*. *Sex Roles, 15*, 279–284.

Hankin, B. L., Abramson, L. Y., Moffitt, T. E., McGee, R., Silva, P., & Angell, K. E. (1998). Development of depression from preadolescence to young adulthood: Emerging gender differences in a 10-year longitudinal study. *Journal of Abnormal Psychology, 107*, 128–140.

Healy, D. (2000). Emergence of antidepressant induced suicidality. *Primary Care Psychiatry, 6*, 23–28.

Healy, D. (2004). *Let them eat Prozac: The unhealthy relationship between the pharmaceutical industry and depression.* New York: New York University Press.

Jack, D. C. (1991). *Silencing the self: Women and depression.* Cambridge, MA: Harvard University Press.

Jack, D. C., & Ali, A. (2010). *Silencing the self across cultures: Depression and gender in the social world.* New York: Oxford University Press.

Kessler, R. C., Berlgund, P., Demler, O., Jin, R., Koretz, D., Merikangas, K. R., . . . Wang, P. S. (2003). The epidemiology of major depressive disorder: Results from the National Comorbidity Survey Replication (NCS-R). *Journal of the American Medical Association, 289*, 3095–4105.

Kirsch, I. (2009). *The emperor's new drugs: Exploding the antidepressant myth.* New York: Basic Books.

Knegtering, H., Eijck, M., & Huijsman, A. (1994). Effects of antidepressants on cognitive functioning of elderly: A review. *Drugs and Aging, 5*, 192–199.

Kutchins, H., & Kirk, S. A. (1997). *Making us crazy: DSM, the psychiatric bible, and the creating of mental disorders.* New York: Free Press.

Mann, J. J., Graham, E., Baldessarini, R. J., Beardslee, W. R., Fawcett, J. A., Goodwin, F. K., . . . Wagner, K. S. (2006). ACNP task force report on SSRIs and suicidal behavior in youth. *Neuropsychopharmacology, 31*, 473–492.

Martinez, R., Johnston-Robledo, I., Ulsh, H. M., & Chrisler, J. C. (2000). Singing "the baby blues": A content analysis of popular press articles about postpartum affective disturbances. *Women & Health, 31*, 37–56.

Mayers, A. G., & Baldwin, D. S. (2005). Antidepressants and their effect on sleep. *Human Psychopharmacology, 20*, 533–559.

Moncrieff, J., & Cohen, D. (2006). Do antidepressants cure or create abnormal brain states? *PLosMed, 3*, 961–965.

Newman, T. B. (2004). A black-box warning for antidepressants in children? *New England Journal of Medicine, 351*, 1595–1598.

Oberlander, T. F., Warburton, W., Misri, S., Aghajanian, J., & Hertzman, C. (2006). Neonatal outcomes after exposure to selective serotonin reuptake inhibitor antidepressants and maternal depression using population-based linked health data. *Archives of General Psychiatry, 63*, 898–906.

Patten, S. B. (2003). Recall bias and major depression lifetime prevalence. *Social Psychiatry and Psychiatric Epidemiology, 38*, 290–296.

Rohde, P., Silva, S. G., Tonev, S. T., Kennard, B. D., Vitello, B., Kratochvil, C. J., . . . March, J. S. (2008). Achievement and maintenance of sustained improvement during the treatment of adolescents with depression: Study continuation and maintenance therapy. *Archives of General Psychiatry, 65*, 447–455.

Sharma, V. (2001). Loss of response antidepressants and subsequent refractoriness: Diagnostic issues in a retrospective case series. *Journal of Affective Disorders, 64*, 99–106.

Shruti, K., & Liebelt, E. (2012). Recognizing serotonin toxicity in the pediatric emergency department. *Pediatric Emergency Care, 28*, 817–821.

Smith, L. (2010). *Psychology, poverty, and the end of social exclusion: Putting our practice to work*. New York: Teachers College Press.

Solomon, D., Leon, A. C., & Mueller, T. I. (2005). Tachyphylaxis in unipolar major depressive disorder. *Journal of Clinical Psychiatry, 66*, 283–290.

Suri, R., Altshuler, L., Helleman, G., Burt, V. K., Aquino, A., & Mintz, J. (2002). Effects of antenatal depression and antidepressant treatment on gestational age at birth and risk of preterm birth. *American Journal of Psychiatry, 164*, 1206–1213.

Tranter, R., Healy, H., Cattell, D., & Healy, D. (2002). Functional effects of agents differentially selective to noradrenergic or serotonergic systems. *Psychological Medicine, 32*, 517–524.

Turner, E. H., Matthews, A. M., Linardatos, E., Tell, R. A., & Rosenthall, R. (2008). Selective publication of antidepressant trials and its influence on apparent efficacy. *New England Journal of Medicine, 358*, 252–260.

Vandell, D. L., Hyde, J. S., Plant, E. A., & Essex, M. J. (1997). Fathers and "others" as infant-care providers: Predictors of parents' emotional well-being. *Merrill-Palmer Quarterly, 43*, 361–385.

Whiffen, V. E. (2004). Myths and mates in childbearing depression. *Women & Therapy, 27*(3–4), 151–164.

Whiffen, V. E. (2006). *A secret sadness*. Oakland, CA: New Harbinger.

Whitaker, R. (2011). *Anatomy of an epidemic: Magic bullets, psychiatric drugs, and the astonishing rise of mental illness in America*. New York: Broadway Books.

Wingen, M., Bothmer, J., Langer, S., & Ramarkers, J. G. (2005). Actual driving performance and psychomotor function in healthy subjects after acute and subchronic treatment with escitalopram, mirtazapine, and placebo: A crossover trial. *Journal of Clinical Psychiatry, 64*, 436–443.

Worell, J., & Remer, P. (2002). *Feminist perspectives in therapy: Empowering diverse women*. Hoboken, NJ: Wiley.

Chapter 13

Mourning Matters: Women and the Medicalization of Grief

Leeat Granek

In the last book of the dystopian trilogy by Margaret Atwood, the main character remarked, "There's the story, then there's the real story, then there's the story of how the story came to be told. Then there's what you leave out of the story. Which is part of the story too" (Atwood, 2013, p. 56). The way in which we understand our grief today is a compilation of layered stories, some explicit, some implicit, some visible, and some hidden, all of which affect the way we experience, understand, and engage with mourning. This chapter is an archaeological dig into the *gendered* narrative of medicalized grief in 21st-century Western industrialized countries. It is one story of many that can be told about grief, but it is an important story, and an important site for a dig, because gender, unlike other social identifiers, affects every aspect of our lives. This is particularly true in the context of expression of emotions such as grief.

I argue in this chapter that the recent historical trend to pathologize grief disproportionally affects women, as they tend to be overdiagnosed with bereavement-related disorders, such as *complicated grief* and *clinical depression*. I suggest that this overdiagnosis is a result of many individual and social factors that are situated in gender inequalities, such as diagnostic bias, social norms for expression of emotion by women and men, and social circumstances, such as poverty, that affect more women than men and that subsequently lead to worse mental (and physical) health outcomes for women.

Ultimately, however, I suggest that women's tendency to express their grief more explicitly and intensely than men do is not a new phenomenon and has historical precedent in a long lineage of women who were expected to carry the heavy load of grief for their families, their communities, and their countries. Although the expectation that women carry the emotional load of mourning for the collective through the expression of their affect has not changed, today, for the first time in recent history, women are being pathologized for doing this "job" too well.

I begin by describing the move toward the pathologization and medicalization of grief and the consequences such actions have on us as a society of mourners. I then review the social psychological literature on the gender differences in grieving followed by a detailed discussion of alternative explanations as to why this overdiagnosis has occurred. I conclude by offering some thoughts on the medicalization of women's grief and why a critical look at mourning matters in contemporary society.

THE PATHOLOGIZATION OF GRIEF

Medicalizing or psychologizing grief means, quite simply, turning what was once considered a normal human reaction to the loss of a loved one, or in some cases grief caused by other losses (e.g., a job, an opportunity), into a mental or medical disorder that necessitates psychological or medical intervention. Because I have written extensively about the pathologization of grief elsewhere, I refer readers to those publications for a thorough historical, cultural, and social account of the ways in which grief has become pathologized in the past century (Granek, 2008, 2010a, 2013a, 2013b). What is important to understand in the current context is that, today, especially in Western industrialized countries, grief is considered to be a psychological process that has a starting point, a middle point, and an end point. The task of grievers is to do their "grief work" and get back to the job of living full, productive lives as soon as possible. If the grievers are not able to "move on" "fast enough" or "well enough," it is their responsibility to seek professional help, which often takes the shape of a therapist or a prescription for medication.

What constitutes "well enough," "fast enough," or "moving on" when it comes to grief has become the domain of the mental health disciplines. In recent years, all grief has come to be understood as potentially pathological (Granek, 2010a), and some forms of grief are understood as a mental disorder that requires interventions, such as therapy or medications

(Forstmeier & Maercker, 2007; Horowitz, 2006; Prigerson & Jacobs, 2001; Prigerson et al., 2009; Shear & Frank, 2006; Shear et al., 2011). These forms of pathological grief have various names; some researchers call it *complicated grief*, others *prolonged grief disorder*, and still others *traumatic grief* (for a review of symptoms of pathological grief, please see Table 13.1). Some of these variants of grief have been proposed as diagnostic categories in the *Diagnostic and Statistical Manual of Mental Disorders* (*DSM*). Although these forms of pathological grief are not official diagnoses, they are often used to diagnose patients who see a therapist or physician for help with emotional difficulties after a major loss. The diagnosis is a justification and a rationale for the medicalization of grief.

Table 13.1 Proposed Criteria for Pathological Grief

Pathological Grief Proponents	Criteria	Cutoff from Time of Bereavement
Prigerson et al. (2009)	A) Chronic yearning, pining, and longing for the deceased; B) Five out of nine symptoms such as: confusion in one's role in life, difficulty accepting the loss, avoidance of reminders of the loss, inability to trust others, bitterness or anger about the loss, difficulty about moving on, numbness/detachment, feeling that life is unfulfilling, and feeling dazed or shocked about the loss; C) The symptom disturbance must cause marked and persistent dysfunction in the social and occupational domain; D) The symptom disturbance must last at least 6 months; E) The disturbance is not better accounted for by major depressive disorder, generalized anxiety disorder, or posttraumatic stress disorder. In order for complicated grief to be diagnosed, all criteria must be met.	6 months

(continued)

Table 13.1 Continued

| Shear and Colleagues (2011) | At least one of the following four symptoms should be present; the symptoms should cause significant distress or impairment in social, occupational, or other important areas of functioning; and should not be better accounted for as a culturally appropriate response:
1. Persistent intense yearning or longing for the person who has died;
2. Frequent intense feelings of loneliness;
3. Recurrent thoughts that it is unfair, meaningless, or unbearable to have lived when the loved one has died;
4. Preoccupying thoughts or images about the person who has died.

In addition, at least two of the following symptoms are present for at least a month:
1. Frequent troubling rumination about circumstances or consequences of the death (e.g., concerns about how or why the person died, worries about not being able to manage without their loved one, or thoughts of having let the deceased person down);
2. Recurrent feeling of disbelief or inability to accept the death, such as the person cannot believe or accept that the loved one is really gone;
3. Persistent feeling of being shocked, stunned, dazed, or emotionally numb since the death;
4. Recurrent feelings of anger or bitterness related to the death;
5. Persistent difficulty trusting or caring about other people or feeling intensely envious of others who have not experienced a similar loss; | 6 months |

6. Frequently experiencing pain or other symptoms that the deceased person had, or hearing the voice or seeing the deceased person;
7. Experiencing intense emotional or physiological reactivity to memories of the person who died or to reminders of the loss;
8. Change in behavior due to excessive avoidance or the opposite—excessive proximity seeking (e.g., refraining from going places, doing things, or having contact with things that are reminders of the loss; or feeling drawn to reminders of the person, such as wanting to see, touch, hear, or smell things).

| Horowitz et al. (1997) | Any three of the following seven symptoms with a severity that interferes with daily functioning:
Intrusive symptoms:
1. Unbidden memories or intrusive fantasies related to the lost relationship;
2. Strong spells or pangs of severe emotion related to the lost relationship;
3. Distressingly strong yearnings or wishes that the deceased were there;

Signs of avoidance and failure to adapt:
4. Feelings of being alone too much or personally empty;
5. Excessively staying away from people, places, or activities that remind the person of the deceased;
6. Unusual levels of sleep interference;
7. Loss of interest in work, social, caretaking, or recreational activities to a maladaptive degree. | 14 months |

A new edition of the *DSM* (American Psychiatric Association, 2013) was released recently and, although a variant of complicated grief was included in the appendix as a category that requires further study, it was not sanctioned as an official diagnosis. What was altered, however, was a diagnostic caveat called the "bereavement exclusion," which was once a part of the criteria for making a diagnosis of major depressive disorder, better known simply as clinical depression. Because the American Psychiatric Association (the publishers of the *DSM*) recognized for many years that grieving and clinical depression often look identical when it comes to symptom presentation, it included the bereavement exclusion, which stipulated that two months had to pass after a major loss before a diagnosis of clinical depression could be given to a bereaved person. What this means for contemporary mourners is that anyone showing sufficient symptoms of depression after a major loss can now be diagnosed with clinical depression by a psychiatrist, a psychologist, or a family doctor even if the symptoms are directly caused by bereavement-related losses (Granek, 2013a).

WHY DOES MOURNING MATTER? CONSEQUENCES OF MEDICALIZING GRIEF

What are the consequences of thinking of grief as a medical or psychological disorder? Why does it matter to people in Western industrialized countries today? In my view, there are three major impacts of pathologizing grief. The first is that it puts unrealistic expectations on people for how grief should look and feel and how long it should last. This, in turn, results in people feeling shame, embarrassment, or as somehow inadequate when they are not able to move on "fast enough" or "well enough." To understand grief as a disease, or a mental disorder, or to think of oneself as in a condition that requires psychological help can be embarrassing (Gilbert, 2006). The connotation of disease, disorder, or illness is contrary to the Western ideal of being healthy and taking care of oneself (Seale, 1998). Although it is now more acceptable to admit to having a mental illness than it has been in the past, there is still a stigma that makes people feel inadequate or marginalized if they are diagnosed with mental illness (Horwitz & Wakefield, 2007).

The psychological construction of grief as a diseased state has had a similar effect on contemporary mourners. For example, Gorer (1967) has suggested that death and, subsequently, mourning are treated with the same prudery as sexual impulses and sexual expression were a century ago. In his famous book *A Grief Observed*, C. S. Lewis (1961) wrote of his "embarrassing" state as a grieving man. Lewis described the reactions of those around him to his desire to speak of his dead wife. "The moment I try [to bring up his wife] there appears on their faces neither grief, nor

love, nor fear, nor pity, but the most fatal of all non-conductors, embarrassment. They look as if I were committing an indecency" (p. 21). He
went on to suggest that perhaps the bereaved "ought to be isolated in special settlements like lepers" (p. 23).

The leper analogy is a good one. In the Old Testament, people were said
to become afflicted with leprosy as a result of gossiping or speaking badly
about others behind their backs. The "punishment" was visceral and visible (Scherman, 1993). Lepers were separated and excommunicated for a
period of time, which caused a deep sense of embarrassment and shame
for those afflicted. When Lewis (1961) mused about being "isolated in a
special settlement like a leper" (p. 23) because of his bereavement, he was
talking not only about the interpersonal isolation that happens when one
is grieving, but also about the shamefulness, embarrassment, and sense of
personal responsibility he was made to feel due to his sadness.

The second major consequence of pathologizing grief is that, as is implied in the term *medicalization*, turning grief into pathology means treating it with medications, such as antidepressants, antianxiety drugs, or
sleeping pills (Granek, 2013a). The number of people who are given pharmaceuticals to treat their grief is difficult to measure. Even though (complicated, pathological, prolonged, or traumatic) grief is not an official
disorder, some psychiatrists and other physicians have explicitly prescribed medications to treat grief. Although these medical professionals
have focused specifically on grief treatment, countless other bereaved
people have been put on antidepressants and antianxiety medications to
treat major depressive disorder, which can be diagnosed in the grief
stricken as soon as *two weeks* after a major loss (American Psychiatric
Association, 2013). The diagnostic system is decontextual, which makes it
impossible to glean *why* people are depressed and prescribed antidepressants (Horwitz & Wakefield, 2007). It is highly plausible that many of the
millions of patients on antidepressants could have been suffering from
context-specific depression that may have had to do with a loss. Indeed
there is evidence to suggest that complicated grief and clinical depression
look similar in presentation, and it is all too easy to conflate them (Granek,
2013a, 2013b). This is an especially salient issue for women and is discussed in more detail in the next section of this chapter.

Finally, the third consequence has to do with the pressure on people to
seek psychological counseling to deal with their grief (Granek, 2013a, for
a review of the efficacy of grief counseling). There is absolutely nothing
wrong with seeking professional help when one is in distress, but the emphasis on "treating grief" in counseling sends two messages to the public.
The first is that grief is a disease that needs to be cured or treated (rather
than a part of life that one learns to live with and integrate into one's life),
and the second is that the proper place to deal with one's grief is in therapy, in private, and with professional help. As psychological counselors

take over this domain, grief becomes a more private event, and public tolerance, public places, and collective mourning rituals diminish in frequency and importance.

GENDER DIFFERENCES IN GRIEVING

Before I discuss how medicalizing grief impacts women specifically, it is necessary to review what the literature on grief claims when it comes to gender differences between women and men regarding grief. The literature is highly variable on this issue. There are studies that indicate no differences between men and women in regard to grief, and still others that indicate significant differences between them (see Stroebe, Stroebe, & Schut, 2001, for a review). Because the focus of this chapter is on the medicalization of grief and how it affects women, I focus my review of the research on the school of thought that there are gender differences in grieving so as to better articulate how and why the medicalization of grief may affect women more than men.

Women and Psychological Distress

The social psychological literature has robustly documented that women are diagnosed more frequently and with higher levels of anxiety, depression, and psychosomatic problems than are men (Davis, Matthews & Twamley, 1999; Nolen-Hoeksema, 2001; Nolen Hoeksema, Larson, & Grayson, 1999; Wool & Barsky, 1994). As such, the basic starting assumption in much of the psychological research on grief is that women have a higher risk of psychological problems, such as clinical depression, prior to experiencing bereavement (Stroebe et al., 2001).

Bereaved Women, Psychological Distress, and Complicated Grief

More specifically in the context of bereavement, there are some studies to indicate that women demonstrate more psychological symptoms in response to bereavement than men do (Chen et al., 1999; Gilbar & Ben-Zur, 2002; Neria et al., 2007; Summers, Zisook, Sciolla, Patterson, & Atkinson, 2004). One study of complicated grief in a representative population-based survey (n = 2,520) showed that women were more likely than men to be diagnosed with complicated grief and that women older than 61 showed a higher prevalence of complicated grief symptoms than did men of the same age (Kersting, Brähler, Glaesmer, & Wagner, 2011). Another study of 432 caregivers who cared for terminal cancer patients in a hospice ward showed that the scores for depression, anxiety, and complicated grief were significantly higher among the women than among the men (Chiu et al., 2011). Finally, Ayuso-Mateos and colleagues (2001) found a higher overall prevalence of depressive disorders in women than men in a European community sample.

WOMEN AND THE MEDICALIZATION OF GRIEF

How, and in what ways, does the medicalization of grief affect women as compared to men? First, as should be evident from the review above, some of the research indicates that women have more intense grieving reactions; report higher levels of anxiety, depression, and complicated grief reactions; and, in general, are more predisposed to psychological distress than are men. If these studies are accurate, then it is logical to conclude that women suffer from grief more than men do and therefore should be treated with medications and therapies to help them to cope with their grief. If this were the case, it might even make sense to conclude that the pathologization of grief could potentially help women to cope with their grieving because they would have more resources available to support them. Before making this assessment, however, it is also necessary to understand the social, clinical, cultural, and research contexts in which these studies took place.

As a critical health psychologist and scholar of grief, the questions that interest me when I read this literature go beyond looking at the studies themselves and extend to asking questions. Who conducted this research? What was the social context in which the research was conducted? What are some alternative explanations of the findings? Are the authors' conclusions valid based on the data they provided? What is the impact of these conclusions on women's lives? And, finally, what other social aspects could explain the higher incidence of distress among grieving women? In the following section, I offer some alterative ways of thinking of the bereavement literature in the context of the medicalization of grief and its impact on women.

Femininity, Masculinity, and Grieving

First, and most important, it is necessary to state that grieving is profoundly affected by the social context in which we live. Grief must always be understood, spoken about, and reflected on within its social, cultural, and historical contexts (Granek, 2010a). Gender is an important part of the social context, and, like all expressions of emotion, the expression of grief is a gendered phenomenon. Men and women are expected, encouraged, and permitted to grieve in gendered ways (Field, Hockey, & Small, 1997; Gerstel & Gallagher, 2001; Hallam, 1997; Littlewood, Cramer, Hoekstra, & Humphrey, 1991; Martin & Doka, 2000; Riches & Dawson, 1996; Schwab, 1996; Sidmore, 1999; Zinner, 2000). Women in general, and bereaved women in particular, tend to acknowledge and express their emotions openly (Derlega, Metts, Petronio, & Margulis, 1993; Notarious & Johnson, 1982; Pennebaker & Roberts, 1992; Shields, 1991). Men, on the other hand, tend to suppress their emotional response to grieving in order to appear stoic and "strong" (Pickard, 1994; Tudiver, Permaul-Woods, Hilditch, & Saini, 1995), which Pickard (1994) has called "bottling up" emotions. Moreover, the socially sanctioned ways that men can express their grief, besides stoicism, are through anger or by "acting out," such as engaging in risk-taking behavior or self-medicating with alcohol (Creighton, Oliffe, Butterwick, & Saewyc, 2013; Kilmartin, 2007). As Creighton and colleagues (2013) have noted, "because expressions of grief are deeply gendered, they are also powerfully policed and men who grieve in ways that do not embody socially assigned masculine practices (such as stoicism and rationality) can feel judged and alienated" (p. 35). In other words, whereas it is acceptable (and encouraged) for women to show outward expressions of grief, such as crying and talking about their emotions of grieving, yearning, and physical and emotional pain, for men the opposite is the case (Archer, 1999; Creighton et al., 2013; Martin & Doka, 2000; Versalle & McDowell, 2005). The split between how women and men are allowed to grieve and show their emotions has a profound effect on how grieving is viewed by the mental health community and the ways in which the distinctions between pathological grief and normal grief are made.

Diagnostic Bias in Clinical Settings and in Research Studies

Although few studies of grief exist in the diagnostic bias context, feminist researchers have pointed out that clinicians tend to overdiagnose women and underdiagnose men with depression (Stoppard, 2000). This is partly due to the normative gender roles described in the previous section where women tend to be more expressive of their emotions, and they are, therefore, more likely to meet criteria or to acknowledge experiencing emotional symptoms of disorders, such as complicated grief and clinical depression. The evidence also indicates that, as a result of their greater frequency of diagnoses of clinical depression, women are also the primary recipients of prescriptions for antidepressant medications (Aston, 1991; Olfson & Klerman, 1993). This does not mean that men experience less clinical depression or suffer less from grief-related distress, but simply that they express less overt emotion or acknowledge fewer "symptoms," and, therefore, they are diagnosed less frequently with these disorders.

For example, there is research to indicate that men may be as depressed as women but report less depressive symptomatology as listed in the *DSM* criteria (Meshot & Leitner, 1992; Stoppard, 2000). In the context of bereavement, a number of studies have indicated that men's bereavement distress may be more likely to be expressed in alcoholism or anger, whereas women may be more likely to show typical depressive symptoms (Cramer,

1993; Stroebe & Stroebe, 1987; Williams, Takeuchi, & Adair, 1992). Research on general distress in mothers and fathers has shown that the current techniques used by clinicians to assess psychosocial distress and to elicit emotional concerns are more conducive to capturing mothers' than fathers' distress (Chesler & Parry, 2001; Goodman, 2004). What these studies indicate is that, in the clinical context, women and men may be equally distressed over a major loss, but women report more symptoms of grief-related distress, and are, therefore, more likely than men to be formally diagnosed with disorders, such as clinical depression and complicated grief.

A similar diagnostic bias can be found in the research context. On the whole, women participate in research more than men do (Chesler & Parry, 2001; Polit & Beck, 2008). Some research has indicated that data collection via interview methods is more conducive to women's than to men's preferred styles of communication (Macdonald, Chilibeck, Affleck, & Cadell, 2010; Rochlen, Land, & Wong, 2004).

This is an especially salient issue in the bereavement context where speaking about one's grief may be particularly difficult for men. One study showed that widowed men who refused bereavement interviews (but who filled out surveys sent in the mail) were significantly more depressed than those who accepted the invitation to do the interview, whereas the opposite pattern was found for women (Stroebe & Stroebe, 1989). In other words, the more distressed the men were, the less likely they were to participate in the research, whereas the more distressed women were, the more likely they were to participate.

As with the clinical context, these patterns of participation in research significantly skew our knowledge about how frequently and intensely distressed men are as compared to women in the bereavement context. The fact that women are more likely to participate in research and more likely to talk about and openly acknowledge their distress does not mean that they are necessarily more distressed or suffering more from grief than are men. Moreover, the finding that the most distressed women are also the most likely to participate in bereavement research, whereas the opposite is true for men, implies that a large swath of the bereavement literature may be based on extreme cases of highly distressed women and highly functioning men.

Leaving Out the (Gendered) Social Economic Context

Few bereavement studies have examined the socioeconomic conditions of their participants, but some research has indicated that those who are living in low-income circumstances are more likely than higher-income people to suffer from grief-related disorders. Kersting and colleagues (2011) studied complicated grief (CG) in a representative population-based survey (n = 2,520) and found that women were more likely to be diagnosed with CG and that the prevalence rate of the disorder was 13% among low-income participants, as compared to 3% to 5% among higher-income participants. This indicates that socioeconomic status is a significant factor in postbereavement distress. Widowhood also increases economic hardship (Lillard & Waite, 1995; Stimpson, Kuo, Ray, Raji, & Peek, 2007; Utz, 2006), which affects psychological well-being. Women are especially likely to suffer from economic strains when widowed (Lee, Willetts, & Seccombe, 1998), which leads some to live in poverty after a major loss.

The American Psychological Association has characterized poverty as the "pathway to depression" for women (Mazure, Keita, & Blehar, 2002). Adults living in poverty are twice as likely to experience major depression as adults who are not poor, and women are three times more likely than men are to live in poverty (Mazure et al., 2002; Stoppard, 2000). Poverty, given its relation to clinical depression, may predispose women to more difficulties when bereaved, particularly if they have become unexpectedly widowed and were dependent on their spouses' income to meet their basic needs.

Single mothers are more likely to experience significant social and economic disadvantage than are mothers in two-parent families (Holden & Smock, 1991; Lipman, Offord, & Boyle, 1997; McQuillan, 1990). Moreover, single mothers must balance the strains of work and family life while sometimes living on the margins of poverty (Avison, 1995), which makes coping with grief particularly challenging. Low-income adults have higher rates of morbidity, disability, mortality, psychological distress, and mental disorders than do their peers with a higher socioeconomic status (Hayward, Crimmins, Miles, & Yang, 2000; House, Lantz, & Herd, 2005; Mirowsky & Ross, 2003a, 2003b; Wilkinson & Pickett, 2009). Chronic stress and hardships, such as poor housing, being unable to meet basic needs, lower social status, and being more socially secluded or isolated, lead to poorer health outcomes (Wilkinson & Pickett, 2009). All of these contextual financial and social factors disproportionately affect women and may explain the imbalance in diagnoses of complicated grief and bereavement-related depression in women as compared to men.

WOMEN AND THE HEAVY LOAD OF GRIEF

> Both men and women weep for their dead, [but] it is women who tend to weep longer, louder, and it is they who are thought to communicate directly with the dead through their wailing songs.
>
> Gilbert, 2006, p. 30, paraphrasing Holst-Warhaft, 2000

The review of the psychological literature on gender differences in grieving and the overdiagnosis of women with psychological distress as a result of their expressed grief is the modern equivalent of a very old sociocultural story. Women have historically been charged with holding, expressing, and containing the collective grief for their families, for their communities, and for their countries. Perhaps for the first time in history, they are now being pathologized for doing their job too well.

Historically, in Europe and the Middle East, professional mourners, who were always women, were hired to keen, to beat their breasts, to weep loudly and dramatically, to tear their hair out at funerals, and to lament expressively at the grave or bedside. Holst-Warhaft (2000) described such a scene as follows:

> In rural villages of Greece, Romania, Bulgaria, and many parts of the developing world, the scene is repeated with minor variations. A man lies dying. The female relatives gather around this beside. When he has taken his last breath, they close his eyes and begin to wail and sob. A woman or group of older women begin to transform their weeping into a song . . . the women may beat their breasts, tear their hair in gestures of mourning so ancient that we recognize them from Egyptian hieroglyphs and ancient Greek vases. (p. 30)

To this day, the practice of hiring professional female lamenters continues in many parts of the world (Host-Warhaft, 2000).

Similarly, in the 19th century, women (but not men) wore mourning clothing, such as black dresses and mourning jewelry (e.g., the deceased's hair was made into a locket or a broach) in public and private spaces for a year or even years after a death. This practice served to display their grief openly and visibly to those around them. Women were particularly involved in grieving rituals, such as postmortem photographs, writing extensive and labored condolence letters on mourning stationery, and participating in condolence calls in the community to comfort the bereaved (Tobin & Goggin, 2013). As Tobin and Goggin (2013) noted:

> Historically, women in many cultures have had a central role in crafting objects to commemorate the dead, such as weaving shrouds, creating mourning clothes, crafting death masks, designing grave markers, stitching memorial samplers, creating hair jewellery, to name but a scant few. Women's engagement with the material culture of death goes well beyond traditional forms of mourning and commemoration to include practices that involve handling dead bodies, with sculptresses making death masks and wax effigies. (p. 4)

In contemporary Western industrialized countries, we no longer have many of the expressive grieving rituals in which women in the past engaged, or, as I suggested earlier in this chapter, many public places where it is acceptable to express, talk about, and experience our grief. As has historically been the case, however, women continue to carry the emotional load of grieving for the collective in contemporary society as is evidenced by their tendency to express their grief symptoms more openly than men do. Indeed, historically the female lamenters described earlier were charged with going temporarily "mad" in the wake of loss in order to symbolically keep their community in order. As temporary insanity was an accepted part of the cultural and societal grieving process, the lamenter's role was to perform this grief-stricken madness publically so that those around her could remain sane (Holst-Warhaft, 2000). This was an acceptable, expected, and encouraged mourning ritual where women played a significant public role. Thus, whereas in the past the expression of grieving by women was expected, required, and even socially and professionally sanctioned, today these very same expressions of grief often result in a diagnosis of complicated grief or bereavement-related clinical depression.

MOURNING MATTERS: LIVING WITH GRIEF AS AN ALTERNATIVE TO MEDICALIZING

I began this chapter by noting that there are many stories one could tell about grief. Although I am a self-proclaimed feminist in my scholarship and in my personal life, and although I have always intuitively known, and even experienced, my own personal grief in gendered ways (Granek, 2010b), this is the first time I have refracted the scholarly light on grief to look at how gender plays an important role in determining the types of stories we can tell about grief. In my previous work, I argued that mourning matters because the types of stories we have about grief affect how we experience ourselves, and our losses, but, as should be evident from this chapter, some stories have particular repercussions for women.

The dominant narrative about grieving in the past 150 years has been one of pathologization and medicalization (Granek, 2010a, 2013a). For women in particular, there is a danger of excessive medicalization when it comes to their grief. Women are more vulnerable to these diagnoses for a number of social and cultural reasons that have to do with the inequalities between the genders, as outlined earlier in this chapter. For all of us, however—women and men alike—this medicalized story has consequences for our personhood.

Thinking of grief as a pathology diminishes the range of what is considered acceptable human emotion. It puts arbitrary limits on how long our grief can last, how intensely we can feel it, and the modes by which we can express our mourning. It claims that the totally normal response to feeling intense sadness over a major loss is a disorder that needs to be eradicated and treated with medication and with therapy in private and as quickly as possible. It means that the bereaved are afforded less time, less compassion, and less public space to mourn their losses. It results in mourners feeling shame and embarrassment over their sadness, and, perhaps most distressingly, it curbs our ability to grieve all of our losses—those that come from death, but also from divorce, from unemployment, from incarceration, from violence, from loss of a dream or a hope, and all the other infinite painful losses that define our humanity.

REFERENCES

American Psychiatric Association. (2013). *Diagnostic and statistical manual of mental disorders* (5th ed.). Arlington, VA: Author.

Archer, J. (1999). *The nature of grief: The evolution and psychology of reactions to loss.* New York: Oxford University Press.

Aston, H. (1991). Psychotropic-drug prescribing for women. *British Journal of Psychiatry, 158,* 30–35.

Atwood, M. (2013). *MaddAddam.* New York: Nan A Talese Publishers.

Avison, W. R. (1995). Roles and resources: The effects of family structure and employment on women's psychological resources and psychological distress. *Research in Community and Mental Health, 8,* 233–256.

Ayuso-Mateos, J. L., Vázquez-Barquero, J. L., Dowrick, C., Lehtinen, V., Dalgard, O. S., Casey, P., . . . & Wilkinson, G. (2001). Depressive disorders in Europe: Prevalence figures from the ODIN study. *British Journal of Psychiatry, 179,* 308–316.

Chen, J. H., Bierhals, A. J., Prigerson, H. G., Kasl, S. V., Mazure, C. M., & Jacobs, S. (1999). Gender differences in the effects of bereavement-related psychological distress in health outcomes. *Psychological Medicine, 29,* 367–380.

Chesler, M. A., & Parry, C. (2001). Gender roles and/or styles in crisis: An integrative analysis of the experiences of fathers of children with cancer. *Qualitative Health Research, 11,* 363–384.

Chiu, Y. W., Yin, S. M., Hsieh, H. Y., Wu, W. C., Chuang, H. Y., & Huang, C. T. (2011). Bereaved females are more likely to suffer from mood problems even if they do not meet the criteria for prolonged grief. *Psycho-Oncology, 20,* 1061–1068.

Cramer, D. (1993). Living alone, marital status, gender, and health. *Journal of Community & Applied Social Psychology, 3*(1), 1–15.

Creighton, G., Oliffe, J. L., Butterwick, S., & Saewyc, E. (2013). After the death of a friend: Young men's grief and masculine identities. *Social Science & Medicine, 84,* 35–43.

Davis, M. C., Matthews, K. A., & Twamley, E. W. (1999). Is life more difficult on Mars or Venus? A meta-analytic review of sex differences in major and minor life events. *Annals of Behavioral Medicine, 21,* 83–97.

Derlega, V. J., Metts, S., Petronio, S., & Margulis, S. T. (1993). *Self-disclosure.* Newbury Park, CA: Sage.

Field, D., Hockey, J. L., & Small, N. (Eds.). (1997). *Death, gender, and ethnicity*. London: Psychology Press.

Forstmeier, S., & Maercker, A. (2007). Comparison of two diagnostic systems for complicated grief. *Journal of Affective Disorders, 99*, 203–211.

Gerstel, N., & Gallagher, S. K. (2001). Men's caregiving, gender, and the contingent character of care. *Gender & Society, 15*, 197–217.

Gilbar, O., & Ben-Zur, H. (2002). Bereavement of spouse caregivers of cancer patients. *American Journal of Orthopsychiatry, 72*, 422–432.

Gilbert, S. (2006*). Death's door: Modern dying and the ways we grieve*. New York: Norton.

Goodman, J. H. (2004). Paternal postpartum depression, its relationship to maternal postpartum depression, and implications for family health. *Journal of Advanced Nursing, 45*(1), 26–35.

Gorer, G. (1967). *Death, grief, and mourning*. Garden City, NY: Doubleday.

Granek, L. (2008). *Bottled tears: The pathologization, psychologization, and privatization of grief*. Unpublished doctoral dissertation, York University.

Granek, L. (2010a). Grief as pathology: The evolution of grief theory in psychology from Freud to the present. *History of Psychology, 13*, 46–73.

Granek, L. (2010b). "The cracks are where the light shines in": Grief in the classroom. *Feminist Teacher, 20*(1), 42–49.

Granek, L. (2013a).The complications of grief: The battle to define modern mourning. In E. Miller (Ed.), *Stories of complicated grief: A critical anthology* (pp. 30–53). Washington, DC: NASW Press.

Granek, L. (2013b). Disciplinary wounds: Has grief become the identified patient for a field gone awry? *Journal of Loss and Trauma, 18*, 275–288.

Hallam, E. (1997). Death and the transformation of gender in image and text. In D. Field, J. Hockey, & M. Small (Eds.), *Death, gender and ethnicity* (pp. 108–123). London: Routledge.

Hayward, M. D., Crimmins, E. M., Miles, T. P., & Yang, Y. (2000). The significance of socioeconomic status in explaining the racial gap in chronic health conditions. *American Sociological Review, 65*, 910–930.

Holden, K. C., & Smock, P. M. (1991). The economic costs of marital dissolution: Why do women bear a disproportionate cost? *Annual Review of Sociology, 17*, 51–78.

Holst-Warhaft, G. (2000). *The cue for passion: Grief and its political uses*. Cambridge, MA: Harvard University Press.

Horowitz, M. (2006). Meditating on complicated grief disorder as a diagnosis. *Omega-Journal of Death and Dying, 52*(1), 87–89.

Horowitz, M. J., Siegel, B., Holen, A., Bonanno, G. A., Milbrath, C., & Stinson, C. H. (1997). Diagnostic criteria for complicated grief disorder. *American Journal of Psychiatry, 154*, 904–910.

Horwitz, A. V., & Wakefield, J. C. (2007). *The loss of sadness: How psychiatry transformed normal sorrow into depressive disorder*. New York: Oxford University Press.

House, J. S., Lantz, P. M., & Herd, P. (2005). Continuity and change in the social stratification of aging and health over the life course: Evidence from a nationally representative longitudinal study from 1986 to 2001/2002. *Journals of Gerontology: Series B, 60,* 15–26.

Kersting, A., Brähler, E., Glaesmer, H., & Wagner, B. (2011). Prevalence of complicated grief in a representative population-based sample. *Journal of Affective Disorders, 131,* 339–343.

Kilmartin, C. T. (2007). *The masculine self.* Cornwall-on-Hudson, NY: Sloan.

Lee, G. R., Willetts, M. C., & Seccombe, K. (1998). Widowhood and depression gender differences. *Research on Aging, 20*(5), 611–630.

Lewis, C. S. (1961). *A grief observed.* San Francisco, CA: HarperCollins.

Lillard, L. A., & Waite, L. J. (1995). 'Til death do us part: Marital disruption and mortality. *American Journal of Sociology, 100,* 1131–1156.

Lipman, E. L., Offord, D. R., & Boyle, M. H. (1997). Single mothers in Ontario: Sociodemographic, physical, and mental health characteristics. *Canadian Medical Association Journal, 156,* 639–645.

Littlewood, J. L., Cramer, D., Hoekstra, J., & Humphrey, G. B. (1991). Gender differences in parental coping following their child's death. *British Journal of Guidance and Counselling, 19,* 139–148.

Macdonald, M. E., Chilibeck, G., Affleck, W., & Cadell, S. (2010). Gender imbalance in pediatric palliative care research samples. *Palliative Medicine, 24,* 435–444.

Martin, T., & Doka, K. J. (2000). *Men don't cry, women do: Transcending gender stereotypes of grief.* Philadelphia, PA: Brunner Mazel.

Mazure, C., Keita, G., & Blehar, M. (2002). *Summit on women and depression: Proceedings and recommendations.* Washington, DC: American Psychological Association.

McQuillan, K. (1990). Family change and family income in Ontario. In L. C. Johnson & D. Barnhorst (Eds.), *Children, families, and public policy in the '90s* (pp. 153–174). Toronto: Thompson Educational.

Meshot, C. M., & Leitner, L. M. (1992). Adolescent mourning and parental death. *Omega-Journal of Death and Dying, 26,* 287–299.

Mirowsky, J., & Ross, C. (2003a). *Education, social status, and health.* New York: Aldine de Gruyter.

Mirowsky, J., & Ross, C. (2003b). *Social causes of psychological distress* (2nd ed.). New York: Aldine de Gruyter.

Neria, Y., Gross, R., Litz, B., Maguen, S., Insel, B., Seirmarco, G., . . . & Marshall, R. D. (2007). Prevalence and psychological correlates of complicated grief among bereaved adults 2.5–3.5 years after September 11th attacks. *Journal of Traumatic Stress, 20,* 251–262.

Nolen-Hoeksema, S. (2001). Gender differences in depression. *Current Directions in Psychological Science, 10,* 173–176.

Nolen-Hoeksema, S., Larson, J., & Grayson, C. (1999). Explaining the gender difference in depressive symptoms. *Journal of Personality and Social Psychology, 77,* 1061.

Notarious, C., & Johnson, J. (1982). Emotional expression in husbands and wives. *Journal of Marriage and the Family, 44*, 483–489.

Olfson, M. D., & Klerman, G. L. (1993). Trends in prescription of antidepressant by office-based psychiatrists. *American Journal of Psychiatry, 150*, 571–577.

Pennebaker, J. W., & Roberts, T. A. (1992). Toward a his and hers theory of emotion: Gender differences in visceral perception. *Journal of Social and Clinical Psychology, 11*, 199–212.

Pickard, S. (1994). Life after a death: The experience of bereavement in South Wales. *Ageing and Society, 14*, 191–217.

Polit, D. F., & Beck, C. T. (2008). Is there gender bias in nursing research? *Research in Nursing & Health, 31*, 417–427.

Prigerson, H. G., Horowitz, M. J., Jacobs, S. C., Parkes, C. M., Aslan, M., & Goodkin, K., & Maciejewski, P. K. (2009). Prolonged grief disorder: Psychometric validation of criteria proposed for *DSM-V* and *ICD-11*. *PLoS Medicine, 6*(8), e1000121.

Prigerson, H. G., & Jacobs, S. C. (2001). *Traumatic grief as a distinct disorder: A rationale, consensus criteria, and a preliminary empirical test*. Washington, DC: American Psychological Association.

Riches, G., & Dawson, P. (1996). "An intimate loneliness": Evaluating the impact of a child's death on parental self-identity and marital relationships. *Journal of Family Therapy, 18*(1), 1–22.

Rochlen, A. B., Land, L. N., & Wong, Y. J. (2004). Male restrictive emotionality and evaluations of online versus face-to-face counseling. *Psychology of Men & Masculinity, 5*, 190–200.

Scherman, N. (Ed.). (1993). *Stone Chumash. The Torah*. New York: Mesorah Publications.

Schwab, R. (1996). Gender differences in parental grief. *Death Studies, 20*, 103–113.

Seale, C. (1998). *Constructing death: The sociology of dying and bereavement*. Cambridge: Cambridge University Press.

Shear, K., & Frank, E. (2006). *Treatment of complicated grief: Integrating cognitive-behavioral methods with other treatment approaches*. New York: Guilford.

Shear, M. K., Simon, N., Wall, M., Zisook, S., Neimeyer, R., Duan, N., . . . Keshaviah, A. (2011). Complicated grief and related bereavement issues for *DSM-5*. *Depression and Anxiety, 28*, 103–117.

Shields, S. A. (1991). Gender in the psychology of emotion: A selective research review. In K. T. Strongman (Ed.), *International review of studies on emotion* (Vol. 1, pp. 227–245). Chichester, UK: Wiley.

Sidmore, K. V. (1999). Parental bereavement: Levels of grief as affected by gender issues. *Omega-Journal of Death and Dying, 40*, 351–374.

Stimpson, J. P., Kuo, Y. F., Ray, L. A., Raji, M. A., & Peek, M. K. (2007). Risk of mortality related to widowhood in older Mexican Americans. *Annals of Epidemiology, 17*, 313–319.

Stoppard, J. (2000). *Understanding depression: Feminist social constructionist approaches*. London: Routledge.

Stroebe, M., Stroebe, W., & Schut, H. (2001). Gender differences in adjustment to bereavement: An empirical and theoretical review. *Review of General Psychology, 5*, 62–83.

Stroebe, M. S., & Stroebe, W. (1989). Who participates in bereavement research? A review and empirical study. *Omega-Journal of Death and Dying, 20*, 1–29.

Stroebe, W., & Stroebe, M. (1987). *Bereavement and health*. New York: Cambridge University Press.

Summers, J., Zisook, S., Sciolla, A. D., Patterson, T., & Atkinson, J. H. (2004). Gender, AIDS, and bereavement: A comparison of women and men living with HIV. *Death Studies, 28*, 225–241.

Tobin, B., & Goggin, M. (2013). *Women and the material culture of death*. Surrey, UK: Ashgate.

Tudiver, F., Permaul-Woods, J. A., Hilditch, J., Harmina, J., & Saini, S. (1995). Do widowers use the health care system differently? *Canadian Family Physician, 41*, 392–400.

Utz, R. L. (2006). Economic and practical adjustments to late life spousal loss. In D. S. Carr, R. M. Nesse, & C. B. Wortman (Eds.), *Spousal bereavement in late life* (pp. 167–192). New York: Springer.

Versalle, A., & McDowell, E. E. (2005). The attitudes of men and women concerning gender differences in grief. *Omega-Journal of Death and Dying, 50*, 53–67.

Wilkinson, R., & Pickett, K. (2009). *The spirit level: Why more equal societies almost always do better*. New York: Bloomsbury Press.

Williams, D. R., Takeuchi, D. T., & Adair, R. K. (1992). Marital status and psychiatric disorders among Blacks and Whites. *Journal of Health and Social Behavior, 33*, 140–157.

Wool, C. A., & Barsky, A. J. (1994). Do women somaticize more than men? Gender differences in somatization. *Psychosomatics, 35*, 445–452.

Zinner, E. S. (2000). Being a man about it: The marginalization of men in grief. *Illness, Crisis, & Loss, 8*, 181–188.

Index

Abramson, J., 2, 4–7
Adams, T. D., 209
adoption, 45, 53
Affordable Care Act, 68
age, 3, 6, 134–135, 227; media messages about, 226
Ahlberg, C. E., 27
Ailshire, J. A., 205
Ali, Alisha, 12, 239–252
Almeling, R., 46, 51, 206
American Congress of Obstetricians and Gynecologists, 22, 62, 79
American Psychiatric Association, 79, 262
American Psychological Association, 268
American Society for Metabolic and Bariatric Surgery, 208
American Society for Reproductive Medicine (ASRM), 40, 46, 48, 50–51; Ethics Committee, 46; Practice Committee for Assisted Reproductive Technology, 48
American Society of Plastic Surgeons, 221

Amy, N. K., 188
Anatomy of an Epidemic, 248
Andrist, L. C., 65, 69–70
anemia, 63, 67
aneuploidy conditions, 48–49
anorexia nervosa, xiv, 169
anti-depressants, 239–252; side effects, 245–247
anxiety, 208, 264
Aphramor, L., 187, 193
Arias, R. D., 65, 70
assisted reproductive technologies (ARTs), 38–39, 42, 44
Association for Reproductive Health Professionals (AHRP), 68
Association for Women in Psychology, xiv
Atwood, Margaret, 257
Australia, 47, 85, 104, 126
Ayuso-Mateos, J. L., 264–265

Babycenter. com, 37
Bacon, L., 3–4, 184–187, 190–195, 204, 206–207, 213
Baiocchi, M., 27

About the Editors and Contributors

MAUREEN C. McHUGH, PhD, is Professor of Psychology at Indiana University of Pennsylvania (IUP) where she teaches graduate and undergraduate courses in gender and in diversity. She has had many leadership roles in feminist psychology, including chair of the Committee on Women in Psychology (CWP) of the American Psychological Association (APA), president of APA Division 35 (Society for Psychology of Women), and national coordinator of the Association for Women in Psychology (AWP). She was awarded the Christine Ladd Franklin Award for her contributions to feminist psychology, and the Florence Denmark Distinguished Mentoring Award for feminist mentoring, both from AWP. She has published dozens of journal articles and book chapters in the areas of feminist research methods, feminist psychology, gender differences, violence against women, women's sexuality, and older women, including chapters in psychology of women textbooks and handbooks. She has recently focused on the critical response to the medicalization of women's bodies and experiences. Working with her graduate student Ashley Kasardo, she challenged the "war on obesity" as an inappropriate, ineffective, and oppressive approach to women's weight. McHugh and Kasardo published a book review and a commentary about fat prejudice in the journal *Sex Roles* and conducted a series of presentations and workshops on weight bias. She has also returned to her earlier work that critically examined the medicalization of women's sexuality. She presented a paper titled "Enough Is Enough" as part of a symposium on "The Wrong Prescription" at the

International Congress of Psychology in Cape Town, South Africa, and published a chapter with her graduate student Camille Interligi, that critically examined the impact of media and medicalization on older women's sense of desire and desirability

JOAN C. CHRISLER, PhD, is The Class of 1943 Professor of Psychology at Connecticut College, where she teaches courses in gender, health, and social psychology. She has served as chair of the Committee on Women in Psychology (CWP) of the American Psychological Association (APA), as president of APA Divisions 1 (General Psychology) and 35 (Psychology of Women), the New England Psychological Association, the Society for Menstrual Cycle Research (SMCR), the Connecticut State Conference of the American Association of University Professors, and as national coordinator of the Association for Women in Psychology (AWP). She has received a number of honors for her work, including the Christine-Ladd Franklin Award (AWP), the Carolyn Wood Sherif Award (APA Division 35), the Ann Voda Distinguished Career Award (SMCR), a Distinguished Leader for Women in Psychology Award (CWP), and Distinguished Publication Awards (AWP) for her books *Lectures on the Psychology of Women* (McGraw-Hill, 1996) and *Reproductive Justice: A Global Concern* (Praeger, 2012). She has published dozens of articles, chapters, books, and reviews in her areas of interest: women's health, menstruation and menopause, reproductive rights and health, body image, women and weight, eating disorders, women and aging, and professional women's careers. She is especially known for her research and theoretical work on premenstrual syndrome, which illustrates its social construction and the medicalization of normal experience. She was an early contributor to the antidieting movement, has continued to write in that area from time to time, and has served on the editorial board of the journal *Fat Studies*. She previously served as editor of *Sex Roles* and is the current editor of the new journal *Women's Reproductive Health*. Other recent books coedited by Chrisler include *Women and Aging* (Springer, 2015), the two-volume *Handbook of Gender Research in Psychology* (Springer, 2010), and *Women Over 50: Psychological Perspectives* (Springer, 2007).

ALISHA ALI, PhD, is Associate Professor of Applied Psychology at New York University, where she conducts research on the psychological effects of violence, abuse, discrimination, and racism. She has written about alternative approaches to mainstream mental health treatment, including programs aimed at poverty reduction, economic empowerment, and the visual and performing arts. She is coeditor of the book *Silencing the Self Across Cultures: Depression and Gender in the Social World* (Oxford University Press, 2010).

JESSICA BARNACK-TAVLARIS, PhD, MPH, is Assistant Professor of Psychology at The College of New Jersey, where she teaches courses in health psychology and social psychology. Her research interests include attitudes toward menstruation, perceived sexual risk, and public perceptions of health disparities. She is the book/media review editor for *Women's Reproductive Health*, the official journal of the Society for Menstrual Cycle Research.

EMILY BREITKOPF, MA, is a doctoral candidate in clinical psychology at The New School for Social Research. In her research, she examines how medicalization, reproductive technologies, and media engagement impact the ways we interact with issues of gender, sexuality, race, and class. She integrates poststructuralist critical theory and feminist psychology to explore topics such as infertility, fetal sex assertion, and reprogenetic testing.

PAULA J. CAPLAN, PhD, is an associate of the DuBois Institute at Harvard University. She is a clinical psychologist, a social justice activist and mental health advocate, and a playwright, screenwriter, book author, and blogger for *Psychology Today*. Much of her work concerns the unwarranted pathologizing of women, including her books *The Myth of Women's Masochism, Don't Blame Mother: Mending the Mother-Daughter Relationship,* and *They Say You're Crazy: How the World's Most Powerful Psychiatrists Decide Who's Normal.*

HEATHER DILLAWAY, PhD, is Associate Professor of Sociology at Wayne State University. Her scholarly interests concern the study of women's reproductive health, women's aging, and health disparities. She is best known for her qualitative studies of women's experiences of menopause and the gynecological health experiences of women with spinal cord injuries. In both projects, she explored the everyday meanings and experiences of health and examined how individuals' definitions of and experiences with health and illness are affected by biomedical perspectives.

MINDY J. ERCHULL, PhD, is Associate Professor of Psychology at the University of Mary Washington. She is a social psychologist who studies feminist identity, women's reproductive health, and the objectification and sexualization of women by both society and women themselves. In both her research and her teaching, she focuses on raising awareness of cultural messages about health and well-being, as well as the need to challenge and critique these messages

RUTHBETH D. FINERMAN, PhD, is Professor of Anthropology and chair of the department at the University of Memphis. She is a medical anthropologist with 30 years of national and international research experience focused on family and maternal-child health. She has been a technical adviser or consultant for the World Health Organization, the U.S. Agency for International Development, and diverse U.S. health organizations. She has served on the executive boards of the Society for Applied Anthropology and the Society for Medical Anthropology.

JENNIFER A. GORMAN, MA, is Senior Lecturer in Psychology at Connecticut College, where she teaches courses on general psychology and research methods. She publishes frequently in her areas of interest, including women's health, menstruation, premenstrual syndrome, and body image. She is the treasurer of the Society for Menstrual Cycle Research.

LEEAT GRANEK, PhD, is Assistant Professor of Public Health at Ben Gurion University of the Negev. She is a critical health psychologist who studies grief and loss; cancer patients, their families, and their professional caregivers; and women's mental health. Recent research projects include examinations of oncologists' grief when patients die, the impact of pre-clinical oncology courses on medical students, and the normal trajectory of grief processes among mourners. She has published extensively in academic journals and in the popular press, including essays in the *New York Times*, *Huffington Post*, and *Slate*.

ASHLEY E. KASARDO, MA, is a doctoral candidate in clinical psychology at Indiana University of Pennsylvania. She is an advocate of body acceptance and health at every size and has organized outreach presentations and discussion groups regarding these paradigms across multiple college campuses. Her research interests include eating and emotions, body image, psychologists' role in size acceptance, weight bias in psychology texts, and size as a diversity issue.

JULIE KONIK, PhD, is Assistant Professor of Psychology at the University of Wisconsin–Sheboygan. She is a personality/social psychologist with interests in gender and sexuality studies.

CHARLOTTE N. MARKEY, PhD, is Professor of Psychology and director of the Healthy Development Lab at Rutgers University. Her research concerns interpersonal influences on body image, eating behaviors, and weight management.

PATRICK M. MARKEY, PhD, is Associate Professor and director of the Interpersonal Research Laboratory at Villanova University. His research concerns ways that the media affect interpersonal and intrapersonal behaviors.

CHLOE PARTON, PhD, is a postdoctoral researcher at the Centre for Health Research at the University of Western Sydney. Her research interests include women's negotiation and experience of sexual change after cancer, families and homelessness, Aboriginal women's experience of motherhood, and sexual changes experienced by gay and bisexual men after treatment for prostate cancer.

JANETTE PERZ, PhD, is Professor of Health Psychology and director of the Centre for Health Research at the University of Western Sydney. She is well known for her research on reproductive and sexual health with a focus on gendered experiences, subjectivity, and identity. Her work includes studies of the experience of premenstrual syndrome (PMS) in the context of heterosexual and lesbian relationships; the development and evaluation of a couple-based psychological intervention for PMS; sexual well-being and reproductive needs of culturally and linguistically diverse populations; and sexual and psychological well-being during menopause and midlife.

LISA R. RUBIN, PhD, is Associate Professor of Psychology and assistant director of Clinical Training at The New School for Social Research. Her research interests include infertility/assisted and selective reproductive technologies, psycho-oncology, and eating and weight concerns. In her work she explores how intersections of gender, objectification, and biomedicalization shape the ways in which these matters are constructed, experienced, and managed. She has served as chair of the American Psychological Association Division 35's Reproductive Issues Committee.

LYNDA M. SAGRESTANO, PhD, is Professor of Psychology and director of the Center for Research on Women at the University of Memphis. Her research is oriented toward applying psychological theory to understand (and intervene to prevent) social problems and to advance theory development that highlights the role of contextual factors in health processes and outcomes. She has developed numerous constructive relationships with local nonprofit organizations to address issues related to infant mortality, adolescent pregnancy, economic security for women, and the empowerment of girls. She has served on the board of directors of the National Council for Research on Women.

ADRIANE M. F. SANDERS, PhD, is Assistant Professor of Psychology and a core faculty member of the industrial-organizational master's program at Austin Peay State University. She studies work-life interaction, stress, and quality of life and promotes the dissemination of timely empirical research to empower women (and men) to make informed decisions about their health, safety, well-being, and work life. She is affiliated with the Center for Research on Women at the University of Memphis.

CHRISTINE A. SMITH, PhD, is Associate Professor of Psychology, Human Development, and Gender & Women's Studies at the University of Wisconsin–Green Bay. She is a social psychologist. Her recent research concerns are fat stigma, LGBT issues, and interpersonal relationships.

LEONORE TIEFER, PhD, a psychologist and activist, is Clinical Associate Professor of Psychiatry at the New York University School of Medicine. Her professional experiences in sexology include research, clinical practice, college and medical school teaching, and extensive organizational work. She has published several books and dozens of empirical and theoretical articles and book chapters on sexuality. In 2000 she founded the New View Campaign (newviewcampaign.org), a feminist activist campaign to challenge the medicalization of sex.

JANE M. USSHER, PhD, is Professor of Women's Health Psychology, at the University of Western Sydney. She has published widely on the construction and lived experience of health, with a focus on women's mental health, the reproductive body, and sexuality. She is the editor of Routledge's "Women and Psychology" book series and the author of a number of books, including *The Psychology of the Female Body* (1989), *Women's Madness: Misogyny or Mental Illness?* (1991), *Managing the Monstrous Feminine: Regulating the Reproductive Body* (2006), and *The Madness of Women: Myth and Experience* (2011).Index for The Wrong Prescription for Women